PHYSIOLOGICAL BASES OF
Sports Performance

PHYSIOLOGICAL BASES OF
Sports Performance

Edited by MARK HARGREAVES and JOHN HAWLEY

Sydney   New York   St.Louis   San Francisco   Auckland   Bogotá
Caracas   Lisbon   London   Madrid   MexicoCity   Milan   Montreal
New Delhi   SanJuan   Singapore   Tokyo   Toronto

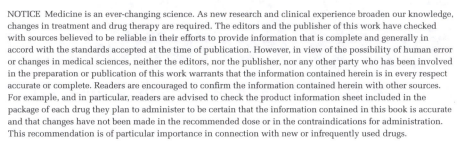

McGraw·Hill Australia

A Division of The McGraw·Hill Companies

Text © 2003 Mark Hargreaves and John Hawley
Illustrations and design © 2003 McGraw-Hill Australia Pty Ltd

National Library of Australia Cataloguing-in-Publication data:

Hargreaves, Mark, 1961-.
Physiological bases of sports performance.

Includes index.
ISBN 0 074 71101 6.

    1. Sports – Physiological aspects.
    I. Hawley, John, 1957-.
    II. Title.

612.044

Published in Australia by
McGraw-Hill Australia Pty Ltd
Level 2, 82 Waterloo Road, North Ryde NSW 2113
Publishing Manager: Meiling Voon
Production Editor: Rosemary McDonald
Editor: Carolyn Pike
Proofreader: Tim Learner
Indexer: Diane Harriman
Designer (interior and cover): Jenny Pace Design
Cover image: gettyimages.com
Illustrator: Alan Laver
Typeset in Melior by Jenny Pace Design
Printed on 80 gsm woodfree by Pantech Limited, Hong Kong.

Foreword

Australia is a world leader in sports performance setting new standards in a wide range of sporting events. Its fourth placing among over 200 nations at the 2000 Sydney Olympics gave clear evidence of such leadership.

Therefore when a group of our sports scientific leaders come together to produce a book about the athlete's body and performance, the reader can be assured that they are at the leading edge of sports science.

I was amazed and then, as an Aussie, reassured to see the encyclopaedic list of references and bibliographies supporting each subject. It seemed to me that the writers had scanned the world for reliable, breakthrough, sports-science research with the aim of assimilating, using and, hopefully, surpassing what it already known.

The book also made me realise how complex the challenge is that confronts the coach and athlete that want to be the best of the elite. I am a scientist by education, but very quickly found myself floundering in strange scientific language. And yet the modern coach and athlete must be aware of much of this science. Therefore the successful athlete of today almost certainly needs a coach and scientist working in harmony to ensure that the athlete is not disadvantaged by a competitor who is using new methods that have emerged from scientific investigation.

The book contains the latest information on many subjects including sports foods and supplements, proteins, carbohydrate loading, creatine, overtraining, heat stress, hydration, altitude training and much more that top coaches need to be aware of to take their athletes to the top of the world of sport.

Herb Elliott AC, MBE, MA(Cantab.)

Acknowledgements

The authors thank Sue, Christopher and James, and Louise for their love and support over the years. They dedicate this book to Professor David Costill whose passion and inspiration brought them, and many others, to the field of exercise and sports physiology and who remains a great mentor and friend.

Mark Hargreaves & John Hawley (Melbourne, 2003)

Contents

Introduction

Accomplished performance in any sport requires that athletes possess the necessary genetic attributes for success; that they apply scientifically proven training principles to their physical preparation; that they adhere to optimal nutritional practices; that they are highly motivated and execute sound tactical strategies; and that on the day of competition, environmental conditions are favourable. It is difficult to partition the contribution of each of these factors to any given performance outcome because of the wide-ranging demands of different sports. Accordingly, the general factors affecting sports performance can be viewed as a series of interrelated input variables that, depending on the specific requirements of a sport, contribute to a greater or lesser extent to the final performance outcome (Fig. I.1).

While recognising the contribution of biomechanical and psychological factors, the focus of this book is on the physiological bases underlying sport and the applications of specific strategies to enhance sports performance.

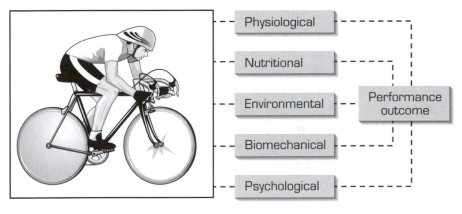

FIG. I.1 General factors affecting sports performance

Fundamental principles of sports performance

The successful performance of any sport depends on the skilful and coordinated activation of an athlete's skeletal muscles to produce power to overcome resistance (or drag) due to air, surface friction (water, snow or asphalt) or an opponent. While sports are diverse in terms of the surface on which they are contested, the equipment required, the activity patterns and the subsequent energy demands, there are several universal principles underlying movement. These principles are briefly discussed. The reader is referred to other reviews for a more comprehensive introduction to the physiology of competitive sport (Coyle et al. 1994; Hawley & Burke 1998; Knuttgen 2000).

Successful performance in athletic events in which a competitor has to complete a set distance in the shortest time possible (i.e. running, cycling, swimming, speed skating, rowing, cross-county skiing) is determined by the ability of an athlete to produce and sustain the highest power output throughout the duration of a race. This, in turn, is determined by how effectively an athlete can overcome the resistance that impedes movement. The resistance (or drag) athletes encounter during training and competition is principally determined by the medium in which they compete: cyclists must produce power to overcome air resistance, rolling resistance (surface friction between road/track and wheels) and resistance to the friction of the moving components of the bike; swimmers encounter large drag forces from the water as well as from the turbulence at the water–swimmer interface; weight-lifters must apply power to overcome gravitational forces offered by the mass of the bar; judo players must apply force to overcome both gravitational forces and those muscular contractions of their opponent.

As the velocity of movement increases, air drag offers the most resistance to impede progress, such that a doubling of speed means a fourfold increase in air drag (Kyle 1991). For cyclists, a twofold increase in velocity requires an eightfold increase in power output (Kyle 1991). In practical terms this means that air drag accounts for approximately 90% of the total resistance to movement for a cyclist riding at speeds above 40 km/h (Kyle 1998). In sports that require a competitor to move at relatively high velocities (i.e. >15 km/h), the speed of movement can only be improved by significantly reducing the resistance or drag of the athlete (and his/her equipment) or by increasing the rate of energy production (i.e. power output). While a variety of ergogenic aids are used by athletes to exert a favourable effect upon energy utilisation and subsequent exercise capacity (i.e. aerodynamic equipment), performance improvements ultimately require an increase in the ability to produce power output aerobically and/or anaerobically.

Performance power output/speed

Several theoretical models of the major physiological factors likely to contribute to the successful performance of endurance-trained athletes have previously been proposed (Coyle 1995; Hawley & Stepto 2001). The working premise is that the sum of adaptations within the various physiological, morphological and functional components of these models ultimately acts synergistically to exert a major influence on the performance capacity of an athlete at any given time (Hawley & Stepto 2001). While such models remain, for the most part, hypothetical, in some sports (e.g. cycling) there is a reasonably good relationship between the theoretical and experimental basis and subsequent performance outcomes (Coyle 1995, 1999). Figures I.2 and I.3 show theoretical models of some of the physiological, morphological and biochemical factors determining performance power/speed capability for athletes competing in sprint (Fig. I.2) and endurance (Fig. I.3) events.

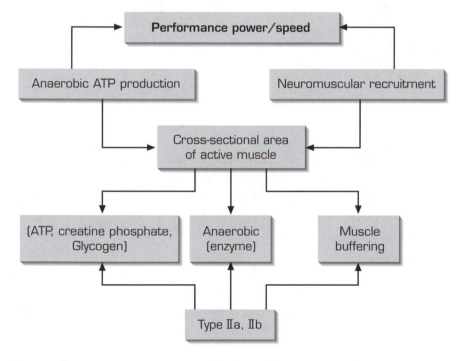

FIG. I.2 Theoretical model of some of the factors determining performance power/speed capability for athletes competing in sprint events

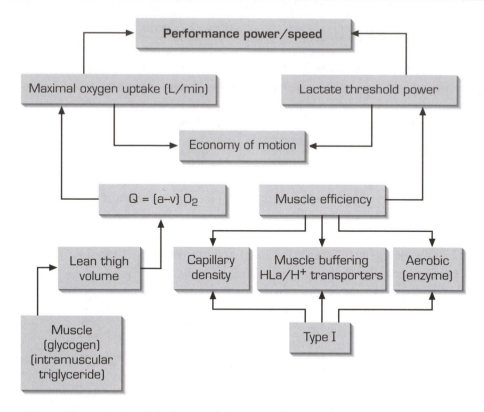

FIG. I.3 Theoretical model of some of the factors determining performance power/speed capability for athletes competing in endurance events

Q = cardiac output. (a–v) O_2 = arterio-venous oxygen difference.

The aim of this book is to provide a 'physiological perspective' of sports performance. The first part summarises recent research on the physiological bases of sports performance, with an emphasis on skeletal muscle metabolism, the oxygen transport system, temperature regulation and fluid balance during exercise, and mechanisms of fatigue. The second part examines some of the factors that exert a major influence on sports performance, such as physical training, nutrition, environment and gender. Ultimately, a greater understanding of the physiological determinants underlying sports performance and how they can be modified by various interventions can facilitate the development of effective strategies to enhance performance.

References

Coyle EF. Integration of the physiological factors determining endurance performance ability. In: Holloszy JO, ed. *Exercise and Sport Sciences Reviews*. 1995;23:25–63.

Coyle EF. Physiological determinants of endurance exercise performance. *Journal Sci Med Sport* 1999;2:181–9.

Coyle EF, Spriet L, Gregg S, Clarkson P. Introduction to physiology and nutrition for competitive sport. In: Lamb DR, Knuttgen HG, Murray R, eds. *Perspectives in Exercise Science and Sports Medicine*. Vol. 7. *Physiology and Nutrition for Competitive Sport*. Carmel, IN: Cooper Publishing Group, 1994: xv–xxxix.

Hawley JA, Burke LM. *Peak Performance: Training and Nutritional Strategies for Sport*. Sydney: Allen & Unwin, 1998.

Hawley JA, Stepto NK. Adaptation to training in endurance-trained cyclists. Implications for performance. *Sports Med* 2001;31:511–20.

Knuttgen HG. Basic exercise physiology. In: Maughan RJ, ed. *Nutrition in Sport*. Oxford: Blackwell Science, 2000: 3–16.

Kyle CR. Ergogenics of bicycling. In: Lamb DR & Williams MH, eds. *Perspectives in Exercise Science and Sports Medicine*. Vol. 4. *Ergogenics: Enhancement of Performance in Exercise and Sport*. Carmel, IN: Brown & Benchmark, 1991: 373–413.

Kyle CR. The mechanics and aerodynamics of cycling. In: Burke EM & Newshom MN, eds. *Medical and Scientific Aspects of Cycling*. Champaign, IL: Human Kinetics, 1988.

PART 1
EXERCISE AND SPORTS PHYSIOLOGY

CHAPTER 1

Skeletal muscle

Rodney SNOW

Introduction

This chapter provides an overview of the structure and function of human skeletal muscle, with special consideration of the different muscle fibre types and the various metabolic, morphological, contractile and fatigue characteristics of each fibre type. Some of the factors influencing the recruitment of the various fibres during exercise are examined, as is the relationship between sports performance and muscle fibre type composition. Finally, this chapter briefly examines the influence of endurance, sprint and resistance training on the morphological and metabolic profile of skeletal muscle.

Function and structure of skeletal muscle

Skeletal muscle accounts for as much as 40–45% of the total body mass and is the tissue responsible for generating the forces required for joint movement during physical activity. The ultrastructure of skeletal muscle and the processes involved in activation and contraction of muscle fibres have been well described and can be gleaned from most physiology textbooks. Consequently, only a brief summary will be given here.

Muscle fibres are multinucleated, long, cylindrical-shaped cells (Fig. 1.1). The cell membrane of a muscle fibre includes the sarcolemma and transverse tubules. Lying either side of each transverse tubule, within the fibre itself, is a calcium-containing membranous network or organelle called the sarcoplasmic reticulum. This organelle is found along the length of the fibre and surrounds the cylindrical-shaped myofibrils that contain the contractile proteins. The myofibrils contain the contractile apparatus, which consists of thick and thin protein filaments organised into repeating

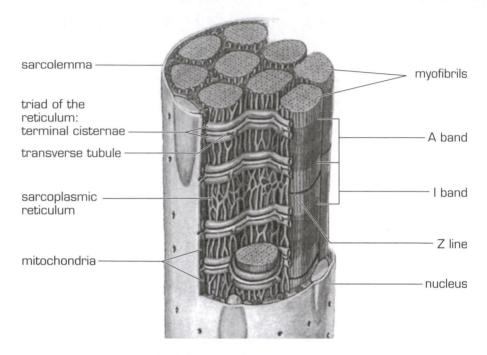

FIG. 1.1 Microstructure of a skeletal muscle fibre (reproduced from Powers & Howley 2001, p. 132)

contractile units called sarcomeres. The thick filaments are located in the central region of each sarcomere and are surrounded by thin filaments projecting from both ends of the sarcomere towards its centre.

Thick filaments are highly organised aggregations of the contractile protein myosin, whereas the thin filament consists of the contractile protein actin and the regulatory proteins troponin and tropomyosin. Myosin consists of two heavy-chain subunits and four light-chain subunits (Fig. 1.2; Schiaffino & Reggiani 1996). Importantly, both the heavy and light chains may exist in various isoforms, thereby influencing contractile function.

Skeletal muscle fibres are stimulated to contract by the somatic nervous system via alpha motor neurons. Once stimulated, action potentials are propagated over the sarcolemma and along the transverse-tubular membranes of the fibre (see Fig. 1.3). This transverse-tubular charge movement triggers the release of calcium from the sarcoplasmic reticulum (Stephenson 1996). The released calcium subsequently binds to troponin, allowing the troponin–tropomyosin complex to shift position, thus exposing the myosin binding site on actin. This shift allows the myosin head to attach to actin (forming a cross-bridge) and begin the process known as cross-bridge cycling.

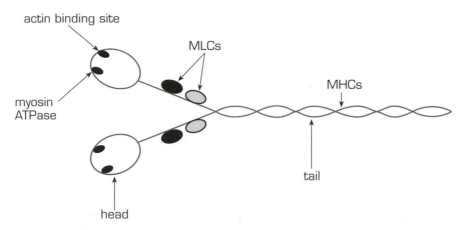

FIG. 1.2 A myosin molecule. Myosin consists of six protein chains: two intertwined myosin heavy chains (MHCs) and four light chains (MLCs). The myosin ATPase is located in the heads of the MHC. The head of the MHC also contains an actin binding site (modified from Schiaffino & Reggiani 1996, p. 377)

This process results in the sliding of thin filaments over the thick filaments and produces sarcomere shortening. To relax the muscle, the sarcoplasmic reticulum re-sequesters the released calcium via the activity of calcium ATPase pumps, restoring sarcoplasmic calcium levels to resting levels. This permits tropomyosin to return to its blocking position, preventing cross-bridge cycling and allowing the sarcomere to recoil to resting length.

Muscle force and power

Since each myosin cross-bridge attached to actin acts as an independent force generator, the overall force produced by a muscle is dependent upon the number of attached cross-bridges in the strong-binding or force-producing state. Factors that influence this include the number and size of the active motor units, motor neuron firing frequency, muscle length, velocity of shortening or lengthening, total active muscle cross-sectional area and muscle fibre type. Muscle power is determined by muscle force multiplied by shortening velocity (Fig. 1.4). For a typical human muscle of average muscle fibre composition, maximal power occurs at about one-third of maximal velocity and one-third of maximal force. Muscle power is markedly affected by fibre type composition mainly as a result of differences in shortening velocity; however, differences in maximal force development between fibre types also contribute (Stienen et al. 1996).

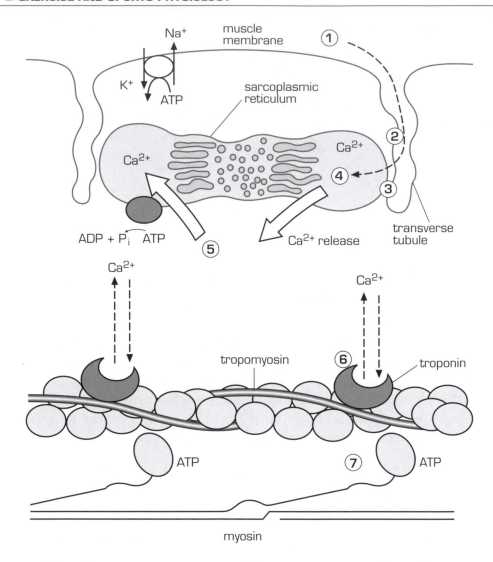

FIG. 1.3 A diagrammatic representation of the major components of a muscle cell. The numbers indicate the processes occurring during activation and contraction of skeletal muscle and include: (1) propagation of the action potential along the sarcolemma; (2) transverse-tubular charge movement; (3) coupling of transverse-tubular charge movement with sarcoplasmic reticulum calcium release; (4) sarcoplasmic reticulum calcium release; (5) sarcoplasmic reticulum calcium reuptake; (6) calcium binding to troponin; (7) actomyosin hydrolysis of ATP and cross-bridge force development and cycling rate (reproduced from Fitts & Metzger 1988, p. 214)

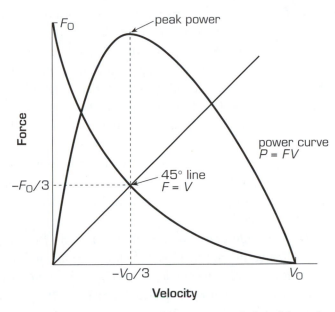

FIG. 1.4 Muscle force–velocity curve and power curve deduced from the force velocity curve (reproduced from Maughan 1999, p. 26)

Classification of muscle fibre types

Skeletal muscle is made up of functional units called motor units, defined as a group of muscle fibres and the neuron that innervates them. Within a motor unit the muscle fibres have similar contractile and biochemical properties that are determined primarily by the motor neuron, either via the pattern of activation (e.g. tonic, low frequency or phasic, high frequency) or by special chemicals (trophic factors) released by the neuron. Superimposed on the type of innervation is the normal activity pattern of the motor unit; that is, the extent to which it is used or recruited during contractile activity. The fibres in a motor unit are distributed in a fairly large cross-sectional area of the muscle and are rarely positioned immediately proximal to each other (Saltin & Gollnick 1983).

Although there is likely to be a continuum of fibre types (and motor units) from slow to fast (Pette 1998), there are generally considered to be two main types: slow twitch (type I) and fast twitch (type II) fibres. Under zero load, type II fibres shorten at velocities about threefold faster than type I fibres (Table 1.1). The type II fibres in mammalian muscle have been further classified into three functional subtypes—types IIa, IIb and IIx. The speed characteristics of these subtypes decreases in the order of: IIb is faster than

IIx, which is faster than IIa. Speed of contraction is determined by the rate of cross-bridge cycling, which in turn is affected by the type of myosin heavy chain (MHC) isoform expressed in each fibre (Fig. 1.2). In addition to the MHC isoform, the type of myosin light chain (MLC) isoforms expressed also fine tunes shortening velocity capability (Pette 1998). Type I fibres express slow MHCIβ, whereas type IIa, IIb and IIx fibres express fast MHCIIa, IIb and IIx, respectively. In human skeletal muscle, very few fibres express the fast MHCIIb isoform, and therefore some researchers (Ennion et al. 1995; Sant'Ana Pereira et al. 1996) suggest that human fibres should be classified as type I, type IIa and type IIx. At present, this classification system has not been widely adopted, with most researchers still preferring to use type IIb instead of IIx (Staron 1997).

There are several techniques for identifying muscle fibre types from samples obtained using the muscle biopsy technique. One of these involves sectioning the tissue and subsequent histochemical determination of myosin ATPase activity following incubation of sections in either an acid or alkaline medium. MHCs from type I fibres are acid stable but alkaline labile, while the opposite is true for MHCs expressed in type II fibres (Fig. 1.5). Another approach is to use gel electrophoresis and immunoblotting (or silver staining) to separate and identify the MHC isoforms that are expressed in single fibres (Pette et al. 1999). Using this technique, it has been demonstrated that muscle fibres can simultaneously express more than one MHC isoform and perhaps a number of MLC isoforms. The most

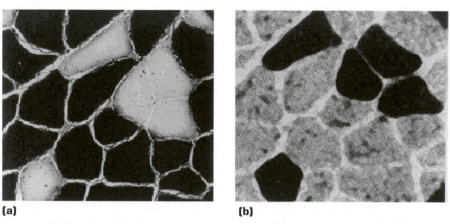

(a)   **(b)**

FIG. 1.5 Myosin ATPase activity in transverse sections of muscle obtained from the vastus lateralis after pre-incubation in either (a) acidic (darkly stained fibres are type I) or (b) alkaline (lightly stained fibres are type I) buffer. Note reversal of staining with different pre-incubation buffers (courtesy of Ian Newey)

common coexpression is that of MHCIIa and IIx, forming type IIax or IIab fibres (Sant'Ana Pereira et al. 1996).

There are many other differences between fibre types in addition to the contractile properties. These differences include metabolic, morphological and fatigue characteristics. Untrained human type I fibres contain similar levels of ATP, higher triglyceride content but lower stores of creatine phosphate (PCr) and glycogen compared with type II fibres (Table 1.1; Casey et al. 1996; Saltin & Gollnick 1983). In addition, untrained human type I fibres display greater maximal activity of enzymes in the tricarboxylic acid cycle and β-oxidation pathways but lower activity of key enzymes associated with glycogen breakdown, glycolysis and PCr metabolism (Table 1.1; Saltin & Gollnick 1983). Furthermore, the number of capillaries per fibre area is significantly greater in human type I compared with type II fibres (Table 1.1; Saltin et al. 1977). This enhanced capillarisation is likely to augment the diffusion of substrates and oxygen into type I fibres. Taken together, the different metabolic and morphological profile enables type I fibres

TABLE 1.1 Contractile, metabolic and morphological characteristics of the various fibre types in the human vastus lateralis muscle of untrained males

	TYPE I	TYPE II	TYPE IIA	TYPE IIB
Contractile characteristics				
Myosin ATPase activity	0.16	0.48		
Time to peak tension (msec)	80	30		
Substrates[a]				
ATP	23.7 ± 0.7	25.2 ± 0.6		
Creatine phosphate	79.4 ± 2.1	89.6 ± 5.2		
Glycogen	364 ± 23	480 ± 24		
Triglyceride	30.9 ± 7.4	18.2 ± 5.2		
Enzymes[b]				
Creatine kinase	13.1	16.6		
Phosphorylase	2.8		5.8	8.8
Phosphofructokinase	7.5		13.7	17.5
Lactate dehydrogenase	94		179	211
3-Hydroxyl-CoA dehydrogenase	14.8		11.6	7.1
Succinate dehydrogenase	7.1		4.8	2.5
Morphological characteristics				
Fibre area (μm^2)	5310		6110	5600
Capillaries per fibre	4.2		4.0	3.2
Fibre area per capillary (μm^2)	1014		1335	1338

(a) Substrate content in mmol/kg dry muscle ± SE. (b) Enzyme activity units in mmol/kg/min, except for creatine kinase where units are mmol/min/mg. Data from Greenhaff et al. (1999); Saltin & Gollnick (1983); Saltin et al. (1977)

to produce ATP more readily from the aerobic metabolism of lipids and carbohydrates than type II fibres. In contrast, type II fibres rely to a greater extent on anaerobic pathways such as PCr degradation and glycolysis to fuel contractile activity (Greenhaff et al. 1999).

The precise cause of muscle fibre fatigue is currently unknown (Fitts 1994; Westerblad et al. 1998); however, there is a strong positive correlation between resistance to fatigue and muscle fibre oxidative capacity. This finding suggests that fibres capable of matching ATP demand with aerobic ATP production are able to sustain contractile activity. Research has clearly demonstrated that type I fibres are resistant to fatigue, whereas type IIb fibres fatigue rapidly (Burke & Edgerton 1975). Type IIa fibres display a fatigue profile that lies between the other fibre types. On the basis of the contractile, metabolic, morphometric and fatigue characteristics of each fibre type outlined, it is not surprising that type I fibres are designed for low power, sustained contractile activity in contrast to type IIb fibres, which are recruited to perform short duration, high force (or power) activities.

Motor unit recruitment

The use of skeletal muscle fibre types during exercise is determined by the intensity and duration of contractile activity. The size principle (Henneman et al. 1974) proposes that motor unit recruitment is directly related to the size of the motor neuron innervating the motor unit. Small motor neurons that innervate type I motor units have a low recruitment threshold and are involved whenever the muscle is producing any force (Fig. 1.6; Sale 1987). In contrast, large-diameter motor neurons innervating type IIb motor units display a high recruitment threshold and are only involved when high forces are required.

Type IIa motor units become active to aid type I fibre activity when intermediate forces are needed. Force production by each active motor unit is also modulated by altering motor neuron firing frequency. The order of motor unit recruitment (type I to IIa to IIb) appears to hold for most types of concentric muscle contractions; however, there is evidence that preferential recruitment of type II fibres may occur during eccentric contractions (Enoka 1996).

The patterns of recruitment in skeletal muscle during exercise can be studied using electromyography or by assessing the utilisation of glycogen within the muscle fibre type populations either histochemically or

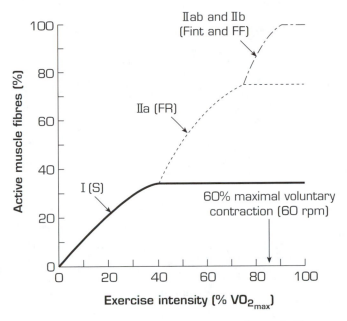

FIG. 1.6 The relationship between exercise intensity and muscle fibre type recruitment pattern in the vastus lateralis muscle during cycling exercise. S, FR, Fint and FF denote slow, fast-twitch fatigue resistant, fast-twitch intermediate and fast-twitch fatigable fibres respectively (reproduced from Sale 1987, p. 99)

biochemically. Using the latter technique, studies in humans have shown a primary reliance upon type I fibres during low-intensity exercise, whereas all fibre types are recruited during high-intensity exercise (Gollnick et al. 1974). During exercise at moderate submaximal intensities, type I and IIa fibres are initially recruited, with type IIab and IIb fibres being increasingly recruited as the other fibres become depleted of glycogen, and presumably fatigue (Fig. 1.7; Vøllestad 1987). This data indicates that exercise duration, in addition to exercise intensity, also affects motor unit recruitment.

Fibre type and performance

Successful athletic performance is dependent upon the complex interaction of psychological, biological and biomechanical factors. One biological factor that is likely to play a role in athletic performance is muscle fibre type composition. Several studies have demonstrated that elite endurance athletes have a high proportion of type I fibres, while athletes involved

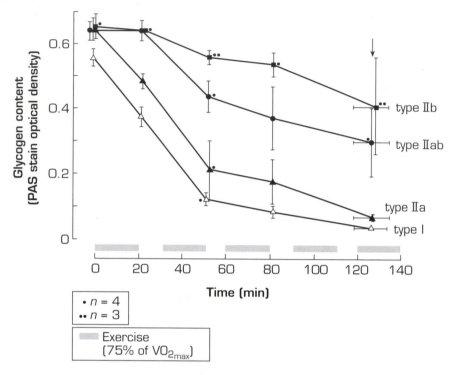

FIG. 1.7 The glycogen content (as determined by PAS stain) of type I (Δ), IIa ($\blacktriangle$), IIab ($\bullet$), and IIb ($\blacksquare$) at rest and during submaximal cycling exercise to exhaustion (reproduced from: Vøllestad 1987, p. 132)

in short-duration sprint events have a greater proportion of type II fibres (Table 1.2; Gollnick et al. 1972; Green et al. 1979; Saltin & Gollnick 1983). Given the various characteristics of each of the fibre types (see above), the predominance of type I fibres in elite endurance athletes and type II fibres in elite sprint athletes is perhaps not surprising.

TABLE 2.2 Typical muscle fibre composition in untrained, sprint and endurance runners

	TYPE I (%)	TYPE II (%)
Endurance runners	59–79	21–41
Sprint runners	24–39	61–76
Untrained	45–55	45–55

Data modified from Saltin & Gollnick (1983)

In the context of muscle fibre composition and athletic performance, it is worth mentioning that at any given speed of movement, muscles that contain a large percentage of type II fibres will produce more power than muscles containing a large proportion of type I fibres (Coyle et al. 1979; Harridge et al. 1996). This finding implies that athletes who have a high proportion of type II fibres would have an advantage in power type events. Indeed, research has demonstrated that the proportion of type II fibres or the relative type II to type I area positively correlates with high-intensity exercise performance (Fig. 1.8; Bar-Or et al. 1980; Kaczkowski et al. 1982; Esborjnsson et al. 1993). Conversely, a high proportion of type I fibres has been associated with superior performance in 10 km running (Fink et al. 1977) and a 1-hour cycling test (Horowitz et al. 1994). One reason why a high proportion of type I fibres may be advantageous during endurance events is that they are more efficient at the muscle contraction speeds required during such events (Horowitz et al. 1994).

It should be noted, however, that there is considerable variation in the fibre composition of skeletal muscle within groups of elite athletes. This means that athletes can be highly successful in endurance or sprint events even if their muscles contain relatively high percentages of type II or I fibres, respectively (Gollnick & Matoba 1984). This fact highlights that high-level

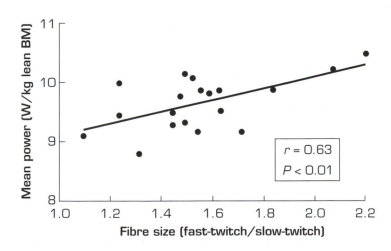

FIG. 1.8 Relationship between mean power on the Wingate anaerobic test and relative fibre size (reproduced from Bar-Or et al. 1980)

performance is a multifactorial phenomenon and is not reliant on one factor, such as muscle fibre type composition.

The question commonly raised by the data presented in Table 1.2 is 'Do elite athletes have a predominant muscle fibre type expression due to training or are they born with this type of composition?' The answer appears to be that both factors are contributing to the final outcome. Results from the dizygotic and monozygotic twin study conducted by Komi et al. (1977) elegantly demonstrated that human muscle fibre type composition was predominantly genetically determined. Nevertheless, several studies have reported that sprint, resistance and endurance training (Adams et al. 1993; Andersen et al. 1994; Dawson et al. 1998; Jacobs et al. 1987; Pette 1998; Schantz 1986) can lead to fibre type transformations, in particular from IIb to IIa fibres, and therefore a small shift in muscle fibre type composition from the genetic template is possible.

The influence of training on skeletal muscle

There has been considerable research on the influence of training on muscle energy stores. Apart from a few exceptions (e.g. MacDougall et al. 1977), most studies have found that high-energy phosphagen stores in resting skeletal muscle are unaltered by most types of training (Saltin & Gollnick 1983; Sahlin & Henriksson 1984). In contrast, endurance (Gollnick et al. 1973), resistance (MacDougall et al. 1977) and sprint training (Parra et al. 2000) result in a marked increase in resting muscle glycogen content. The effect of training on muscle triglyceride stores is unclear, with reports indicating that with endurance training they either remain unaltered or increase (Saltin & Gollnick 1983; Suter et al. 1995).

Cross-sectional studies have demonstrated that endurance-trained athletes typically have higher aerobic and similar, or lower, glycolytic enzyme activity compared with untrained control subjects (Salmons & Henriksson 1981). Endurance-trained athletes also display a marked increase in the number of capillaries per type I, IIa and IIb fibres compared with untrained individuals (Saltin et al. 1977). The higher aerobic enzyme activity in elite endurance athletes is observed in both type I and II fibres (Table 1.3; Jansson & Sylven 1985; Saltin & Gollnick 1983). Longitudinal endurance training experiments usually report a marked increase in muscle mitochondrial enzyme activity (e.g. half- to twofold increase) and an increase in muscle fibre capillarity (Andersen & Henriksson 1977). The effect endurance training has on muscle fibre cross-sectional area is unclear.

TABLE 1.3 Succinate dehydrogenase activity[a] of thigh muscle fibre types in untrained and endurance trained individuals

	TYPE I	TYPE IIA	TYPE IIB
Untrained	9.2	5.8	4.9
Endurance trained	23.2	22.1	22

[a] An enzyme involved with aerobic metabolism. Units are mmol/kg/min.
Adapted from Saltin & Gollnick (1983)

For example, Gollnick et al. (1973) observed a 23% increase in type I fibre area but no change in type II fibre area after endurance training. In contrast, Schantz et al. (1983) found no change in type I area and a 12% decrease in type IIa area with training. The discrepancy is probably dependent on the training protocol employed and pre-training strength status.

Increases in aerobic enzyme activity in type I and/or II fibres are also dependent upon the training protocol (Henriksson & Reitman 1976) and probably reflect fibre recruitment patterns. For example, continuous exercise at moderate intensities favour an increase in aerobic enzyme activities (about 30%) in type I fibres with little or no change in type II fibres, whereas intermittent, more intense activity promotes the opposite response. The effect of endurance training on skeletal muscle glycolytic enzyme activity is unclear, with studies reporting an increase (Gollnick et al. 1973), no change (Henriksson & Reitman 1976; Schantz et al. 1983) or a decrease (Green et al. 1979) with training. The increased capillary supply and mitochondrial enzyme activity in endurance-trained muscle is thought to be largely responsible for the enhanced muscle oxygen extraction and oxidation of fuels, in particular lipids (Martin et al. 1993). These adaptations increase the ability to perform prolonged exercise at a higher percentage of maximal oxygen consumption for longer.

Cross-sectional studies have reported that sprint-trained athletes display a higher glycolytic capacity but similar oxidative capacity to untrained controls (Boros-Hatfaludy et al. 1986; Mackova et al. 1986). The effect of sprint training on muscle capillarity is currently unknown. Sprint training has no influence on either type I or type II muscle fibre cross-sectional area in men but increases type IIb fibre area by 25% in females (Esborjnsson-Liljedahl et al. 1996). Unfortunately, longitudinal sprint training experiments have utilised quite different training protocols (e.g. number of repetitions, sprint and recovery durations), making it difficult to generalise about the metabolic adaptations that occur (Parra et al. 2000). Nevertheless, sprint training can increase the activity of myokinase, creatine kinase and various glycolytic (in particular, phosphofructokinase) and mitochondrial enzymes (Jacobs et al. 1987; MacDougall et al. 1998; Parra et al. 2000; Thorstensson et al. 1975). The performance improvements normally observed with sprint training may be due, at least in part, to the enhanced anaerobic and/or aerobic capacity of the contracting muscle (Harmer et al. 2000; MacDougall et al. 1998; Nevill et al. 1989).

Cross-sectional experiments investigating the effects of resistance training on metabolic enzymes have found that resistance-trained individuals display a reduced mitochondrial enzyme activity but an elevated activity of enzymes associated with anaerobic metabolism compared with untrained controls (Tesch et al. 1989). Some of these differences were specific to a particular muscle fibre type (Tesch et al. 1989). The lower oxidative enzyme activity in resistance-trained muscle is probably the result of a reduced mitochondrial volume density caused by muscle fibre hypertrophy (Chilibeck et al. 1999; MacDougall et al. 1979). In this regard, the area of type I and II fibres in body builders is about 65% and 120% greater, respectively, than control subjects (Tesch et al. 1989). Cross-sectional studies comparing body builders with controls also report an increased number of capillaries per fibre; however, when expressed per fibre area either a decrease (MacDougall 1986) or no (Bell & Jacobs 1990) training adaptation was found. Longitudinal resistance-training studies, in which significant muscle hypertrophy has occurred, have reported a training-induced reduction in muscle creatine kinase, myokinase and certain glycolytic and mitochondrial enzyme activities (Tesch et al. 1987). Resistance training has also been shown to cause an enlargement of the cross-sectional area (about 30%) of both type I and II fibres (Chilibeck et al. 1999; Tesch 1987), with most (MacDougall et al. 1979; MacDougall et al. 1980; Tesch 1987) but not all (Chilibeck et al. 1999) research indicating that the greatest relative increase in area occurs in type II fibres.

Summary

This chapter has provided an overview of skeletal muscle structure and function. The metabolic, morphological, contractile and fatigue characteristics of the various human muscle fibre types have been discussed. Metabolic and morphological adaptations of skeletal muscle to various training stimuli have also been addressed. Finally, evidence has been provided that fibre type composition and metabolic capacity may influence athletic performance.

References

Adams GR, Hather BM, Baldwin KM, Dudley GA. Skeletal muscle myosin heavy chain composition and resistance training. *J Appl Physiol* 1993;74:911–15.

Andersen P, Henriksson J. Capillary supply of the quadriceps femoris muscle of man: adaptive response to exercise. *J Physiol* 1977;270:677–90.

Andersen JL, Klitgaard H, Saltin B. Myosin heavy chain isoforms in single fibres from m. vastus lateralis of sprinters: influence of training. *Acta Physiol Scand* 1994;151: 135–42.

Bar-Or O, Dotan R, Inbar O, Rothstein A, Karlsson J, Tesch P. Anaerobic capacity and muscle fiber type distribution in man. *Int J Sports Med* 1980;1:82–5.

Bell DG, Jacobs I. Muscle fibre area, fibre type and capillarization in male and female body builders. *Can J Sports Sci* 1990;15:115–19.

Boros-Hatfaludy S, Fekete G, Apor P. Metabolic enzyme patterns in muscle biopsy samples in different athletes. *Eur J Appl Physiol* 1986;55:334–8.

Burke RE, Edgerton VR. Motor unit properties and selective involvement in movement. *Exerc Sports Sci Rev* 1975;3:31–81.

Casey A, Constantin-Teodosiu D, Howell S, Hultman E, Greenhaff P. Metabolic responses of type I and II fibres during repeated bouts of maximal exercise in humans. *Am J Physiol* 1996;271:E38–E43.

Chilibeck PD, Syrotuik DG, Bell GJ. The effect of strength training on estimates of mitochondrial density and distribution throughout muscle fibres. *Eur J Appl Physiol* 1999;80:604–9.

Coyle E, Costill D, Lesmes G. Leg extension power and muscle fibre composition. *Med Sci Sports Exerc* 1979;11:12–15.

Dawson B, Fitzsimons M, Green S, Goodman C, Carey M, Cole K. Changes in performance, muscle metabolites, enzymes and fibre types after short sprint training. *Eur J Appl Physiol* 1998;78:163–9.

Enoka RM. Eccentric contractions require unique activation strategies by the nervous system. *J Appl Physiol* 1996;81:2339–46.

Ennion S, Sant'Ana Pereira JAA, Sargeant AJ. Characterisation of human skeletal muscle fibres according to the myosin heavy chains they express. *J Muscle Res Cell Motility* 1995;16:35–43.

Esborjnsson-Liljedahl M, Holm I, Sylven C, Jansson E. Different responses of skeletal muscle following sprint training in men and women. *Eur J Appl Physiol* 1996;74: 375–83.

Esbjornsson M, Slyven C, Holm I, Jansson E. Fast twitch fibres may predict anaerobic performance in both males and females. *Int J Sports Med* 1993;14:257–63.

Fink WJ, Costill DL, Pollock MJ. Submaximal and maximal work capacity of elite distance runners. Part II. Muscle fiber composition and enzyme activity. *Ann NY Acad Sci* 1977;301:323–7.

Fitts R. Cellular mechanisms of muscle fatigue. *Physiol Rev* 1994;74:49–94.

Fitts RH, Metzger JM. Mechanisms of muscle fatigue. In: Poortmans JR, ed. *Principles of Exercise Biochemistry: Medicine and Sport Science*. Basel: Karger, 1988;27: 214.

Gollnick PD, Armstrong RB, Saltin B, Saubert CW 4th, Sembrowich WL, Shepherd RE. Effect of training on enzyme activity and fibre type composition of human skeletal muscle. *J Appl Physiol* 1973;34:107–11.

Gollnick PD, Armstrong RB, Saubert CW 4th, Piehl K, Saltin B. Enzyme activity and fiber composition in skeletal muscle of untrained and trained men. *J Appl Physiol* 1972;33:312–19.

Gollnick PD, Matoba H. The muscle fibre composition of skeletal muscle as a predictor of athletic success: an overview. *Am J Sports Med* 1984;12:212–17.

Gollnick PD, Piehl K, Saltin B. Selective glycogen depletion pattern in human muscle fibres after exercise of varying intensity and at varying pedalling rates. *J Physiol* 1974;241:45–57.

Green H, Thomson JA, Daub WD, Houston ME, Ranney DA. Fiber composition, fiber size and enzyme activities in vastus lateralis of elite athletes involved in high intensity exercise. *Eur J Appl Physiol* 1979;41:109–17.

Greenhaff P, Casey A, Constantin-Teodosiu D, Tzintas K. Energy metabolism of skeletal muscle fibre types and the metabolic basis of fatigue in humans. In: Hargreaves M, Thompson M, eds. *Biochemistry of Exercise X*. Champaign, IL: Human Kinetics, 1999: 275–87.

Harmer A, Mckenna MJ, Sutton JR, Snow RJ, Ruell PA, Booth J, Thompson MW, Mackay NA, Stathis CG, Crameri RM, Carey MF, Eager DM. Skeletal muscle metabolic and ionic adaptations during intense exercise following sprint training in humans. *J Appl Physiol* 2000;89:1793–803.

Harridge SD, Bottinelli R, Canepari M, Pellegrino MA, Reggiani C, Esborjnsson M, Saltin B. Whole-muscle and single fibre contractile properties and myosin heavy chain isoforms in humans. *Pflugers Arch* 1996;432:913–20.

Henriksson J, Reitman JS. Quantitative measures of enzyme activities in type I and type II muscle fibres of man after training. *Acta Physiol Scand* 1976;97:392–7.

Henneman E, Clamann HP, Gillies JD, Skinner RD. Rank order of motorneurons within a pool, law of combination. *J Neurophysiol* 1974;37:1338–49.

Horowitz JF, Sidosis LS, Coyle EF. High efficiency of type I muscle fibres improves performance. *Int J Sports Med* 1994;15:152–7.

Jacobs I, Esborjnsson M, Sylven C, Holm I, Jansson E. Sprint training effects on muscle myoglobin, enzymes, fiber types, and blood lactate. *Med Sci Sports Exerc* 1987;19: 368–74.

Jansson E, Sylven C. Creatine kinase MB and citrate synthase in type I and type II muscle fibres in trained and untrained men. *Eur J Appl Physiol* 1985;54:207–9.

Kaczkowski W, Montgomery DL, Taylor AW, Klissouras V. The relationship between muscle fiber composition and maximal anaerobic power and capacity. *J Sports Med* 1982;22:407–13.

Komi PV, Vitasalo JHT, Havu M, Thorstennsson A, Sjodin B, Karlsson J. Skeletal muscle fibres and muscle enzyme activities in monozygous and dizygous twins of both sexes. *Acta Physiol Scand* 1977;100:385–92.

MacDougall JD. Morphological changes in human skeletal muscle following strength and immobilization. In: Jones NL, et al., eds. *Human Muscle Power*. Champaign, IL: Human Kinetics, 1986: 269–88.

MacDougall JD, Elder GC, Sale DG, Moroz JR, Sutton JR. Effects of strength training and immobilization on human muscle fibres. *Eur J Appl Physiol* 1980;43:25–34.

MacDougall JD, Hicks AL, MacDonald JR, McKelvie RS, Green HJ, Smith KM. Muscle performance and enzymatic adaptations to sprint interval training. *J Appl Physiol* 1998;84:2138–42.

MacDougall JD, Sale DG, Moroz JR, Elder GC, Sutton JR, Howald H. Mitochondrial volume density in human skeletal muscle following heavy resistance training. *Med Sci Sports* 1979;11:164–6.

MacDougall JD, Ward GR, Sale DG, Sutton JR. Biochemical adaptation of human skeletal muscle to heavy resistance training and immobilization. *J Appl Physiol* 1977;43:700–3.

Mackova E, Melichna J, Havlickova L, Placheta Z, Blahova D. Skeletal muscle characteristics of sprint cyclists and nonathletes. *Int J Sports Med* 1986;7:295–7.

Martin WH, Dalsky GP, Hurley BF, Mathews DE, Bier DM, Hagberg JO, Holloszy JO. Effect of endurance training on plasma FFA turnover and oxidation during exercise. *Am J Physiol* 1993;265:E708–E714.

Maughan RJ, ed. *Basic and Applied Sciences for Sports Medicine.* Oxford: Butterworth & Heinemann, 1999: 26.

Nevill ME, Boobis LH, Brooks S, Williams C. Effect of training on muscle metabolism during treadmill sprinting. *J Appl Physiol* 1989;67:2376–82.

Parra J, Cadefau JA, Rodas G, Amigo N, Cusso R. The distribution of rest periods affects performance and adaptations of energy metabolism induced by high-intensity training in human muscle. *Acta Physiol Scand* 2000;169:157–65.

Pette D. Training effects on the contractile apparatus. *Acta Physiol Scand* 1998;162: 367–76.

Pette D, Peuker H, Staron RS. The impact of biochemical methods for single muscle fibre analysis. *Acta Physiol Scand* 1999;166:261–77.

Powers SK, Howley ET. *Exercise Physiology: Theory and Application to Fitness and Performance.* New York: McGraw-Hill, 2001.

Sahlin K, Henriksson J. Buffer capacity and lactate accumulation in skeletal muscle of trained and untrained men. *Acta Physiol Scand* 1984;122:331–9.

Sale DG. Influence of exercise and training on motor unit activation. *Exerc Sports Sci Rev* 1987;15:95–151.

Salmons S, Henriksson J. The adaptive response of skeletal muscle to increased use. *Muscle & Nerve* 1981;4:94–105.

Saltin B, Gollnick P. Skeletal muscle adaptability: significance for metabolism and performance. In: Peachey LD, Adrian RH, Geiger SR, eds. *Handbook of Physiology 10.* Bethesda, MD: American Physiological Society, 1983: 555–631.

Saltin B, Henriksson J, Nygaard E, Andersen P. Fibre types and metabolic potentials of skeletal muscles in sedentary man and endurance runners. *Ann NY Acad Sci* 1977;301:3–29.

Sant'Ana Pereira J, Sargeant AJ, Rademaker AC, de Haan A, van Mechelen W. Myosin heavy chain isoform expression and high energy phosphate content in human muscle fibres at rest and post-exercise. *J Physiol* 1996;496:583–8.

Schantz PG. Plasticity of human skeletal muscle with reference to effects of physical training on enzyme levels of the NADH shuttles and phenotypic expression of slow and fast myofibrillar proteins. *Acta Physiol Scand* 1986;558(suppl.):1–62.

Schantz PG, Henriksson J, Jansson E. Adaptation of human skeletal muscle to endurance training of long duration. *Clin Physiol* 1983;3:141–51.

Schiaffino S, Reggiani C. Molecular diversity of myofibrillar proteins: gene regulation and functional significance. *Physiol Rev* 1996;76:371–423.

Staron RS. The classification of human skeletal muscle fiber types. *J Strength Cond Res* 1997;11:62.

Steinen GJ, Kiers JL, Bottinelli R, Reggiani C. Myofibrillar ATPase activity in skinned human skeletal muscle fibres: fibre type and temperature dependence. *J Physiol* 1996;493:299–307.

Stephenson DG. Molecular cogs in machina carnis. *Clin Exp Pharm Physiol* 1996;23:898–907.

Suter E, Hoppeler H, Claassen H, Billeter R, Aebi U, Horber F, Jaeger P, Marti B. Ultrastructural modification of human skeletal muscle tissue with 6-month moderate-intensity exercise training. *Int J Sports Nutr* 1995;16:160–6.

Tesch PA. Acute and long-term metabolic changes consequent to heavy resistance exercise. *Med Sport Sci* 1987;26:67–89.

Tesch PA, Thorsson A, Essen-Gustavsson B. Enzyme activities of FT and ST muscle fibres in heavy resistance trained athletes. *J Appl Physiol* 1989;67:83–7.

Tesch PA, Komi PV, Hakkinen K. Enzymatic adaptations consequent to long-term strength training. *Int J Sports Med* 1987;8(suppl.):66–9.

Thorstensson A, Sjodin B, Karlsson J. Enzyme activities and muscle strength after 'sprint training' in man. *Acta Physiol Scand* 1975;94:313–18.

Vøllestad NK. Motor unit recruitment: a histochemical approach. In: Marconnet P, Komi P, eds. *Muscular Function in Exercise and Training: Medicine and Sport Science.* Basel: Karger, 1987;26:128–41.

Westerblad H, Allen D, Bruton J, Andrade F, Lannergren J. Mechanisms underlying the reduction of isometric force in skeletal muscle fatigue. *Acta Physiol Scand* 1998;162:253–60.

CHAPTER 2

Exercise metabolism: fuels for sport

Mark HARGREAVES

Success in athletic competition is critically dependent upon the ability to provide energy to contracting skeletal muscle in order to generate maximal power and/or force for short periods, or to maintain a high average power output for fixed distances or time periods. The immediate energy source for muscle cross-bridge cycling and the associated cellular processes is derived from the hydrolysis of adenosine triphosphate (ATP):

$$ATP + H_2O \rightarrow ADP + P_i + H^+ + energy$$

Since the intramuscular stores of ATP are small (~5 mmol/kg wet muscle) other metabolic pathways must be activated to regenerate ATP at a rate sufficient to maintain the required level of contractile activity during exercise. These include the degradation of creatine phosphate (PCr), the breakdown of muscle glycogen to lactate (oxygen-independent, substrate-level phosphorylation) and the oxidative metabolism of carbohydrate (CHO) and lipid (oxidative phosphorylation). These metabolic processes are summarised in Figure 2.1.

The relative importance of these pathways is primarily determined by the prevailing intensity and duration of exercise. The anaerobic energy systems are able to generate ATP at a high rate but have a relatively small capacity; in contrast, the aerobic energy system has an almost infinite capacity, in practical terms, but lower rates of ATP generation.

Metabolism during high-intensity exercise

During high-intensity exercise of short duration, ATP and PCr hydrolysis and the degradation of muscle glycogen to lactate are the predominant

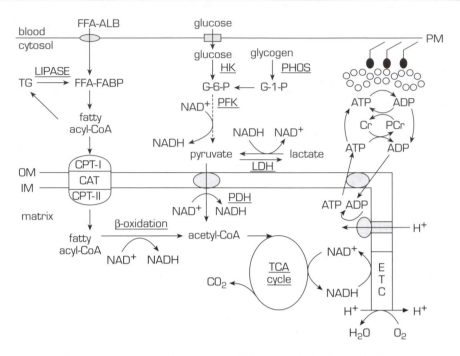

FIG. 2.1 Schematic overview of energy metabolism in skeletal muscle (from Spriet & Howlett 1999, with permission)

Abbreviations: PM—plasma membrane; OM, IM—outer and inner mitochondrial membranes; FFA—free fatty acid; ALB—albumin; FABP—fatty acid binding protein; CoA—coenzyme A; CPT 1, 11—carnitine palmitoyltransferase 1 and 11; CAT—carnitine acyl-translocase; NAD+, NADH—oxidised and reduced nicotinamide adenine dinucleotide; HK—hexokinase; PFK—phosphofructokinase; PHOS—glycogen phosphorylase; LDH—lactate dehydrogenase; PDH—pyruvate dehydrogenase; G-6-P, G-1-P—glucose-6- and glucose-1-phosphate; ATP, ADP—adenosine diphosphate and triphosphate; PCr—creatine phosphate; Cr—creatine; TCA—tricarboxylic acid; TG—triglyceride; ETC—electron transport chain.

energy-yielding pathways (Withers et al. 1991), although there can be a significant contribution from oxidative metabolism (Medbø & Tabata 1989). Muscle ATP levels are usually reduced by 30–50% following intense exercise (Söderlund & Hultman 1991; Spriet et al. 1987), whereas PCr levels can be completely depleted following such activity (Söderlund & Hultman 1991). Muscle glycogen levels are reduced by 50–60% depending upon exercise intensity and duration (Spriet et al. 1989) but muscle glycogen availability is not thought to be a major limiting factor during this type of exercise. Accompanying the decline in these substrates are marked increases in the intramuscular concentrations of inorganic phosphate (P_i), lactate and hydrogen ions. ATP can also be produced in the adenylate kinase reaction and adenosine monophosphate (AMP) is used to produce inosine monophosphate (IMP) and ammonia in a reaction catalysed by AMP deaminase.

Activation of muscle phosphagen and glycogen degradation occurs with the onset of exercise. Although the capacity for ATP generation is greater for the glycolytic system (190–300 mmol ATP/kg dry muscle) than for the phosphagen system (55–95 mmol ATP/kg dry muscle), the power output is lower (4.5 vs 9 mmol ATP/kg dry muscle/s). For this reason, when the levels of PCr decline with maximal activity, the anaerobic ATP turnover cannot be sustained (Fig. 2.2) and this contributes to the decline in power output that is observed during 'all-out' exercise.

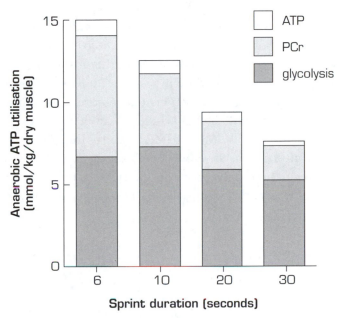

FIG. 2.2 Anaerobic ATP utilisation during maximal cycling exercise of varying duration (from Nevill et al. 1996, with permission)

Metabolism during endurance exercise

The oxidative metabolism of CHO and lipid substrates, derived from both intra- and extramuscular sources, provides almost all of the required ATP during prolonged, strenuous endurance exercise. Although amino acids can be utilised, their contribution to overall energy metabolism is small.

Carbohydrate metabolism

Muscle glycogen and blood-borne glucose, derived from liver glycogenolysis and gluconeogenesis (and the gastrointestinal tract when glucose in ingested), are important substrates for contracting skeletal muscle. Fatigue during prolonged strenuous exercise is often associated with depletion of these CHO reserves (Coyle et al. 1986). Increased muscle glycogen availability prior to exercise and CHO ingestion during exercise enhance endurance exercise performance (Coyle et al. 1986; Hawley et al. 1997) due to maintenance of CHO availability and oxidation during exercise.

Muscle glycogen degradation during exercise is primarily dependent upon exercise intensity (Romijn et al. 1993; Van Loon et al. 2001; Fig. 2.3) and is most rapid during the early stages of exercise (Gollnick et al. 1974; Vøllestad & Blom 1985). As exercise at a given intensity continues, the rate of muscle glycogenolysis declines as a function of reduced glycogen levels and glycogen phosphorylase activity, and increased blood-borne substrate availability. The increase in glycogenolysis during exercise occurs due to activation of glycogen phosphorylase in response to increased sarcoplasmic calcium levels with muscle contractions and β-adrenergic stimulation by adrenaline (Johnson 1992; Richter et al. 1982; Watt et al. 2001). In addition, allosteric modulators such as AMP and IMP, as well as the substrates inorganic phosphate and glycogen itself, influence glycogen phosphorylase activity. This complex regulation of glycogen phosphorylase activity ensures that the rate of muscle glycogenolysis is closely coupled to the ATP demand.

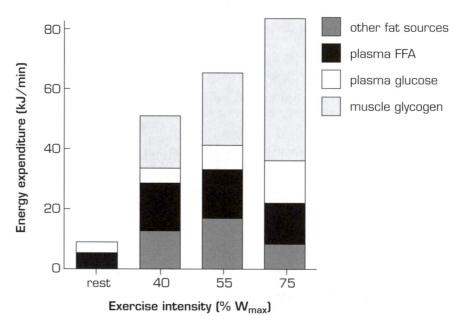

FIG. 2.3 The relative contribution of intramuscular and extramuscular CHO and lipid oxidation to energy metabolism during exercise of increasing intensity (Van Loon et al. 2001, with permission)

Increased muscle glycogen availability results in a greater rate of glycogenolysis during submaximal exercise (Hargreaves et al. 1995). Despite the increase in muscle glycogen utilisation, increased pre-exercise muscle glycogen availability is associated with enhanced endurance exercise performance (Hawley et al. 1997). Blood glucose availability appears to have little effect on muscle glycogen degradation, at least during prolonged cycling exercise (Hargreaves 1997). In contrast, alterations in plasma free fatty acid (FFA) levels influence muscle glycogen metabolism. Inhibition of FFA mobilisation lowers plasma FFA levels and increases muscle glycogen use, whereas an increase in plasma FFA levels has been shown to reduce net muscle glycogen utilisation during exercise (Costill et al. 1977; Dyck et al. 1996; Vukovich et al. 1993).

Exercise is a powerful stimulus for skeletal muscle glucose uptake, the magnitude of the exercise-induced increase in muscle glucose uptake being related to both the exercise intensity (Katz et al. 1986; Fig. 2.3) and duration (Ahlborg et al. 1974; Katz et al. 1991). At a given exercise intensity, there is an increase in muscle glucose uptake with increasing exercise duration. This is the result of a progressive increase in sarcolemmal glucose transport (Kristiansen et al. 1997) and an increase in glucose metabolism due to a lower glucose-6-phosphate level as the rate of muscle glycogenolysis decreases (Katz et al. 1991).

Glucose and insulin delivery to contracting skeletal muscle are increased during exercise as a consequence of the large increase in muscle blood flow, but this cannot fully explain the exercise-induced increase in muscle glucose uptake and local factors within the contracting muscle play the major role (Zinker et al. 1993). These include increased sarcolemmal transport of glucose and activation of the glycolytic and oxidative enzymes responsible for glucose metabolism. Sarcolemmal glucose transport occurs by facilitated diffusion, with the GLUT-4 isoform being responsible for contraction and insulin-stimulated glucose transport. GLUT-4 translocation from an intracellular storage site to the plasma membrane is the major mechanism responsible for the increase in sarcolemmal glucose transport during exercise of skeletal muscle (Kristiansen et al. 1996, 1997; Thorell et al. 1999). The intracellular distribution of GLUT-1, the isoform responsible for basal glucose transport, is unaltered by exercise (Kristiansen et al. 1996). The increase in muscle glucose uptake and GLUT-4 translocation can occur in the absence of insulin (Gao et al. 1994; Ploug et al. 1984). This is consistent with observations that contractions stimulate muscle glucose uptake via a mechanism that is different from insulin stimulation (Lee et al. 1995; Lund et al. 1995) and that the effects of contractions and insulin are additive. Despite these observations, the prevailing plasma insulin level has an important influence on skeletal muscle glucose uptake during exercise (Wasserman et al. 1991).

Substrate availability also influences muscle glucose uptake during exercise. In general, there is an inverse relationship between muscle glycogen availability and muscle glucose transport and metabolism (Hargreaves 1997). Increased blood glucose availability results in enhanced glucose uptake and oxidation during exercise (Ahlborg & Felig 1976; McConell et al. 1994), whereas a decline in arterial blood glucose levels may limit muscle glucose uptake during the latter stages of prolonged exercise (Ahlborg & Felig 1982; Ahlborg et al. 1974). There are conflicting reports in the literature on the effect of elevated plasma FFA levels on muscle glucose uptake (Hargreaves et al. 1991; Odland et al. 1998).

Accompanying the increase in muscle glucose uptake is an increase in liver glucose output so that blood glucose levels stay at or slightly above resting levels. During intense exercise, a greatly increased liver glucose output results in hyperglycaemia; in contrast, during prolonged moderate-intensity exercise, peripheral glucose uptake may exceed liver glucose output, resulting in hypoglycaemia. The magnitude of increase in liver glucose output during exercise is determined by both exercise intensity and duration. Most of the liver glucose output is derived from liver glycogenolysis, and the decline in liver glycogen availability during prolonged, strenuous exercise results in a reduced liver glucose output since gluconeogenesis, although increasing due to increased liver gluconeogenic enzyme activity and precursor availability, is unable to compensate fully for the decrease in liver glycogenolysis.

The regulation of liver glucose output during exercise is complex. During low-intensity exercise, it is thought that alterations in the plasma levels of the pancreatic hormones, insulin and glucagon, are crucial for the increase in liver glucose output. Even in the absence of large changes in the systemic plasma levels of these hormones, it is possible that small fluctuations in the portal vein concentrations exert a major effect on liver metabolism. Glucagon is likely to be most important during prolonged exercise and is known to stimulate liver gluconeogenesis. At higher exercise intensities (> 70% $\dot{V}O_{2max}$), increased plasma adrenaline levels and sympathetic activity play a greater role but cannot fully account for the increased liver glucose output that is observed (Coggan et al. 1997; Howlett et al. 1999). For many years it was thought that liver glucose output responded to a fall in blood glucose during the early stages of exercise (classical feedback regulation). It is now apparent that stimulation of the liver may also occur in parallel with activation of the contracting skeletal muscles, the cardiorespiratory responses and the neuroendocrine centres that modulate many metabolic processes, such that there is 'feed-forward' stimulation of the liver, particularly at higher exercise intensities. This does not diminish the importance of feedback regulation. Indeed, increased blood glucose availability can inhibit (McConell et al. 1994) or completely abolish (Howlett et al. 1998; Jeukendrup et al. 1999) the exercise-induced rise in liver glucose output. In addition, afferent feedback from contracting skeletal muscle may also influence liver glucose output during exercise (Kjær et al. 1996). It has even been suggested that a 'factor' released from contracting skeletal muscle may act to stimulate liver glucose output in proportion to the intensity of muscle contraction. Finally, there is evidence that the liver glycogen level may influence liver glucose output in much the same way that the pre-exercise muscle glycogen level determines its subsequent rate of utilisation.

The complex and redundant nature of the regulation of liver glucose output only serves to emphasise the crucial role of the liver in glucose homeostasis during exercise. Nevertheless, during prolonged strenuous exercise liver glucose output can fall behind peripheral glucose uptake, resulting in the development of a relative hypoglycaemia which may contribute to fatigue. Under such exercise conditions, ingestion of CHO has been shown to be an effective strategy to enhance endurance performance by maintaining blood glucose availability and a high rate of CHO oxidation at a time when muscle glycogen stores are low (Coyle et al. 1986).

Although most of the glycogen/glucose used during prolonged, submaximal exercise is fully oxidised, lactate is also produced and there is growing evidence that it is an important metabolic intermediate during and after exercise, being a substrate for oxidative metabolism in contracting skeletal and cardiac muscle and a gluconeogenic precursor. During incremental exercise, there is an exponential rise in blood lactate concentrations and the lactate threshold has been generally defined as that workload eliciting an increase in blood lactate levels.

There is considerable debate in the exercise literature physiology on the underlying causes of this threshold phenomenon and the link between blood lactate levels and ventilatory control (the classical 'anaerobic threshold'). The classical view has been that lactate production by contracting skeletal muscle is the consequence of oxygen deficiency (Katz & Sahlin 1988) and there continues to be debate on this issue. Simplistically, it can be suggested that lactate will be produced whenever there is an imbalance between the rates of pyruvate production from glycolysis and oxidation within the mitochondria (Spriet et al. 2000). An increase in pyruvate (and sarcoplasmic calcium ions) stimulates flux through pyruvate dehydrogenase (PDH, which catalyses the first step in the oxidation of pyruvate) but also has a mass-action effect on lactate dehydrogenase (LDH), the enzyme that catalyses the reaction that produces lactate and regenerates cytosolic NAD$^+$, which is crucial for the maintenance of glycolysis. A reduction in oxygen delivery to contracting skeletal muscle during exercise (e.g. under conditions of hypoxia, anaemia, carbon monoxide poisoning) is associated with higher rates of muscle and blood lactate production; however, as mentioned above, there is ongoing debate as to whether this is a direct consequence of muscle hypoxia. Other factors that influence lactate production during exercise include plasma adrenaline levels and muscle glycogen availability via their effects on the rate of pyruvate formation. Without question, however, an increase in blood lactate concentration must be due to the rate of lactate production and release into the circulation exceeding the rate of lactate removal from the circulation.

Irrespective of the debate surrounding the regulation of lactate metabolism, measurement of blood lactate levels during exercise has become widespread in the evaluation of endurance athletes and indeed, lactate variables such as lactate threshold and onset of blood/plasma lactate accumulation are often better predictors of endurance exercise performance than maximal oxygen uptake. This probably reflects the close associations between lactate threshold, muscle oxidative capacity and the rate of CHO utilisation (Coyle et al. 1988). During exercise above the lactate threshold there is a continuous rise in blood lactate levels, indicating a sustained rate of lactate production and a greater reliance on CHO; in contrast, during exercise below the lactate threshold a steady-state blood lactate level is achieved due to a balance between the rates of lactate production and removal.

Lipid metabolism

Free fatty acids (FFAs), derived from the breakdown of adipose tissue and intramuscular triglyceride stores (lipolysis), are a major oxidative substrate during exercise lasting several hours. As exercise intensity increases, the rate appearance of FFAs derived from adipose tissue into the circulation decreases, but fat oxidation is maintained due to oxidation of FFAs derived from intramuscular triglyceride stores, although their contribution and regulation is not well described. During intense exercise, both adipose tissue and intramuscular lipolysis are inhibited and CHO oxidation is dominant. With increasing duration of low-intensity exercise

(30% $\dot{V}O_{2max}$), the plasma FFA concentration increases progressively and this is associated with enhanced FFA uptake in the leg, such that after 4 hours of exercise, oxidation of plasma FFAs can account for 60% of oxygen uptake in the leg.

The oxidation of fatty acids during exercise involves a number of steps, the first being the hydrolysis of intramuscular and/or adipose tissue triglycerides (lipolysis) and the transport of FFAs in either the plasma or cytosol to the skeletal muscle mitochondria for oxidation. During exercise in the fasted state, the rate of lipolysis exceeds the rate of fat oxidation both at rest and during moderate-intensity exercise, suggesting that FFA availability may not limit fat oxidation under these conditions. In contrast, during intense exercise, or following inhibition of lipolysis (e.g. following nicotinic acid administration or carbohydrate ingestion), FFA availability may be rate-limiting.

Adipose tissue lipolysis is mediated via hormone-sensitive lipase. Activation of this lipase occurs via protein-kinase-mediated phosphorylation, secondary to increased intracellular cyclic AMP levels following hormone-receptor interaction. The stimulatory effects of adrenaline on lipolysis are β-receptor mediated, while adenosine is inhibitory. Insulin is also a powerful inhibitor of lipolysis, although its mechanism of action is not fully clear. During exercise, β-adrenergic stimulation (Arner et al. 1990) and a decrease in plasma insulin are the major factors responsible for the increased rate of lipolysis. An increase in plasma insulin following carbohydrate ingestion results in inhibition of lipolysis (Horowitz et al. 1997). In addition to the rate of lipolysis, the mobilisation of FFAs into the systemic circulation is determined by adipose tissue blood flow and the balance between FFA and albumin levels (since FFAs are bound to albumin). It has been suggested that vasoconstriction in adipose tissue may explain the reduction in plasma FFA mobilisation during intense exercise (Romijn et al. 1993).

The regulation of intramuscular lipolysis is much less understood and there is even debate as to whether muscle triglycerides are utilised during exercise at all. Tracer studies and measurement of glycerol release from contracting skeletal muscle indicate significant intramuscular lipolysis, particularly at higher exercise intensities where plasma FFA mobilisation is reduced. On the other hand, direct measurement of muscle triglyceride concentrations before and after exercise has often yielded conflicting results. Recently, it has been demonstrated that the rate of intramuscular triglyceride synthesis from fatty acids is reduced during exercise and in the absence of a reduction in triglyceride hydrolysis, there was a net reduction in muscle triglyceride concentration (Sacchetti et al. 2002). A hormone-sensitive lipase has been found in skeletal muscle and is thought to be under both local control by sarcoplasmic calcium levels and hormonal regulation by adrenaline (Langfort et al. 1999, 2000). Much more work is required to fully understand intramuscular lipolysis and its regulation during exercise.

In order to be oxidised, FFAs must enter the mitochondria where they undergo β-oxidation, the sequential removal of two-carbon units in the form of acetyl-CoA for entry into the tricarboxylic acid (TCA) cycle. The mitochondrial uptake of FFAs from the sarcoplasm involves the carrier carnitine, which is combined with fatty acyl-CoA in a reaction catalysed by carnitine acyl-translocase (CAT). There has been some interest in the potential of dietary carnitine supplementation to enhance fat oxidation but little experimental evidence to support such a practice (Vukovich et al. 1994). In the cytosol, FFAs (derived from either the plasma or intramuscular lipolysis) are converted to the CoA derivative by fatty acyl-CoA synthetase (also known as thiokinase). Although muscle FFA uptake from plasma has long been thought to occur by simple diffusion, recent results in perfused rat hind limbs and exercising humans suggest a carrier-mediated process and attention has focused on various putative sarcolemmal and cytosolic fatty acid transport proteins (Turcotte 2000).

During exercise in the fasted state, FFA availability, as determined by the rate of lipolysis and FFA mobilisation, is not thought to limit FFA oxidation within contracting skeletal muscle. There are circumstances, however, where FFA availability may be limiting. During intense exercise, a reduction in FFA appearance into the plasma, due to vasoconstriction in adipose tissue, is thought to contribute to a decline in fat oxidation (Romijn et al. 1993). In addition, hyperglycaemia and hyperinsulinaemia following CHO ingestion inhibit lipolysis and fat oxidation during subsequent exercise (Coyle et al. 1997; Horowitz et al. 1997). Restoring plasma FFA availability, by infusing Intralipid and heparin, only partially overcomes the decrease in fat oxidation seen under these conditions (Horowitz et al. 1997; Romijn et al. 1995), suggesting that there may be factors within skeletal muscle that limit fat oxidation.

Results from studies comparing the relative rates of oxidation of long-chain and medium-chain fatty acids during low- and high-intensity exercise (Sidossis et al. 1997) and following carbohydrate ingestion (Coyle et al. 1997) have suggested that the limitation may be entry of long-chain fatty acids into the mitochondria in the step catalysed by CAT. Increases in CHO flux, as seen during intense exercise or following CHO ingestion, are believed to result in higher intramuscular levels of malonyl-CoA, an inhibitor of CAT activity. While this is an attractive hypothesis and there are good experimental data demonstrating a role for malonyl-CoA in rat skeletal muscle, the single study in exercising humans is less convincing (Odland et al. 1996). Since medium-chain fatty acids can bypass the mitochondrial barrier that exists for long-chain fatty acids, there has been interest in the potential benefits of medium-chain triglyceride (MCT) ingestion on endurance exercise performance, especially in combination with CHO ingestion which would normally inhibit lipolysis and fat oxidation; however, the experimental results obtained so far do not convincingly support their use.

Plasma triglycerides can be hydrolysed by capillary-bound lipoprotein lipase in skeletal muscle but make a minor contribution (< 10%) to overall lipid metabolism during exercise. Exercise activates capillary bound lipoprotein lipase in skeletal muscle (Kiens et al. 1989) and exercise training results in adaptations in muscle lipoprotein metabolism that contribute to the higher levels of high-density lipoprotein (HDL) cholesterol seen following training (Kiens & Lithell 1989). Glycerol, the breakdown product of lipolysis, cannot be utilised directly by skeletal muscle but can serve as a gluconeogenic precursor, although glycerol turnover during exercise in humans is slow (Miller et al. 1983). Ketone bodies (acetoacetate and β-hydroxybutyrate) can be oxidised by skeletal muscle but their contribution to oxidative metabolism during exercise is small (1–2%).

Protein metabolism

Amino acids, derived from muscle protein reserves, can be oxidised during exercise, especially under conditions of reduced CHO availability (Wagenmakers et al. 1991). However, their contribution to energy metabolism during exercise is minor (1–5%) compared with that from CHO and lipid. The branched-chain amino acids (BCAA: valine, leucine, isoleucine) are the major amino acids used for oxidation and the activity of the branched-chain oxo-acid dehydrogenase, the rate-limiting enzyme in BCAA oxidation, is increased with exercise (Wagenmakers et al. 1991). While the carbon skeletons of the amino acids are oxidised, the nitrogen-containing amino groups must be removed.

Alanine and glutamine are the major amino acids involved in the transfer of nitrogen between tissues, the former being able to be used as a gluconeogenic substrate by the liver, the so-called glucose-alanine cycle. Another potential function of amino acid catabolism during exercise may be in anaplerotic reactions that generate TCA cycle intermediates (Gibala et al. 1997b), the most important of these being the alanine aminotransferase reaction (Gibala et al. 1997a). Another nitrogen carrier released from contracting skeletal muscle is ammonia and it is thought that a major part of the ammonia produced is derived from the deamination of BCAA (Van Hall et al. 1995). Increased plasma BCAA availability following BCAA ingestion results in increased skeletal muscle BCAA uptake and ammonia production (MacLean et al. 1996). Furthermore, increased blood glucose availability after CHO ingestion, which decreases leucine oxidation during exercise, results in lower plasma and muscle ammonia accumulation during prolonged exercise (Snow et al. 2000). At higher exercise intensities the story is more complicated since ammonia (and IMP) can be produced from AMP deamination in the purine nucleotide cycle.

Factors influencing exercise metabolism

The major factors determining the metabolic responses to exercise are the intensity and duration of exercise. As exercise intensity is increased, there is a greater reliance on CHO oxidation, in particular of muscle glycogen (Romijn et al. 1993; Van Loon et al. 2001; Fig. 2.3). With increasing exercise duration at a given exercise intensity there is increasing reliance on lipid oxidation (Ahlborg et al. 1974; Romijn et al. 1993), primarily of plasma FFAs, as muscle glycogen and blood glucose levels decline. The ingestion of CHO does not significantly affect this general pattern of substrate utilisation (Angus et al. 2002; Fig. 2.4) but does maintain a relatively higher CHO oxidation and increases endurance capacity. Because of the heavy reliance on CHO during strenuous training and competition, and the relatively small endogenous CHO reserves and their depletion during exercise, nutritional strategies designed to enhance sports performance have focused on ingestion of sufficient CHO before, during and after exercise (see Chapter 8).

Other factors that influence the metabolic response to exercise include training status, preceding diet, environmental temperature and gender. The major adaptations to endurance training are reductions in CHO utilisation and lactate accumulation during exercise, with a concomitant increase in lipid oxidation (Coggan 1997). These effects of training are manifested as lower rates of muscle glycogen and blood glucose oxidation, reduced liver glycogenolysis and gluconeogenesis and attenuation of muscle and blood lactate accumulation during exercise, together with increased oxidation of FFAs derived from both muscle and adipose tissue triglyceride stores. The major mechanisms responsible for these changes are an enhanced muscle oxidative capacity, increased levels and activities of key proteins involved

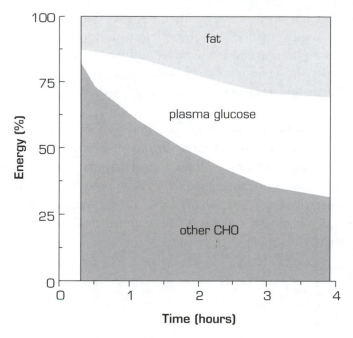

FIG. 2.4 Estimated percentage contributions from fat, plasma glucose and other CHOs to total aerobic energy expenditure during exercise to fatigue at 68 ± 2% VO_{2peak} until fatigue. Subjects ingested an 8% glucose solution at a rate of 1 L/h throughout the trial (Angus et al. 2002, with permission)

in substrate transport and utilisation, alterations in substrate availability and a blunting of the hormonal response to exercise. These effects of training are most apparent when comparisons between trained and untrained subjects are made at the same absolute power output. In response to exercise at the same relative power output, the effects of training are less apparent and may be determined by the relative magnitude of increases in maximal oxygen uptake and muscle oxidative capacity. Nevertheless, the increased capacity for metabolic energy provision in the trained state is likely to be an important contributor to the enhanced exercise performance observed after training.

Following consumption of a high CHO diet, CHO utilisation during exercise is increased and lipid utilisation is decreased, while following consumption of a high fat diet the reverse is true (Burke et al. 2000; Galbo et al. 1979; Hargreaves et al. 1995). Alterations in substrate availability and hormonal responses to exercise account for these metabolic changes, although their persistence when muscle glycogen availability is similar (Burke et al. 2000) suggests that other adaptations to diet may be important.

These include, but are not limited to, alterations in the abundance and activities of key proteins involved in substrate transport and utilisation.

An increase in environmental temperature results in a greater reliance on muscle glycogen during exercise (Febbraio et al. 1994) due to increased core and muscle temperature and higher plasma adrenaline levels (see Chapter 10).

Finally, there has been interest in potential gender differences in exercise metabolism and the implications for sports performance. While it is generally suggested that females have a greater reliance on lipid fuel sources during exercise, conflicting results have been reported (Freidlander et al. 1998; Roepstorff et al. 2002; Romijn et al. 2000; Tarnopolsky et al. 1990). More detail on gender differences in exercise metabolism can be found in Chapter 12.

Summary

In summary, the supply of ATP to contracting skeletal muscle during exercise is crucial for successful sports performance. Since the intramuscular stores of ATP are small, other metabolic pathways must be activated in order to regenerate ATP at a rate sufficient to maintain the required level of contractile activity during exercise. During high-intensity, short-duration exercise, these include the degradation of PCr and the breakdown of muscle glycogen to lactate (oxygen-independent, substrate-level phosphorylation), while during prolonged, endurance-type exercise the oxidative metabolism of CHO and lipid (oxidative phosphorylation) predominates, with only a minor contribution from protein. Due to the heavy reliance on CHO at moderate-to-high exercise intensities and the relatively small endogenous CHO reserves, CHO depletion can limit sports performance during prolonged, strenuous exercise.

References

Ahlborg G, Felig P. Influence of glucose ingestion on fuel-hormone response during prolonged exercise. *J Appl Physiol* 1976;41:683–8.

Ahlborg G, Felig P. Lactate and glucose exchange across the forearm, legs, and splanchnic bed during and after prolonged leg exercise. *J Clin Invest* 1982;69:45–54.

Ahlborg G, Felig P, Hagenfeldt L, Hendler R, Wahren J. Substrate turnover during prolonged exercise in man: splanchnic and leg metabolism of glucose, free fatty acids, and amino acids. *J Clin Invest* 1974;53:1080–90.

Angus DJ, Febbraio MA, Hargreaves M. Plasma glucose kinetics during prolonged exercise in trained humans when fed carbohydrate. *Am J Physiol* 2002 (283:E573–E577).

Arner P, Kriegholm E, Engfeldt P, Bolinder J. Adrenergic regulation of lipolysis in situ at rest and during exercise. *J Clin Invest* 1990;85:893–8.

Burke LM, Angus DJ, Cox GR, Cummings NK, Febbraio MA, Gawthorn K, Hawley JA, Minehan M, Martin DT, Hargreaves M. Effect of fat adaptation and carbohydrate restoration on metabolism and performance during prolonged cycling. *J Appl Physiol* 2000;89:2413–21.

Coggan AR. Plasma glucose metabolism during exercise: effect of endurance training in humans. *Med Sci Sports Exerc* 1997;29:620–7.

Coggan AR, Raguso CA, Gastaldelli A, Williams BD, Wolfe RR. Regulation of glucose production during exercise at 80% VO_{2peak} in untrained humans. *Am J Physiol* 1997;273:E348–E354.

Costill DL, Coyle E, Dalsky G, Evans W, Fink W, Hoopes D. Effects of elevated plasma FFA and insulin on muscle glycogen usage during exercise. *J Appl Physiol* 1977: 43:695–9.

Coyle EF, Coggan AR, Hemmert MK, Ivy JL. Muscle glycogen utilization during prolonged strenuous exercise when fed carbohydrate. *J Appl Physiol* 1986;61: 165–72.

Coyle EF, Coggan AR, Hopper MK, Walters TJ. Determinants of endurance in well-trained cyclists. *J Appl Physiol* 1988;64:2622–30.

Coyle EF, Jeukendrup AE, Wagenmakers AJM, Saris WHM. Fatty acid oxidation is directly regulated by carbohydrate metabolism during exercise. *Am J Physiol* 1997;273:E268–E275.

Dyck DJ, Peters SJ, Wendling PS, Chesley A, Hultman E, Spriet LL. Regulation of muscle glycogen phosphorylase activity during intense aerobic cycling with elevated FFA. *Am J Physiol* 1996;270:E116–E125.

Febbraio M, Snow RJ, Hargreaves M, Stathis CG, Martin IK, Carey M. Muscle metabolism during exercise and heat stress in trained men: effect of acclimation. *J Appl Physiol* 1994;76:589–97.

Freidlander AL, Casazza GA, Horning MA, Buddinger TF, Brooks GA. Training-induced alterations of carbohydrate metabolism in women: women respond differently from men. *J Appl Physiol* 1998;85:1175–86.

Galbo H, Holst JJ, Christensen NJ. The effect of different diets and of insulin on the hormonal response to prolonged exercise. *Acta Physiol Scand* 1979;107:19–32.

Gao J, Ren J, Gulve E, Holloszy JO. Additive effect of contractions and insulin on GLUT-4 translocation into the sarcolemma. *J Appl Physiol* 1994;77:1597–601.

Gibala MJ, MacLean DA, Graham TE, Saltin B. Anaplerotic processes in human skeletal muscle during brief dynamic exercise. *J Physiol* 1997a;502:703–13.

Gibala MJ, Tarnopolsky MA, Graham TE. Tricarboxylic acid cycle intermediates in human muscle at rest and during prolonged cycling. *Am J Physiol* 1997b;272: E239–E244.

Gollnick PD, Piehl K, Saltin B. Selective glycogen depletion pattern in human muscle fibres after exercise of varying intensity and at varying pedalling rates. *J Physiol* 1974;241:45–57.

Hargreaves M. Interactions between muscle glycogen and blood glucose during exercise. *Exerc Sports Sci Rev* 1997;25:21–39.

Hargreaves M, Kiens B, Richter EA. Effect of increased plasma free fatty acid concentrations on muscle metabolism in exercising men. *J Appl Physiol* 1991;70: 194–201.

Hargreaves M, McConell G, Proietto J. Influence of muscle glycogen on glycogenolysis and glucose uptake during exercise. *J Appl Physiol* 1995;78:288–92.

Hawley JA, Schabort EJ, Noakes TD, Dennis SC. Carbohydrate-loading and exercise performance: an update. *Sports Med* 1997;24:73–81.

Horowitz JF, Mora-Rodriguez R, Byerley LO, Coyle EF. Lipolytic suppression following carbohydrate ingestion limits fat oxidation during exercise. *Am J Physiol* 1997;273: E768–E775.

Howlett K, Angus D, Proietto J, Hargreaves M. Effect of increased blood glucose availability on glucose kinetics during exercise. *J Appl Physiol* 1998;84:1413–17.

Howlett K, Febbraio M, Hargreaves M. Glucose production during strenuous exercise in humans: role of epinephrine. *Am J Physiol* 1999;276:E1130–E1135.

Jeukendrup AE, Wagenmakers AJM, Stegen JHCH, Gijsen AP, Brouns F, Saris WHM. Carbohydrate ingestion can completely suppress endogenous glucose production during exercise. *Am J Physiol* 1999;276:E672–E683.

Johnson LN. Glycogen phosphorylase: control by phosphorylation and allosteric effectors. *FASEB J* 1992;6:2274–82.

Katz A, Broberg S, Sahlin K, Wahren J. Leg glucose uptake during maximal dynamic exercise in humans. *Am J Physiol* 1986;251:E65–E70.

Katz A, Sahlin K. Regulation of lactic acid production during exercise. *J Appl Physiol* 1988;65:509–18.

Katz A, Sahlin K, Broberg S. Regulation of glucose utilization in human skeletal muscle during moderate dynamic exercise. *Am J Physiol* 1991;260:E411–E415.

Kiens B, Lithell H. Lipoprotein metabolism influenced by training-induced changes in human skeletal muscle. *J Clin Invest* 1989;83:558–64.

Kiens B, Lithell H, Mikines KJ, Richter EA. Effects of insulin and exercise on muscle lipoprotein lipase activity in man and its relation to insulin action. *J Clin Invest* 1989;84:1124–9.

Kjær M, Secher NH, Bangsbo J, Perko G, Horn A, Mohr T, Galbo H. Hormonal and metabolic responses to electrically induced cycling during epidural anesthesia in humans. *J Appl Physiol* 1996;80:2156–62.

Kristiansen S, Hargreaves M, Richter EA. Exercise-induced increase in glucose transport, GLUT-4 and VAMP-2 in plasma membrane from human muscle. *Am J Physiol* 1996;270:E197–E201.

Kristiansen S, Hargreaves M, Richter EA. Progressive increase in glucose transport and GLUT-4 in human sarcolemmal vesicles during moderate exercise. *Am J Physiol* 1997;272:E385–E389.

Langfort J, Ploug T, Ihlemann J, Holm C, Galbo H. Stimulation of hormone-sensitive lipase activity by contractions in rat skeletal muscle. *Biochem J* 2000;351:207–14.

Langfort J, Ploug T, Ihlemann J, Saldo M, Holm C, Galbo H. Expression of hormone-sensitive lipase and its regulation by adrenaline in skeletal muscle. *Biochem J* 1999;340:459–65.

Lee AD, Hansen PA, Holloszy JO. Wortmannin inhibits insulin-stimulated but not contraction-stimulated glucose transport activity in skeletal muscle. *FEBS Lett* 1995;361:51–4.

Lund S, Holman GD, Schmitz O, Pedersen O. Contraction stimulates translocation of the glucose transporter GLUT4 in skeletal muscle through a mechanism distinct from that of insulin. *Proc Nat Acad Sci USA* 1995;92:5817–21.

MacLean DA, Graham TE, Saltin B. Stimulation of muscle ammonia production during exercise following branched-chain amino acid supplementation in humans. *J Physiol* 1996;493:909–22.

McConell G, Fabris S, Proietto J, Hargreaves M. Effect of carbohydrate ingestion on glucose kinetics during exercise. *J Appl Physiol* 1994;77:1537–41.

Medbø JI, Tabata I. Relative importance of aerobic and anaerobic energy release during short-lasting exhausting bicycle exercise. *J Appl Physiol* 1989;67:1881–6.

Miller JM, Coyle EF, Sherman WM, Hagberg JM, Costill DL, Fink WJ, Terblanche SE, Holloszy JO. Effect of glycerol feeding on endurance and metabolism during prolonged exercise in man. *Med Sci Sports Exerc* 1983;15:237–42.

Nevill ME, Bogdanis GC, Boobis LH, Lakomy HKA, Williams C. Muscle metabolism and performance during sprinting. In: Maughan RJ, Shirreffs S, eds. *Biochemistry of Exercise IX*. Champaign, IL: Human Kinetics, 1996: 243–59.

Odland LM, Heigenhauser GJF, Lopaschuk GD, Spriet LL. Human skeletal muscle malonyl-CoA at rest and during prolonged submaximal exercise. *Am J Physiol* 1996;270:E541–E544.

Odland LM, Heigenhauser GJF, Wong D, Hollidge-Horvat MG, Spriet LL. Effects of increased fat availability on fat–carbohydrate interaction during prolonged exercise in men. *Am J Physiol* 1998;274:R894–R902.

Ploug T, Galbo H, Richter EA. Increased muscle glucose uptake during contractions: no need for insulin. *Am J Physiol* 1984;247:E726–E731.

Richter EA, Ruderman NB, Gavras H, Belur ER, Galbo H. Muscle glycogenolysis during exercise: dual control by epinephrine and contractions. *Am J Physiol* 1982;242:E25–E32.

Roepstorff C, Steffensen CH, Madsen M, Stallknecht B, Kanstrup I-L, Richter EA, Kiens B. Gender differences in substrate utilization during submaximal exercise in endurance-trained subjects. *Am J Physiol* 2002;282:E435–E447.

Romijn JA, Coyle EF, Sidossis LS, Gastaldelli A, Horowitz JF, Endert E, Wolfe RR. Regulation of endogenous fat and carbohydrate metabolism in relation to exercise intensity and duration. *Am J Physiol* 1993;265:E380–E391.

Romijn JA, Coyle EF, Sidossis LS, Rosenblatt J, Wolfe RR. Substrate metabolism during different exercise intensities in endurance-trained women. *J Appl Physiol* 2000;88: 1707–14.

Romijn JA, Coyle EF, Sidossis LS, Zhang X-J, Wolfe RR. Relationship between fatty acid delivery and fatty acid oxidation during strenuous exercise. *J Appl Physiol* 1995;79:1939–45.

Sacchetti M, Saltin B, Osada T, Van Hall G. Intramuscular fatty acid metabolism in contracting and non-contracting human skeletal muscle. *J Physiol* 2002;540: 387–95.

Sidossis LS, Gastaldelli A, Klein S, Wolfe RR. Regulation of plasma fatty acid oxidation during low- and high-intensity exercise. *Am J Physiol* 1997;272:E1065–E1070.

Snow RJ, Carey MF, Stathis CG, Febbraio MA, Hargreaves M. Effect of carbohydrate ingestion on ammonia metabolism during prolonged exercise. *J Appl Physiol* 2000;88:1576–80.

Söderlund K, Hultman E. ATP and phosphocreatine changes in single human muscle fibres after intense electrical stimulation. *Am J Physiol* 1991;261:E737–E741.

Spriet LL, Howlett RA. Metabolic control of energy production during physical activity. In: Lamb DR, Murray R, eds. *Perspectives in Exercise Science and Sports Medicine*. Vol. 12. *The Metabolic Bases of Performance in Sport and Exercise*. Carmel: Cooper Publishing Group, 1999: 1–44.

Spriet LL, Howlett RA, Heigenhauser GJF. An enzymatic approach to lactate production in human skeletal muscle during exercise. *Med Sci Sports Exerc* 2000;32:756–63.

Spriet LL, Lindinger MI, McKelvie RS, Heigenhauser GJF, Jones NL. Muscle glycogenolysis and H+ concentration during maximal intermittent cycling. *J Appl Physiol* 1989;66:8–13.

Spriet LL, Söderlund K, Bergstrom M, Hultman E. Anaerobic energy release in skeletal muscle during electrical stimulation in men. *J Appl Physiol* 1987;62:611–15.

Tarnopolsky LJ, MacDougall JD, Atkinson SA, Tarnopolsky MA, Sutton JR. Gender differences in substrate for endurance exercise. *J Appl Physiol* 1990;68:302–8.

Thorell A, Hirshman MF, Nygren J, Jorfeldt L, Wojtaszewski JF, Dufresne SD, Horton ES, Ljungqvist O, Goodyear LJ. Exercise and insulin cause GLUT-4 translocation in human skeletal muscle. *Am J Physiol* 1999;277:E733–E741.

Turcotte LP. Muscle fatty acid uptake during exercise: possible mechanisms. *Exerc Sport Sci Rev* 2000;28:4–9.

Van Hall G, Saltin B, Van Der Vusse GJ, Söderlund K, Wagenmakers AJM. Deamination of amino acids as a source for ammonia production in human skeletal muscle during prolonged exercise. *J Physiol* 1995;489:251–61.

Van Loon LJC, Greenhaff PL, Constantin-Teodosiu C, Saris WHM, Wagenmakers AJM. The effects of increasing exercise intensity on muscle fuel utilisation in humans. *J Physiol* 2001;536:295–304.

Vøllestad NK, Blom PCS. Effect of varying exercise intensity on glycogen depletion in human muscle fibres. *Acta Physiol Scand* 1985;125:395–405.

Vukovich MD, Costill DL, Fink WJ. Carnitine supplementation: effect on muscle carnitine and glycogen content during exercise. *Med Sci Sports Exerc* 1994;26:1122–9.

Vukovich MD, Costill DL, Hickey MS, Trappe SW, Cole KJ, Fink WJ. Effect of fat emulsion infusion and fat feeding on muscle glycogen utilization during cycle exercise. *J Appl Physiol* 1993;75:1513–18.

Wagenmakers AJM, Beckers EJ, Brouns F, Kuipers H, Soeters PO, Van Der Vusse GJ, Saris WHM. Carbohydrate supplementation, glycogen depletion, and amino acid metabolism during exercise. *Am J Physiol* 1991;260:E883–E890.

Wasserman DH, Geer RJ, Rice DE, Bracy D, Flakoll PJ, Brown LL, Hill JO, Abumrad NN. Interaction of exercise and insulin action in humans. *Am J Physiol* 1991;260: E37–E45.

Watt MJ, Howlett KF, Febbraio MA, Spriet LL, Hargreaves M. Adrenaline increases skeletal muscle glycogenolysis, pyruvate dehydrogenase activation and carbohydrate oxidation during moderate exercise in humans. *J Physiol* 2001;534: 269–78.

Withers RT, Sherman WM, Clark DG, Esselbach PC, Nolan SR, Mackay MH, Brinkman M. Muscle metabolism during 30, 60 and 90 s of maximal cycling on an air-braked ergometer. *Eur J Appl Physiol* 1991;63:354–62.

Zinker BA, Lacy DB, Bracy DP, Wasserman DH. Role of glucose and insulin loads to the exercising limb in increasing glucose uptake and metabolism. *J Appl Physiol* 1993;74:2915–21.

CHAPTER 3

Oxygen transport system

Mark HARGREAVES

The provision of energy via oxidative metabolism is critically dependent upon the availability of both CHO and lipid substrates (see Chapter 2) and oxygen (O_2), and the carbon dioxide (CO_2) produced must be removed. The delivery of O_2 to contracting skeletal muscle and CO_2 removal are achieved by the combined abilities of the respiratory and cardiovascular systems. An increase in skin blood flow is also essential to facilitate removal of heat produced by increased muscle metabolism during exercise (see Chapter 4) and this places an additional stress on the cardiovascular system, especially when the environmental temperature is elevated (see Chapter 10). For a given external power output there is a corresponding steady-state O_2 uptake (VO_2), which may vary slightly between individuals due to differences in mechanical efficiency and body mass, resulting in a linear relationship between VO_2 and power output (Fig. 3.1). At higher intensities, there may be loss of linearity and a more pronounced rise in VO_2 (Zoladz et al. 1995).

With the onset of exercise, there is a lag in VO_2 over the first few minutes until the steady-state VO_2 is attained (Fig. 3.1), with aerobic energy provision being supplemented by substrate level phosphorylation (glycolysis and PCr degradation—see Chapter 2). This so-called O_2 deficit has traditionally been attributed to a delayed O_2 delivery to skeletal muscle (Tschakovsky & Hughson 1999), but inertia in mitochondrial oxidative metabolism also plays a role (Bangsbo et al. 2000; Howlett et al. 1999; Timmons et al. 1998). With more prolonged exercise, there is an upward drift in VO_2 that is termed O_2 drift or VO_2 slow component (Poole & Richardson 1997). The increase in pulmonary VO_2 is a function of both time and power output and its origin has not been clearly defined; however, since more than 80% of the increase in pulmonary VO_2 can be accounted for by increases in

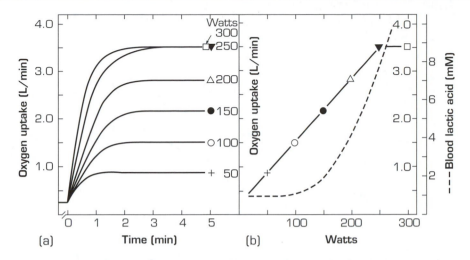

FIG. 3.1 Oxygen uptake over time at a given power output and with increasing power output to maximum (from Åstrand & Rodahl 1986, with permission)

contracting muscle VO_2, interest has focused on factors within contracting muscle. These include changes in mechanical efficiency related to muscle fibre recruitment, muscle temperature, altered substrate metabolism and expression of uncoupling proteins (Poole et al. 1994; Russell et al. 2002).

The increased VO_2 during exercise requires greater ventilation to ensure arterial oxygenation and haemoglobin saturation, as well as increased cardiac output and skeletal muscle blood flow to increase O_2 delivery to mitochondria.

Respiratory responses to exercise

Increased ventilation is achieved by increasing both tidal volume and breathing frequency. The ventilatory response to incremental exercise is characterised by a gradual increase in ventilation at lower intensities, with an abrupt increase at higher intensities, which is often referred to as the ventilatory threshold (Fig. 3.2). There has been considerable debate in the literature on the mechanisms responsible for the hyperventilation at higher exercise intensities. The classic 'anaerobic threshold' theory holds that it arises from the increase in plasma lactic acid, produced as a consequence of muscle hypoxia, which results in increased extracellular buffering and CO_2 production, which stimulates peripheral chemoreceptors (Wasserman 1994). This hypothesis has been challenged by a number of studies that have, by the

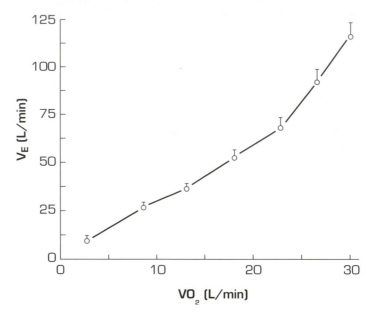

FIG. 3.2 Ventilation relative to oxygen uptake during incremental exercise (Forster & Pan 1991, with permission)

use of various experimental strategies, demonstrated dissociation between the ventilatory and lactate responses to exercise. It is likely that several factors contribute to the hyperventilation of heavy exercise.

During constant-load exercise, there is an initial rapid increase in ventilation (phase 1), a levelling off (phase 2) and a gradual drift upwards over time, especially during more prolonged or intense exercise. Upon cessation of exercise, ventilation rapidly returns towards pre-exercise levels but remains elevated for some time during recovery. The rapid changes in ventilation with the onset and cessation of exercise are most likely the result of neural regulation, linked with motor cortical activation of contracting muscle (Fink et al. 1995). The slower adjustments are probably due to various humoral factors. During prolonged strenuous exercise, increases in body temperature and plasma adrenaline may contribute to the progressive hyperventilation that is often observed.

The challenge for respiratory physiologists in relation to exercise hyperpnoea has been to explain the increase in ventilation in the absence of changes in some of the classic regulators of ventilation under resting conditions (P_aO_2, P_aCO_2, arterial pH). As mentioned, the rapid increase in ventilation with the onset of exercise is likely to be due to concurrent stimulation of the respiratory centres by motor cortical activation (Fink et al.

1995). In addition, afferent fibres in contracting skeletal muscle, sensitive to accumulation of local metabolites (e.g. H^+, CO_2, lactate) have been proposed as mediators of a 'ventilatory metaboreflex' (Evans et al. 1998; Smith et al. 1999). There may also be some input from mechanosensitive afferents.

Despite the large increase in CO_2 production during exercise, arterial PCO_2 remains relatively stable until it is lowered by the hyperventilation of heavy exercise. This has prompted suggestions that CO_2 flux to the lung, possibly detected by a vagally mediated, mixed venous chemoreceptor, is a major stimulator of ventilation during exercise. Other potential humoral stimuli include elevated plasma potassium (Paterson 1992), increased plasma catecholamines, and reduced arterial pH, while elevated body temperature may also play a role.

It is readily apparent that there are multiple controls on ventilation during exercise and their success in matching ventilation to the metabolic demands of exercise is demonstrated by the removal of CO_2 and the maintenance of arterial O_2 saturation during exercise under most circumstances. Having said that, arterial desaturation during strenuous exercise has been demonstrated in a significant number of fit, healthy subjects (Dempsey et al. 1984). Factors contributing to this include inadequate hyperventilation due to mechanical constraints on the lung and an excessive alveolar–arterial PO_2 difference due to ventilation–perfusion maldistribution and diffusion limitation (Dempsey & Wagner 1999). It has been suggested that the greater occurrence of desaturation in highly trained individuals reflects an inability of the pulmonary system to adapt in parallel with the cardiovascular system during strenuous training. Finally, there is evidence of significant respiratory muscle fatigue during strenuous exercise and at high intensities this may impact on exercise performance (Johnson et al. 1996). This has led to interest in the potential of specific respiratory muscle training to enhance exercise performance (Spengler & Boutellier 2000).

Cardiovascular responses to exercise

The effects of exercise on increasing intensity of VO_2, cardiac output and regional blood flows are summarised in Table 3.1.

The rapid increase in skeletal muscle blood flow at the onset of exercise is thought to be due to the mechanical effects of muscle contraction, the so-called muscle pump, which increases the arteriovenous pressure gradient in contracting skeletal muscle (Delp 1999). Skeletal muscle vasodilation results from the relaxing effects of various putative vasodilator metabolites

Table 3.1 Oxygen uptake (VO_2), cardiac output (Q) and regional blood flows, in L/min, during exercise of increasing intensity

CIRCULATION	REST	LIGHT	STRENUOUS	MAXIMAL
Muscle	1.20	4.50	12.50	22.00
Coronary	0.25	0.35	0.75	1.00
Skin	0.50	1.50	1.90	0.60
Splanchnic	1.40	1.10	0.60	0.30
Renal	1.10	1.10	0.60	0.30
Cerebral	0.75	0.75	0.75	0.75
Other	0.60	0.40	0.40	0.10
Q	5.80	9.50	17.50	25.00
VO_2	0.28	0.80	2.40	4.00

(e.g. K^+, adenosine) on vascular smooth muscle (Lott et al. 2001; Saltin et al. 1998). In recent years there has been interest in the potential role of endothelium-derived nitric oxide (NO) in mediating exercise hyperaemia (Hickner et al. 1997), although other studies have failed to support a role for NO, at least during exercise (Frandsen et al. 2001; Rådegran & Saltin 1999). Recently, combined inhibition of NO and prostaglandins reduced skeletal muscle blood flow during exercise in humans, suggesting a synergistic role for these compounds in mediating muscle blood flow during exercise (Boushel et al. 2002). Finally, there is evidence that the vascular bed of contracting skeletal muscle is less sensitive to neurogenic vasoconstriction —'functional sympatholysis'—and this may also contribute to muscle blood flow regulation during exercise (DeLorey et al. 2002; Tschakovsky et al. 2002). Capillary recruitment increases the available cross-sectional area for diffusive exchange, thereby enhancing O_2 and substrate delivery to contracting muscle.

To maintain a relatively constant mean arterial pressure (MAP), in the face of a large decrease in active skeletal muscle vascular resistance, sympathetic-mediated vasoconstriction occurs in the splanchnic, renal and inactive muscle vascular beds (Table 3.1). The cutaneous and active muscle circulations are also targets of vasoconstriction during near-maximal exercise, as demonstrated by increased noradrenaline spillover from skeletal muscle, despite the need to remove heat and supply O_2 to contracting muscle. Another endothelium-derived product, endothelin-1, may contribute to vasoconstriction in non-working muscle beds. Evidence in support of the need for some vasoconstriction in contracting skeletal muscle comes from experiments using the single-leg, knee extension model which demonstrate that the maximal flow capacity of isolated, contracting muscle is larger than could be sustained by the maximal cardiac output during whole-body exercise with a larger active muscle mass (Saltin et al. 1998).

Cardiac output increases as a consequence of increased heart rate and stroke volume. The early increase in heart rate is mediated by vagal withdrawal, while at higher exercise intensities sympathoadrenal activation plays the major role. Patients who have undergone cardiac transplantation rely on increases in plasma adrenaline for their exercise-induced increase in heart rate. Heart rate reaches a maximal level that is age-dependent. Stroke volume increases as a consequence of increased venous return and end-diastolic volume and enhanced ventricular contractility. Ventricular filling is maintained by the action of the muscle and respiratory pumps, which increase venous return. Stroke volume typically increases in proportion to exercise intensity to about 40–60% of maximal capacity, with no further increase thereafter (Gledhill et al. 1994; Zhou et al. 2001). However, in endurance-trained athletes no such plateau is observed and stroke volume increases progressively, thereby accounting for the greater maximal cardiac output in these subjects (Gledhill et al. 1994; Zhou et al. 2001). The greater stroke volume is a consequence of greater ventricular filling (Gledhill et al. 1994), secondary to an expanded blood volume and enhanced myocardial contractility (Jensen-Urstad et al. 1998). A higher stroke volume accounts for the lower heart rate during submaximal exercise, requiring a given O_2 uptake and cardiac output, which is characteristic of the trained state.

Systolic blood pressure increases in proportion to the rise in cardiac output, whereas diastolic blood pressure is determined by the balance between vasodilation and vasoconstriction in the vascular beds (i.e. total peripheral resistance). During dynamic exercise with a large active muscle mass, diastolic blood pressure may decrease at higher exercise intensities. Despite this, the increase in systolic blood pressure results in an elevated MAP during incremental exercise. The simultaneous increase in blood pressure and heart rate occurs due to resetting of the baroreflex during exercise (Norton et al. 1999). The rise in MAP is exaggerated during exercise involving a small muscle mass or during static exercise. The latter form of exercise results in mechanical compression of blood vessels, restriction of muscle blood flow and activation of chemosensitive nerve fibres within skeletal muscle which enhance sympathetic activity and the pressor response to exercise (Gandevia & Hobbs 1990). The cardiovascular response to exercise is primarily determined by the absolute O_2 uptake and the active muscle mass, resulting in a tight coupling between O_2 delivery and metabolic demand (Lewis et al. 1983).

During prolonged exercise, the cardiovascular response is characterised by a progressive increase in heart rate and a decline in stroke volume, which has been termed cardiovascular drift (Fig. 3.3, Coyle & González-Alonso 2001). Factors contributing to cardiovascular drift include progressive dehydration and hyperthermia, increased plasma catecholamines, loss of central blood volume and reduced ventricular filling. These changes are more exaggerated during exercise in the heat and are minimised by attenuating dehydration and hyperthermia by fluid ingestion (McConell et al. 1997).

The overall cardiovascular response to exercise is mediated by descending activation (central command), linked to motor cortical activation of skeletal muscle in direct proportion to the number of motor units required for force output (Mitchell 1990). Central command exerts both cardiac and vasomotor effects by increasing heart rate, cardiac output and blood pressure early in exercise. Feedback from mechanosensitive and chemosensitive type III and IV afferent nerves in contracting muscle (exercise pressor reflex), baroreceptors, volume/osmoreceptors and thermoreceptors interacts with the descending drive to modify cardiovascular responses (Mitchell 1990) as summarised in Figure 3.4. Both central command and exercise pressor reflex activation are involved in resetting of the baroreflex function (Gallagher et

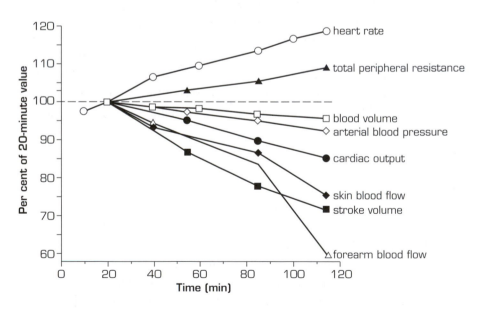

FIG. 3.3 Cardiovascular variables during prolonged strenuous exercise in a warm environment with progressive dehydration and hyperthermia (from Coyle & González-Alonso 2001, with permission)

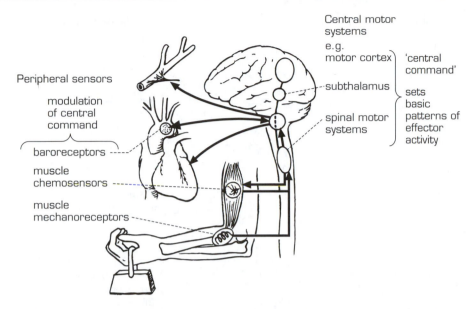

FIG. 3.4 Central and peripheral control of cardiovascular responses to exercise (from Rowell 1986, with permission)

al. 2001a, b). The possibility that contracting muscle releases a humoral factor with direct cardiac effects has also been raised (Kjær et al. 1999).

Maximal oxygen uptake

Maximal O_2 uptake (VO_{2max}) is the most widely accepted measure of aerobic fitness and represents the maximal rate of energy generation by the aerobic energy system. It is determined by the combined abilities of the respiratory and cardiovascular systems to deliver O_2 to contracting skeletal muscle and the ability of that muscle to consume O_2. Values for VO_{2max} range from 30–40 mL/kg/min in inactive sedentary individuals to as high as 80–90 mL/kg/min in highly trained endurance athletes. Such high values reflect a combination of genetic endowment and vigorous physical training. The measurement of VO_{2max} is useful in the assessment of endurance athletes and, together with the ventilatory/lactate threshold, is a strong predictor of endurance exercise performance (Williams 1990).

Although all links in the transport and utilisation of O_2 are potential sites of limitation (Fig. 3.5), and skeletal muscle oxidative capacity is an important determinant of VO_{2max} (Ivy et al. 1980), recent evidence suggests O_2 delivery to contracting skeletal muscle is the most important rate limiting step (Richardson et al. 1999). In a small number of well-trained

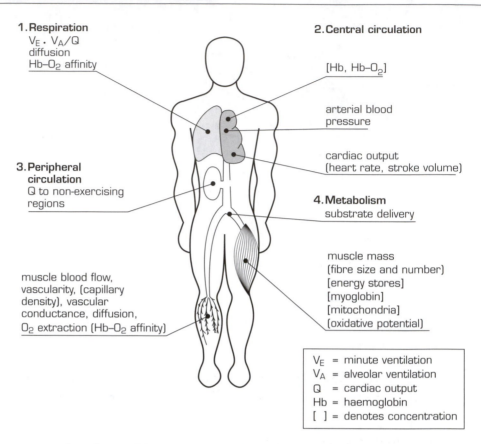

1. Respiration
   $V_E \cdot V_A/Q$
   diffusion
   Hb–O_2 affinity

2. Central circulation

   [Hb, Hb–O_2]

   arterial blood
   pressure

   cardiac output
   (heart rate, stroke volume)

3. Peripheral
   circulation
   Q to non-exercising
   regions

4. Metabolism
   substrate delivery

   muscle mass
   (fibre size and number)
   [energy stores]
   [myoglobin]
   [mitochondria]
   (oxidative potential)

muscle blood flow,
vascularity, (capillary
density), vascular
conductance, diffusion,
O_2 extraction (Hb–O_2 affinity)

V_E	= minute ventilation
V_A	= alveolar ventilation
Q	= cardiac output
Hb	= haemoglobin
[ ]	= denotes concentration

FIG. 3.5 Physiological determinants of maximal oxygen uptake (from Saltin & Rowell 1980, with permission)

athletes, a pulmonary diffusion limitation has been observed and hyperoxia increased VO_{2max} (Powers et al. 1989); however, in most healthy individuals the respiratory system is not thought be a major limiting factor to maximal aerobic exercise performance at sea level. The maximal cardiac output is an important determinant of VO_{2max} (Saltin & Strange 1992) and individuals with high VO_{2max} values show increased stroke volumes during exercise as a result of increased ventricular filling and myocardial contractility (Gledhill et al. 1994; Jensen-Urstad et al. 1998). An expanded blood volume contributes to this enhanced cardiac performance (Hopper et al. 1988; Martino et al. 2002).

The capacity of the blood to transport O_2 (as determined by the haemoglobin level) has an important role for O_2 delivery and this has resulted in interest in blood doping and erythropoietin administration to increase red cell mass (Ekblom 1996) and nutritional factors that are involved in the regulation of erythropoiesis (e.g. dietary iron, vitamin B_{12}, folic acid intake).

Finally, tissue O_2 conductance (capillary blood → muscle mitochondria) appears to have a major role in determining VO_{2max} (Wagner 1995). Of note, rats selectively bred for endurance running performance are characterised by a higher capacity for tissue O_2 transfer when compared with low-capacity runners, while ventilation, pulmonary gas exchange, maximal cardiac output and arterial O_2 content were similar in the two groups (Henderson et al. 2002).

VO_{2max} sets the upper limit for aerobic metabolism and is an important predictor of endurance exercise performance; however, various related variables influencing the submaximal exercise response (e.g. lactate/ ventilatory threshold, muscle oxidative capacity) are often better predictors of endurance success (Farrell et al. 1979). This is related to the association between metabolic adaptations within skeletal muscle, which influence the lactate threshold and reduced CHO utilisation during prolonged exercise (Baldwin et al. 2000; Coyle et al. 1988). Thus, in addition to having a large 'aerobic engine', it is also important to be able to maintain an exercise intensity that requires a large fraction of the aerobic capacity without excessive rates of CHO oxidation and lactate production (Costill et al. 1973). Measurement of the lactate responses to submaximal exercise and determination of the lactate threshold have become an integral part of the assessment of the endurance athlete (Williams 1990).

Summary

In summary, the ability to generate energy via oxidative metabolism during exercise requires the co-ordinated activation of the respiratory and cardiovascular systems. Increased ventilation, cardiac output (heart rate × stroke volume) and skeletal muscle blood flow ensure that O_2 delivery is tightly coupled to O_2 demand during exercise. Maximal O_2 uptake is the most widely accepted measure of aerobic fitness and represents the maximal rate of energy generation by the aerobic energy system, as determined by the combined abilities of the respiratory and cardiovascular systems to deliver O_2 to contracting skeletal muscle and the ability of that muscle to consume O_2. It is a strong predictor of endurance exercise performance, as is the ability to maintain an exercise intensity that requires a large fraction of the aerobic capacity without excessive rates of CHO oxidation and lactate accumulation.

References

Åstrand PO, Rodahl K. *Textbook of Work Physiology: Physiological Bases of Exercise.* New York: McGraw-Hill, 1986.

Baldwin J, Snow RJ, Febbraio MA. Effect of training status and relative exercise intensity on physiological responses in men. *Med Sci Sports Exerc* 2000;32: 1648–54.

Bangsbo J, Krustrup P, González-Alonso J, Boushel R, Saltin B. Muscle oxygen kinetics at onset of intense dynamic exercise in humans. *Am J Physiol* 2000;279: R899–R906.

Boushel R, Langberg H, Gemmer C, Olesen J, Crameri R, Scheede C, Sander M, Kjær M. Combined inhibition of nitric oxide and prostaglandins reduces human skeletal muscle blood flow during exercise. *J Physiol* 2002;543:691–8.

Costill DL, Thomason H, Roberts E. Fractional utilization of the aerobic capacity during distance running. *Med Sci Sports* 1973;5:248–52.

Coyle EF, Coggan AR, Hopper MK, Walters TJ. Determinants of endurance in well-trained cyclists. *J Appl Physiol* 1988;64:2622–30.

Coyle EF, González-Alonso J. Cardiovascular drift during prolonged exercise: new perspectives. *Exerc Sports Sci Rev* 2001;29:88–92.

DeLorey DS, Wang SS, Shoemaker JK. Evidence for sympatholysis at the onset of forearm exercise. *J Appl Physiol* 2002;93:555–60.

Delp MD. Control of skeletal muscle perfusion at the onset of dynamic exercise. *Med Sci Sports Exerc* 1999;31:1011–18.

Dempsey JA, Hanson PG, Henderson KS. Exercise-induced arterial hypoxemia in healthy human subjects at sea level. *J Physiol* 1984;355:161–75.

Dempsey JA, Wagner PD. Exercise-induced arterial hypoxemia. *J Appl Physiol* 1999;87:1997–2006.

Ekblom B. Blood doping and erythropoietin: the effects of variation in hemoglobin concentration and other related factors on physical performance. *Am J Sports Med* 1996;24;S40–S42.

Evans AB, Tsai LW, Oelberg DA, Kazemi H, Systrom DM. Skeletal muscle ECF pH error signal for exercise ventilatory control. *J Appl Physiol* 1998;84:90–6.

Farrell PA, Wilmore JH, Coyle EF, Billing JE, Costill DL. Plasma lactate accumulation and distance running performance. *Med Sci Sports* 1979;11:338–44.

Fink GR, Adams L, Watson JDG, Innes JA, Wuyam B, Kobayashi I, Corfield DR, Murphy K, Jones T, Frackowiak RSJ, Guz A. Hyperpnoea during and immediately after exercise in man: evidence of motor cortical involvement. *J Physiol* 1995;489: 663–75.

Forster HV, Pan LG. Exercise hyperpnea: its characteristics and control. In: Crystal RG, West JB et al., eds. *The Lung: Scientific Foundations.* New York: Raven Press, 1991.

Frandsen U, Bangsbo J, Sander M, Höffner L, Betak A, Saltin B, Hellsten Y. Exercise-induced hyperaemia and leg oxygen uptake are not altered during effective inhibition of nitric oxide synthase with N^G-nitro-L-arginine methyl ester in humans. *J Physiol* 2001;531:257–64.

Gallagher KM, Fadel PJ, Strømstad M, Ide K, Smith SA, Querry RG, Raven PB, Secher NH. Effects of partial neuromuscular blockade on carotid baroreflex function during exercise in humans. *J Physiol* 2001a;533:861–70.

Gallagher KM, Fadel PJ, Strømstad M, Ide K, Smith SA, Querry RG, Raven PB, Secher NH. Effects of exercise pressor reflex activation on carotid baroreflex function during exercise in humans. *J Physiol* 2001b;533:871–80.

Gandevia SC, Hobbs SF. Cardiovascular responses to static exercise in man: central and reflex contributions. *J Physiol* 1990;430:105–17.

Gledhill N, Cox D, Jamnik R. Endurance athletes' stroke volume does not plateau: major advantage is diastolic function. *Med Sci Sports Exerc* 1994;26:1116–21.

Henderson KK, Wagner H, Favret F, Britton SL, Koch LG, Wagner PD, Gonzalez NC. Determinants of maximal O_2 uptake in rats selectively bred for endurance running capacity. *J Appl Physiol* 2002;93:1265–74.

Hickner RC, Fisher JS, Ehsani AA, Kohrt WM. Role of nitric oxide in skeletal muscle blood flow at rest and during dynamic exercise in humans. *Am J Physiol* 1997;273: H405–H410.

Hopper MK, Coggan AR, Coyle EF. Exercise stroke volume relative to plasma-volume expansion. *J Appl Physiol* 1988;64:404–8.

Howlett RA, Heigenhauser GJF, Hultman E, Hollidge-Horvat MG, Spriet LL. Effects of dichloroacetate infusion on human skeletal muscle metabolism at the onset of exercise. *Am J Physiol* 1999;277:E18–E25.

Ivy JL, Costill DL, Maxwell BD. Skeletal muscle determinants of maximum aerobic power in man. *Eur J Appl Physiol* 1980;44:1–8.

Jensen-Urstad M, Bouvier F, Nejat M, Saltin B, Brodin L-Å. Left ventricular function in endurance runners during exercise. *Acta Physiol Scand* 1998;164:167–72.

Johnson BD, Aaron EA, Babcock MA, Dempsey JA. Respiratory muscle fatigue during exercise: implications for performance. *Med Sci Sports Exerc* 1996;28:1129–37.

Kjær M, Pott F, Mohr T, Linkis P, Tornøe P, Secher NH. Heart rate during exercise with leg vascular occlusion in spinal-cord injured humans. *J Appl Physiol* 1999;86: 806–11.

Lewis SF, Taylor WF, Graham RM, Pettinger WA, Schutte JE, Blomqvist CG. Cardiovascular responses to exercise as functions of absolute and relative work load. *J Appl Physiol* 1983;54:1314–23.

Lott ME, Hogeman CS, Vickery L, Kunselman AR, Sinoway LI, MacLean DA. Effects of dynamic exercise on mean blood velocity and muscle interstitial metabolites responses in humans. *Am J Physiol* 2001;281:H1734–H1741.

Martino M, Gledhill N, Jamnik V. High VO_{2max} with no history of training is primarily due to high blood volume. *Med Sci Sports Exerc* 2002;34:966–71.

McConell, GK, Burge CM, Skinner SL, Hargreaves M. Influence of ingested fluid volume on physiological responses during prolonged exercise. *Acta Physiol Scand* 1997;160:149–56.

Mitchell JH. Neural control of the circulation during exercise. *Med Sci Sports Exerc* 1990;22:141–54.

Norton KH, Boushel R, Strange S, Saltin B, Raven PB. Resetting of the carotid baroreflex during dynamic exercise in humans. *J Appl Physiol* 1999;87:332–8.

Paterson DJ. Potassium and ventilation in exercise. *J Appl Physiol* 1992;72:811–20.

Poole DC, Barstow TJ, Gaesser GA, Willis WT, Whipp BJ. VO_2 slow component: physiological and functional significance. *Med Sci Sports Exerc* 1994;26:1354–8.

Poole DC, Richardson RS. Determinants of oxygen uptake: implications for exercise testing. *Sports Med* 1997;24:308–20.

Powers SK, Lawler J, Dempsey JA, Dodd S, Landry G. Effects of incomplete pulmonary gas exchange on VO_{2max}. *J Appl Physiol* 1989;66:2491–5.

Rådegran G, Saltin B. Nitric oxide in the regulation of vasomotor tone in human skeletal muscle. *Am J Physiol* 1999;276:H1951–H1960.

Richardson RS, Grassi B, Gavin TP, Haseler LJ, Tagore K, Roca J, Wagner PD. Evidence of O_2 supply-dependent VO_{2max} in the exercise-trained human quadriceps. J Appl Physiol 1999;86:1048–53.

Rowell LB. *Human Circulation: Regulation during Physical Stress.* Oxford: Oxford University Press, 1986.

Russell A, Wadley G, Snow R, Giacobino J-P, Muzzin P, Garnham A, Cameron-Smith D. Slow component of Vo_2 kinetics: the effect of training status, fibre type, UCP3 mRNA and citrate synthase activity. *Int J Obesity* 2002;26:157–64.

Saltin B, Rådegran G, Koskolou MD, Roach, RC. Skeletal muscle blood flow in humans and its regulation during exercise. *Acta Physiol Scand* 1998;162:421–36.

Saltin B, Rowell LB. Functional adaptations to physical activity and inactivity. *Fed Proc* 1980;39;1506–13.

Saltin B, Strange S. Maximal oxygen uptake: 'old' and 'new' arguments for a cardiovascular limitation. *Med Sci Sports Exerc* 1992;24:30–7.

Smith SA, Gallagher KM, Norton KH, Querry RG, Welch-O'Connor RM, Raven PB. Ventilatory responses to dynamic exercise elicited by intramuscular sensors. *Med Sci Sports Exerc* 1999;31:277–86.

Spengler CM, Boutellier U. Breathless legs? Consider training your respiration. *News Physiol Sci* 2000;15:101–5.

Timmons JA, Gustafsson T, Sundberg CJ, Jansson E, Greenhaff PL. Muscle acetyl group availability is a major determinant of oxygen deficit in humans during submaximal exercise. *Am J Physiol* 1998;274:E377–E380.

Tschakovsky ME, Hughson RL. Interaction of factors determining oxygen uptake at the onset of exercise. *J Appl Physiol* 1999;86:1101–13.

Tschakovsky ME, Sujirattanawimol K, Ruble SB, Valic R, Joyner MJ. Is sympathetic neural vasoconstriction blunted in the vascular bed of exercising human muscle? *J Physiol* 2002;541:623–35.

Wagner PD. Muscle O_2 transport and O_2 dependent control of metabolism. *Med Sci Sports Exerc* 1995;27:47–53.

Wasserman K. Coupling of external to cellular respiration during exercise: the wisdom of the body revisited. *Am J Physiol* 1994;266:E519–E539.

Williams C. Value of physiological measurement in sport. *J R Coll Surg Edinb* 1990;35: S7–S13.

Zhou B, Conlee RK, Jensen R, Fellingham GW, George JD, Fisher AG. Stroke volume does not plateau during graded exercise in elite male distance runners. *Med Sci Sports Exerc* 2001;33:1849–54.

Zoladz JA, Rademaker ACHJ, Sargeant AJ. Non-linear relationship between O_2 uptake and power output at high intensities of exercise in humans. *J Physiol* 1995;488: 211–17.

CHAPTER 4

Thermoregulation and fluid balance

Ron J. MAUGHAN and **Susan M. SHIRREFFS**

Introduction

All metabolic reactions taking place in the body require energy and some of this energy appears as heat. At rest, this heat helps to maintain body temperature at a comfortable level, but the rate of heat production increases during exercise in proportion to the exercise intensity and the rate of heat loss must be increased to limit the rise in body temperature that would otherwise occur. There is clearly an optimum temperature for the function of muscle and other tissues and likewise there is an optimum ambient temperature for exercise. The optimum ambient temperature will depend on many different factors, including the duration and intensity of exercise, the type and amount of clothing worn, and the physiological characteristics of the individual.

Whatever the exercise conditions, some water is inevitably lost from the body, including water loss from the lungs and through the skin in addition to sweat losses. Small losses of water from the body can be ignored but even small losses during exercise will impair performance and will also greatly increase the risk of heat-related illness (Sutton 1990). Keeping core temperature within the optimum range and maintaining an adequate hydration status are, therefore, key aims of the athlete during both training and competition.

Temperature regulation in exercise

About 80% of the energy available from the catabolism of ingested foods appears as heat. In an average (body mass about 70–80 kg) resting individual, the rate of heat production at rest is about 60 W. Energy is required for the work of breathing and of the heart, but most is used for the transport of ions and solutes across membranes and for biosynthetic processes. The energy demand at rest is met entirely by the aerobic metabolism of fats and carbohydrate (CHO), with a small contribution from the oxidation of the carbon skeletons of amino acids. This requires a rate of oxygen consumption of about 3–4 mL/kg of body mass/min, or about 250–300 mL/min.

In the exercise physiology laboratory, cycling is the form of exercise most widely studied. Oxygen uptake, and therefore heat production, are closely related to the power output, and the two can be used interchangeably as an index of physiological stress and the metabolic demand. Well-trained endurance athletes have a maximum aerobic capacity (VO_{2max}) of about 70–80 mL/kg/min, with values being slightly higher for men than for women (Wilmore & Costill 1999). In prolonged exercise, the fraction of VO_{2max} that can be sustained increases with training status but decreases with the time or distance to be covered. In the laboratory, well-trained cyclists can sustain a power output equivalent to about 75–80% of VO_{2max} for 2–3 hours (Wilmore & Costill 1999) and this corresponds to an oxygen cost of 4–5 L/min. The energy available when 1 L of oxygen is used to combust metabolic fuels is about 20 kJ (5 kcal). Elite marathon runners sustain an oxygen uptake of about 4 L/min and therefore a power output of about 1200 W for the entire duration of a race that lasts for a little more than 2 hours.

Taking the heat capacity of human tissue to be 3.47 kJ/°C/kg, and assuming a body mass of 65 kg, a rate of heat production of 1200 W would cause the body temperature to rise by 1°C approximately every 3 minutes. Although the skin temperature is the primary determinant of heat exchange, it is the deep body or core temperature that must be protected. If core temperature were to rise by 1°C every 3 minutes, a runner would exceed the upper limit of the tolerable core temperature within about 10 minutes of the start of the race. The body's thermoregulatory mechanisms ensure that this does not happen and core temperature seldom rises above about 40–41°C even in events held in hot climates (Table 4.1, Cheuvront & Haymes 2001).

Heat exchange—either gain or loss—between the body and the

TABLE 4.1 Thermoregulatory responses to marathon running

FINISH TIME (min)	NUMBER	AMBIENT TEMPERATURE (°C)	HUMIDITY	RECTAL TEMPERATURE (°C)	REFERENCE
–	239	–	–	35.9–41.5	Roth et al. 1966
207 ± 26	30	19–22	68	38.0–40.5	Noakes et al.1991
159 ± 3[a]	1	19.4	–	40.8 ± 0.9	Maron et al. 1977
162 ± 3[a]	1	19.4	–	39.7 ± 0.3	Maron et al. 1977
221 ± 37	57	12	–	35.6–39.8	Maughan 1985
213 ± 48	62	7–12	88	35.6–40.3	Maughan et al. 1985
–	7	20.4	37	38.9±0.5	Buskirk & Beetham 1960

Values are ranges and means ± SD. (a) Average of three marathon races.

environment occurs by the physical processes of conduction, convection and radiation: in addition, evaporation of water from the respiratory tract and skin can cause heat to be lost from the body (Fig. 4.1; Leithead & Lind 1964). Conduction is important only in water immersion as air is a good insulator and physical contact with solid objects in the environment is generally small. Convection and radiation are effective methods of heat loss when the skin temperature is high and the ambient temperature is low. Under these conditions, they account for a major part of the heat loss during intense exercise, especially when the speed of air movement over the skin is high, as in downhill cycling. Convective losses can lead to a rapid drop in body temperature in cyclists on downhill stages, especially if this is preceded by a hard climb. As the ambient temperature rises, however, the gradient from skin to environment falls, and above about 35°C the gradient is reversed so that heat is gained from the environment. Evaporation is, therefore, the only means of heat loss in hot weather conditions. Ignoring the negligible exchange via conduction, the avenues of heat exchange can be quantified as follows:

Convective loss: $C = 8.3(T_{sk} - T_a) \times V$ W/°C/m^2

Radiant loss: $R = 5.2(T_{sk} - T_{mrt})$ W/°C/m^2

Evaporative loss: $E = 124(P_{sk} - P_a) \times V$ W/kPa/m^2

Where:

T_{sk} = mean skin temperature (°C)

T_a = ambient temperature (°C)

T_{mrt} = mean radiant temperature (°C)

P_{sk} = mean skin water vapour pressure (kPa)

P_a = ambient water vapour pressure (kPa)

V = mean air velocity (m/s)

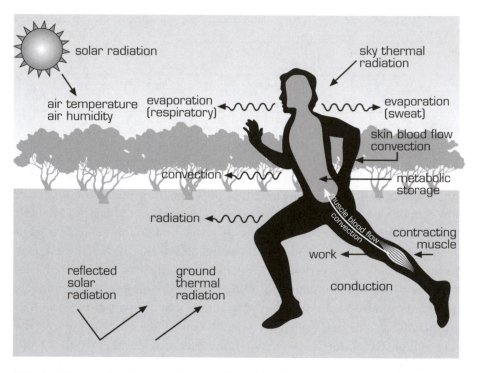

FIG. 4.1 Heat production in active muscle and its dissipation through and from the body (adapted from Gisolfi & Wenger 1984)

These equations may give the impression that heat balance can be precisely measured but they are gross simplifications that ignore several important factors: there is no single value of skin temperature; only a small part of the body surface is exposed to a headwind equivalent to the speed of forward movement; limb movement complicates the calculation of air velocity; and clothing greatly restricts air movement and also raises local humidity. Nonetheless, a high rate of evaporative heat loss is clearly essential when the rate of metabolic heat production is high and when the body is also gaining heat by convection and radiation. The potential for heat loss by evaporation of water from the skin is high but this will not be the case if the sweating rate is insufficient to wet the skin surface or if the vapour pressure gradient between the skin and the environment is low. This latter situation will arise if the skin temperature is low or if the ambient water vapour pressure is high. High ambient humidity or clothing that restricts air flow will, therefore, limit the evaporation of water from the skin surface. A large body surface area and a high rate of air movement over the body surface are also factors that will have a major impact on evaporative heat loss, but these same factors will also promote heat gain by convection when the ambient temperature is higher than skin temperature (Leithead & Lind 1964). The high surface-area-to-volume ratio of children means that they are at particular risk of heat stress in games or sports taking place in the summer months.

The ability of athletes to exercise hard in the heat with relatively little change in body temperature indicates that the thermoregulatory system is normally able to dissipate heat almost as fast as it is being generated. High rates of evaporative heat loss, however, require high rates of sweat secretion onto the skin surface, and the price to be paid for the maintenance of core temperature is a progressive loss of water and electrolytes in sweat.

Sweating: water and electrolyte losses

Evaporation of 1 L of water from the skin surface will remove about 2.4 MJ (580 kcal) of heat from the body. For the marathon runner with a body mass of 70 kg who runs for 2 hours 30 minutes, to balance the rate of metabolic heat production by evaporative loss alone requires about 1.6 L of sweat to evaporate per hour: allowing for some sweat to drip from the skin without evaporating, a sweat secretion rate of about 2 L/h is necessary to achieve this rate of evaporative heat loss. Trained athletes, especially those acclimatised to the heat, can easily sustain such a sweat rate but would lose about 5 L of body water over the course of a marathon, corresponding to a loss of more than 7% of body weight for a 70 kg runner. Some water will also be lost by evaporation from the respiratory tract and this will also contribute to heat dissipation. During hard exercise in a hot dry environment, respiratory water loss can be significant (Mitchell et al. 1972). The rise of 2–3°C in body temperature which normally occurs during marathon running means that some of the heat produced is stored but the effect on heat balance is minimal: for a 70 kg runner a rise in mean body temperature of 3°C—about the maximum tolerable increase—would reduce the total requirement for evaporation of sweat by less than 300 mL. Some rise in body temperature is probably necessary to invoke effective heat loss mechanisms.

The sweat that is secreted onto the skin contains a wide variety of organic and inorganic solutes, and significant losses from the body of some of these components will occur where large volumes of sweat are produced. The electrolyte composition of sweat is variable and the concentration of individual electrolytes as well as the total sweat volume will influence the extent of these losses. A number of factors contribute to the variability in the composition of sweat: methodological problems in the collection procedure, including evaporative loss, incomplete collection and contamination with skin cells, account for at least part of the variability, but there is also a large biological variability (Shirreffs & Maughan 1997). Published values for the normal concentration ranges of the main electrolytes present in sweat are shown in Table 4.2, along with their plasma and intracellular concentrations for comparison.

The composition of sweat varies between individuals but can also vary within the same individual depending on the rate of sweating and the current level of fitness and state of heat acclimatisation. In response to a standard heat stress, the sweat rate is higher after a period of endurance training or heat acclimatisation and the electrolyte content is lower: there is also a redistribution of sweating, with a greater sweat rate on the limbs and relatively less on the trunk. An advantage of decreasing the sodium loss is a disproportionate loss of fluid from the intracellular space, which helps to maintain plasma volume and cardiovascular function (Nadel et al. 1990). The major electrolytes in sweat, as in the extracellular fluid, are sodium

TABLE 4.2 Concentration (mmol/L) of the major electrolytes in sweat, plasma and intracellular water[a]

ELECTROLYTE	SWEAT	PLASMA	INTRACELLULAR WATER
Sodium	20–80	130–155	10
Potassium	4–8	3.2–5.5	150
Calcium	0–1	2.1–2.9	0
Magnesium	< 0.2	0.7–1.5	15
Chloride	20–60	96–110	8
Bicarbonate	0–35	23–28	10
Phosphate	0.1–0.2	0.7–1.6	65
Sulphate	0.2–2.0	0.3–0.9	10

(a) These values are taken from a variety of sources as quoted by Maughan (1994) and the data of Shirreffs & Maughan (1997).

and chloride (Table 4.2). There is conflicting data on the effects of sweating rate, fitness level and acclimatisation status on sweat electrolyte losses (see Maughan 1991 for review) and this may be due to differences in the training status and degree of acclimatisation of the subjects used, as well as differences in the methodology employed for sweat collection and analysis. The use of improved sweat collection techniques will begin to resolve these issues (Shirreffs & Maughan 1997).

Sweat is invariably hypotonic with respect to body fluids, so one of the effects of prolonged sweating is to increase the plasma osmolality, which may have a significant effect on the ability to maintain body temperature. A direct relationship between plasma osmolality and body temperature has been demonstrated during exercise (Greenleaf et al. 1974; Harrison et al. 1978). Increasing the osmolality of plasma prior to exercise has been shown to result in a decreased thermoregulatory effector response: the threshold for sweating is elevated and the cutaneous vasodilator response is reduced (Fortney et al. 1984). In contrast, changes in plasma osmolality during exercise have no effect on the cardiovascular and thermoregulatory responses to short periods (about 30 min) of exercise (Fortney et al. 1988).

There is a large inter-subject variability in the changes in the plasma concentration of individual electrolytes but, except where very large volumes of electrolyte-free solutions are ingested, an increase in the plasma sodium and chloride concentrations is generally observed in response to both running and cycling exercise. There are some reports of differences in sweating function and in sweat composition between men and women (see Brouns et al. 1992 for review), but this apparent gender difference may well reflect differences in training and acclimatisation status. The sweating capacity of children is low when expressed per unit surface area, and the sweat electrolyte content is low relative to that of adults, but the need for fluid and electrolyte replacement is no less important than in adults. Indeed, in view of the evidence that core temperature increases to a greater extent in children than in adults at a given level of dehydration, the need for fluid replacement may well be greater in children (Bar-Or 1989).

Sweat loss: effects on exercise performance

Dehydration leads to impaired exercise performance and failure to replace sweat losses in endurance events will lead to the early onset of fatigue. A fluid deficit of as little as 1.8% of body mass incurred during 1 hour of cycling has been shown to impair exercise tolerance (Walsh et al. 1994). It may be that even smaller fluid deficits can adversely affect performance in competitive sport, where the difference between winning and losing is often measured in fractions of 1%, but the laboratory methods used to assess performance are not sufficiently sensitive to detect small changes. In higher intensity events, such as 1500 m or 10 000 m track running, the duration is too short for substantial sweat losses to occur during the event itself but prior mild (1.5–2% of body mass) dehydration will impair performance (Nielsen et al. 1981; Armstrong et al. 1985). This is a particular concern for individuals living in the heat who may be chronically hypohydrated. These effects on performance are not trivial and reflect a major impairment of cardiovascular capacity.

Some of the water and solutes lost in sweat come from the plasma, some from the extracellular space and some from the intracellular space. The fractions of the total loss that come from each of these compartments are not entirely clear as redistribution over time redresses acute changes that occur. A decrease in plasma volume of 5–10% is not unusual in the early stages of prolonged exercise due to a movement of water into active tissues under the influence of osmotic and hydrostatic forces, and this deficit will increase if sweat losses are high and fluid is not ingested (Maughan 2001). Reductions in plasma volume may be of particular importance in influencing an individual's work capacity: blood flow to the muscles must be maintained at a high level to supply oxygen and substrates, but a high blood flow to the skin is also required to convect heat to the body surface where it can be dissipated (Nadel 1980). Effective heat loss requires that a high skin temperature is maintained, requiring in turn a high skin blood flow. Vasodilatation also occurs in active muscles to promote the delivery of oxygen and substrates and for convection away of heat. Vasoconstriction occurs in the skin vessels to maintain central venous pressure, reducing heat loss and causing body temperature to rise (Rowell 1986).

These factors have been investigated by Coyle and colleagues (Hamilton et al. 1991; Montain et al. 1992a, b). Their results clearly demonstrate that increases in core temperature and heart rate during prolonged exercise are graded according to the level of hypohydration achieved. They also showed, however, that the ingestion of fluid during exercise increases skin blood flow, and therefore thermoregulatory capacity, independent of increases in the circulating blood volume. Plasma volume expansion using a dextran/saline infusion was less effective in preventing a rise in core temperature than was the ingestion of sufficient volumes of a CHO–electrolyte drink to maintain plasma volume at a similar level.

Control of water and electrolyte balance

Water and electrolyte balance are closely coupled to ensure maintenance of total body water content and of tissue osmolality. Regulation is achieved by balancing input and losses.

Renal blood flow at rest of about 1 L/min, or about 20% of total cardiac output, and approximately 15–20% of the renal plasma flow—about 170 L/day—is filtered out by the glomeruli. Most (99% or more) of this is reabsorbed in the tubular system, with only about 1–1.5 L appearing as urine. The volume of urine produced is determined primarily by the action of antidiuretic hormone (ADH), which regulates water reabsorption by increasing the permeability of the distal tubule of the nephron and the collecting duct to water. ADH is released from the posterior lobe of the pituitary in response to an increase in osmolality and a decrease in blood volume. An increased plasma angiotensin concentration will also stimulate ADH output.

Sodium is the main cation of the extracellular space, with sodium salts accounting for about 90% of total osmolality, and plasma sodium concentration is regulated by the reabsorption of sodium from the glomerular filtrate, which occurs primarily in the proximal renal tubule. Aldosterone, which promotes sodium reabsorption in the distal tubules and enhances the excretion of potassium and hydrogen ions, has a major influence on the extent to which this occurs. Aldosterone is released from the kidney in response to a fall in the circulating sodium concentration or a rise in plasma potassium concentration. Its release is also stimulated by angiotensin, which is produced by the renin–angiotensin system in response to a decrease in the plasma sodium concentration. Angiotensin, thus, has a twofold action: on the release of aldosterone as well as ADH. Atrial natriuretic factor (ANF) is a peptide synthesised in and released from the heart in response to atrial distension. It increases the glomerular filtration rate and decreases sodium and water reabsorption, leading to an increase in their loss: this may be important in the regulation of extracellular volume but probably does not play a significant role during exercise.

Changes in renal function during exercise act to conserve water and sodium, but compared with the losses that commonly occur by sweating, the amounts involved are fairly trivial. Likewise, reducing renal blood flow during intense exercise will allow more blood to be diverted to active tissues, but even total renal shutdown would make only an extra 1 L of cardiac output available.

Fluid intake: thirst

The kidneys can help to conserve water and electrolytes during periods of increased loss or restricted intake but they cannot restore a deficit. Fluid intake is required and this is partly a behavioural response initiated in response to physiological signals consequent upon a fluid deficit, but is also partly under conscious control. Thirst is generally a poor indicator of acute hydration status in humans, but the overall stability of the total water volume of an individual indicates that the desire to drink is a powerful regulatory factor over the long term (Adolph et al. 1947). Drinking may not be directly involved with a physiological need for water intake but can be initiated by habit, ritual, or a taste or desire for nutrients, stimulants, or a warm or cooling effect. A number of the sensations associated with thirst are learned, with signals such as dryness of the mouth or throat inducing drinking, while distension of the stomach can stop ingestion before a fluid deficit has been restored. However, the underlying regulation of thirst is controlled separately by both the osmotic pressure and volume of the body fluids and, as such, is regulated by the same mechanisms that affect water and solute reabsorption in the kidneys and control central blood pressure.

Changes in intravascular volume and pressure appear to be less effective in provoking thirst than do changes in plasma osmolality. A rise of 2–3% in plasma osmolality is sufficient to evoke a strong desire to drink (Hubbard et al. 1990). Large variations in blood volume and pressure occur in response to postural changes, as well as modest levels of activity, and this lack of sensitivity presumably serves to dampen the effects of short-term changes. Prolonged exercise, especially in the heat, is associated with a decrease in plasma volume and an increased plasma osmolality, but fluid intake during and immediately following exercise is often less than that required to restore normal hydration status (Ramsay 1989). This appears not to be due to a lack of initiation of the drinking response but rather to a premature termination of the drinking response (Rolls et al. 1980).

Receptors in the mouth, oesophagus and stomach are thought to meter the volume of fluid ingested, while distension of the stomach tends to reduce the perception of thirst (Verbalis 1990). These pre-absorptive signals appear to be behavioural, learnt responses and may be subject to disruption in situations that are essentially novel to the individual. This may partly explain the inappropriate voluntary fluid intake in individuals exposed to an acute increase in environmental temperature or to exercise-induced dehydration. It also suggests that learnt behaviour is important when large volumes of fluid must be ingested to maintain hydration status, as happens when athletes from cool climates move to warm conditions for training or competition.

Fluid and electrolyte replacement during exercise

Limitations to replacement

In any exercise task lasting longer than about 30–40 minutes, CHO depletion, elevation of core temperature and reductions in the circulating fluid volume are likely to be important factors in causing fatigue. All of these can be manipulated by the ingestion of fluids, but the most effective drink composition and the optimum amount of fluid will depend on individual circumstances. Water is not the optimum fluid for ingestion during endurance exercise, and there is compelling evidence that drinks containing added substrate and electrolytes are more effective. Increasing the CHO content of drinks will increase the amount of fuel that can be supplied but will tend to decrease the rate at which water can be made available (Vist & Maughan 1995). Where provision of water is the priority, the CHO content of drinks and their total osmolality should be low, thus restricting the rate at which substrate is provided. The composition of drinks to be taken will thus be influenced by the relative importance of the need to supply fuel and water, which in turn depends on the intensity and duration of the exercise task, on the ambient temperature and humidity, and on the physiological and biochemical characteristics of the individual athlete. CHO depletion will result in fatigue and a reduction in the exercise intensity that can be sustained but is not normally a life-threatening condition. Disturbances in fluid balance and temperature regulation have potentially more serious consequences, and it may be, therefore, that the emphasis for the majority of participants in endurance events should be on proper maintenance of fluid and electrolyte balance.

The optimum type and concentration of sugars to be added to drinks will depend on individual circumstances. High CHO concentrations will delay gastric emptying, thus reducing the amount of fluid that is available for absorption: very high concentrations will also result in secretion of water into the intestine and thus temporarily increase the danger of dehydration (Merson et al. 2002). Perhaps because of this effect, high sugar concentrations (> 10%) may result in an increased risk of gastrointestinal disturbances. Where there is a need to supply an energy source during exercise, however, increasing the sugar content of drinks will increase the delivery of CHO to the site of absorption in the small intestine.

The available evidence indicates that the only electrolyte that should be added to drinks consumed during exercise is sodium, which is usually added in the form of sodium chloride, but which may also be added as sodium citrate or other salts. The use of citrate rather than chloride helps stabilise pH and affects taste. Sodium will stimulate sugar and water uptake in the small intestine and will help to maintain extracellular fluid volume as well as maintaining the drive to drink by keeping plasma osmolality high (Noakes et al. 1985; Maughan 2001).

Most soft drinks of the cola or lemonade variety contain virtually no sodium (1–2 mmol/L), and drinking water is also essentially sodium-free; sports drinks commonly contain 10–25 mmol/L sodium, and oral rehydration solutions intended for use in the treatment of diarrhoea-induced dehydration have higher sodium concentrations, usually 30–90 mmol/L. A high sodium content may be important in stimulating jejunal absorption of glucose and water, but it tends to make drinks unpalatable. Drinks intended for ingestion during or after exercise, when thirst may be suppressed and large volumes must be consumed, should have a pleasant taste in order to stimulate consumption. Sports drinks must strike a balance between the twin aims of efficacy and palatability.

Hyperthermia and hypernatraemia are relatively common in endurance events held in the heat and often affect the less-well-prepared participants. It has, however, become clear that a small number of individuals at the end of very prolonged events may be suffering from hyponatraemia: this may be associated with either hyperhydration or dehydration. The total number of reported cases is rather small and the great majority of these have been associated with ultramarathon or prolonged triathlon events; there are few reports of cases of exercise-associated hyponatraemia where the exercise duration is less than 4 hours. The dangers of ingestion of excessive volumes of fluid without adding salt have long been recognised in various industrial settings, including foundry workers and ships' stokers. It is also well recognised that the inclusion of sodium salts in drinks ingested in these situations is a simple and effective preventive measure. Many of the drinks consumed in endurance events, whether plain water, soft drinks or sports beverages, have little or no electrolyte content. Even among the CHO–electrolyte drinks intended for consumption by sportsmen and women during prolonged exercise, most have a low electrolyte content, with sodium concentrations typically in the range of 10–20 mmol/L. This is adequate in most situations but may not be so when sweat losses and fluid intakes are high. Some supplementation with sodium chloride in amounts beyond those normally found in sports drinks may be required in extremely prolonged events where large sweat losses can be expected and where it is possible to consume large volumes of fluid. It remains true, however, that electrolyte replacement during exercise is not a priority for most participants in most sporting events. Extra salting of food is an effective strategy for athletes living and training hard in hot weather conditions.

Early experimental evidence suggested an advantage to taking chilled (4°C) drinks as this accelerates gastric emptying and thus improves the availability of ingested fluids. More comprehensive studies, however, suggest that the gastric emptying rate of hot and cold beverages is not markedly different (Maughan 1994). In spite of this, there may be advantages in taking chilled drinks, as the palatability of most CHO–electrolyte drinks is improved at low temperatures: this has the effect of stimulating consumption and also helps the exercising athlete to feel better. Such effects on the athlete's sense of well-being cannot be ignored.

Cardiovascular, metabolic and performance effects

Many of the published studies investigating the effects of fluid ingestion on exercise performance have failed to include appropriate control trials that allow the separate effects of water replacement and substrate provision to be assessed. Generally, the studies in the literature have reported either no effect of fluid ingestion on exercise performance or a beneficial effect. In many cases, the absence of a statistically significant effect simply reflects the variability in the assessment methods used and inadequate subject numbers. There seems to be a lessened hyperthermia and cardiovascular drift during prolonged moderate intensity exercise (Hamilton et al. 1991; Montain et al. 1992 a, b) which is attributed to fluid replacement during the exercise. A better maintenance of blood glucose, which can be used by the exercising muscles with a consequent reduction in the need for mobilisation of the limited liver glycogen reserves (e.g. Maughan et al. 1989; McConnell et al. 1994) appears to be the major benefit of CHO consumption during exercise. The studies that have reported adverse effects of fluid ingestion on exercise performance have generally been studies in which the fluid ingestion has resulted in gastrointestinal disturbances.

Drinking plain water can improve performance in endurance exercise but there are further performance improvements when CHO and electrolytes are added (Fig. 4.2). Another study attempted to distinguish between the effects of CHO provision from the water replacement properties of a drink. Below et

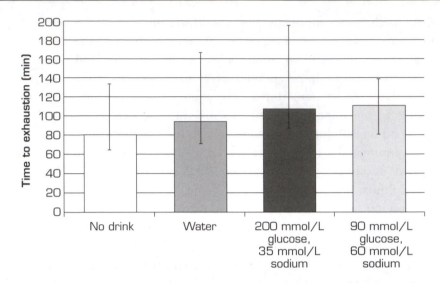

FIG. 4.2 Exercise times to exhaustion (median, minimum and maximum) after consumption of water, an isotonic CHO–electrolyte drink (200 mmol/L glucose, 35 mmol/L sodium), a hypotonic CHO–electrolyte drink (90 mmol/L glucose, 60 mmol/L sodium) and with no drink consumption (data from Maughan et al. 1996)

al. (1995) required eight men to undertake the same cycle ergometer exercise on four separate occasions. After 50 minutes' exercise at 80% of VO_{2max}, a performance test at a higher exercise intensity (completion of set amount of work as quickly as possible) was completed; this test lasted approximately 10 minutes. On each of the four trials, a different beverage consumption protocol was followed during the 50 minutes' exercise; nothing was consumed during the performance tests. The beverages were electrolyte-containing water in a large (1330 mL) and small (200 mL) volume and CHO–electrolyte solutions (79 g) in the same large and small volumes; the electrolyte content of each beverage was the same and amounted to 619 mg (27 mmol) and 141 mg (3.6 mmol) of sodium and potassium, respectively. The results of the study indicated that performance was 6.5% better after consuming the large volume of fluid in comparison to the smaller volume and was 6.3% better after consuming CHO-containing rather than CHO-free beverages; the fluid and CHO each independently improved performance and the two improvements were additive. The mechanism for the improvements in performance with the large fluid replacement versus the small fluid replacement was attributed to a lower heart rate and oesophageal temperature when the large volume was consumed. The authors were unable, however, to identify the mechanism by which CHO ingestion improved performance.

Pre-exercise hydration

Given the limited opportunities for fluid replacement in most exercise situations and the small volumes of fluid that are normally consumed, it is important that individuals should be fully hydrated when exercise begins. This has led to suggestions that hyperhydration before exercise might benefit performance, but the kidneys will normally clear any excess water ingested. Some degree of temporary hyperhydration appears to result when drinks with high (100 mmol/L) sodium concentrations are ingested but this seems unlikely to be beneficial for performance carried out in the heat on account of the high osmolality that ensues (Fortney et al. 1984).

An alternative strategy that has recently been the subject of interest has attempted to induce an expansion of the blood volume prior to exercise by the addition of glycerol to ingested fluids. Glycerol in high concentrations has little metabolic effect, being used only slowly by the liver as a substrate for gluconeogenesis, but exerts an osmotic action: although its distribution in the body water compartments is variable, glycerol will expand the extracellular space and some of the water ingested with the glycerol will be retained rather than lost in the urine (Riedesel et al. 1987). The elevated osmolality of the extracellular space will result in some degree of intracellular dehydration, and the implications of this are, at present, unknown. It might be expected, however, that the raised plasma osmolality will have negative consequences for thermoregulatory capacity (Fortney et al. 1984; Thecomata et al. 1997), although the available evidence at present seems to indicate that this is not the case (Montner et al. 1996; Latzka et al. 1996). The results of studies investigating the effects on exercise performance of glycerol ingestion before or during exercise have shown mixed results: there have been some recent suggestions of improved performance after administration of glycerol and water prior to prolonged exercise (Montner et al. 1996) but some earlier work clearly indicated that it did not improve the capacity to perform prolonged exercise (Gleeson et al. 1986; Miller et al. 1983).

Post-exercise rehydration

Post-exercise replacement of water and electrolyte losses may be of crucial importance when repeated bouts of exercise have to be performed: CHO ingestion at this time is also important when the exercise has resulted in a significant reduction in the body's liver and muscle glycogen stores. The need for replacement of each of these will obviously depend on the extent of the losses incurred during exercise, but will also be influenced by the time and nature of subsequent exercise bouts. Rapid rehydration may also be important in events where competition is by weight category. Competitors in events such as wrestling, boxing and weight-lifting frequently undergo acute thermal and exercise-induced dehydration to make weight. The key issues in achieving complete restoration of fluid losses are the volume of fluid ingested and its electrolyte content.

González-Alonso et al. (1992) have shown that a dilute CHO–electrolyte solution (60 g/L CHO, 20 mmol/L sodium, 3 mmol/L potassium) is more effective in promoting post-exercise rehydration than either plain water or a low-electrolyte diet cola. The difference between the drinks was primarily a result of differences in the volume of urine produced; there was a suggestion in this study that the caffeine content of the diet cola may have exerted a negative effect because of its diuretic properties.

Ingestion of plain water in the post-exercise period results in a rapid fall in the plasma sodium concentration and in plasma osmolality, reducing thirst and stimulating urine output, and both of these will delay the rehydration process (Nose et al. 1988). A systematic evaluation of the effects of replacing a fixed volume of fluid with different sodium concentrations demonstrated that urine output over the few hours following ingestion was inversely related to the sodium content of the ingested fluid (Maughan & Leiper 1995). In this study, subjects were dehydrated by intermittent exercise in the heat until 2% of body mass was lost and then consumed a volume of fluid equivalent to 1.5 times the sweat loss: these drinks contained 0, 25, 50 or 100 mmol/L sodium. Because the sodium content of sweat varies widely between individuals, with acclimatisation status and with other factors, it is not possible to identify a single formulation that will meet the needs of all individuals in all situations. However, it is not necessary that the concentration of drinks should match that of sweat but simply that the total volume ingested and the amount of electrolytes should be sufficient (Shirreffs 2001). The ingestion of the necessary electrolytes need not come from the beverage itself, and if solid food is consumed together with an adequate fluid volume (e.g. with water or a soft drink), effective rehydration can ensue (Maughan et al. 1996).

References

Adolph ED and associates. *Physiology of Man in the Desert*. New York: Interscience, 1947.

Armstrong LE, Costill DL, Fink WJ. Influence of diuretic-induced dehydration on competitive running performance. *Med Sci Sports Exerc* 1985;17:456–61.

Bar-Or O. Temperature regulation during exercise in children and adolescents. In: Gisolfi CV, Lamb DR, eds. *Perspectives in Exercise Science and Sports Medicine*. Vol. 2. *Youth, Exercise, and Sport*. Indianapolis, IN: Benchmark Press, 1989: 335–62.

Below RP, Mora-Rodriguez R, González-Alonso J, Coyle EF. Fluid and carbohydrate ingestion independently improve performance during 1 h of intense exercise. *Med Sci Sports Exerc* 1995;27:200–10.

Brouns F, Saris WHM, Schneider H. Rationale for upper limits of electrolyte replacement during exercise. *Int J Sports Nutr* 1992;2:229–38.

Buskirk ER, Beetham WP. Dehydration and body temperature as a result of marathon running. *Estratto da Medicina Sportiva* 1960;14:493–506.

Cheuvront SN, Haymes EM. Thermoregulation and marathon running. *Sports Med* 2001;31:743–62.

Fortney SM, Vroman NB, Beckett WS, Permutt S, LaFrance ND. Effect of exercise on haemoconcentration and hyperosmolality on exercise responses. *J Appl Physiol* 1988;65:519–24.

Fortney SM, Wenger CB, Bove JR, Nadel ER. Effect of hyperosmolality on control of blood flow and sweating. *J Appl Physiol* 1984;57:1688–95.

Galloway SDR, Maughan RJ. Effects of ambient temperature on the capacity to perform prolonged cycle exercise in man. *Med Sci Sports Exerc* 1997;29:1240–9.

Gisolfi CV, Wenger CB. Temperature regulation during exercise: old concepts, new ideas. *Exerc Sport Sci Rev* 1984;12:339–72.

Gleeson M, Maughan RJ, Greenhaff PL. Comparison of the effects of pre-exercise feeding of glucose, glycerol and placebo on endurance and fuel homeostasis in man. *Eur J Appl Physiol* 1986;55:645–53.

González-Alonso J, Heaps CL, Coyle EF. Rehydration after exercise with common beverages and water. *Int J Sports Med* 1992;13:399–406.

Greenleaf JE, Castle BL, Card DH. Blood electrolytes and temperature regulation during exercise in man. *Acta Physiol Polonica* 1974;25:397–410.

Hamilton MT, González-Alonso J, Montain SJ, Coyle EF. Fluid replacement and glucose during exercise prevent cardiovascular drift. *J Appl Physiol* 1991;71:871–7.

Harrison MH, Edwards RJ, Fennessy PA. Intravascular volume and tonicity as factors in the regulation of body temperature. *J Appl Physiol* 1978;44:69–75.

Hubbard RW, Szlyk PC, Armstrong LE. Influence of thirst and fluid palatability on fluid ingestion. In: Gisolfi CV, Lamb DR, eds. *Perspectives in Exercise Science and Sports Medicine*. Vol. 3. *Fluid Homeostasis during Exercise*. Indianapolis, IN: Benchmark Press, 1990: 39–95.

Latzka WA, Sawka MN, Matott RP, Staab JE, Montain SJ, Pandolf KB. Hyperhydration: physiologic and thermoregulatory effects during compensable and uncompensable exercise-heat stress. *US Army Tech Rep* 1996:T96–6.

Leithead CS, Lind AR. *Heat Stress and Heat Disorders*. London: Cassell, 1964.

Maron MB, Wagner JA, Horvath SM. Thermoregulatory responses during competitive marathon running. *J Appl Physiol* 1977;42:909–14.

Maughan RJ. Thermoregulation and fluid balance in marathon competition at low ambient temperature. *Int J Sports Med* 1985;6:15–19.

Maughan RJ. Effects of CHO-electrolyte solution on prolonged exercise. In: Lamb DR, Williams MH, eds. *Perspectives in Exercise Science and Sports Medicine*. Vol. 4. *Ergogenics—Enhancement of Performance in Exercise and Sport*. Carmel, IN: Cooper Publishing Group, 1991: 35–85.

Maughan RJ. Physiology and nutrition for middle distance and long distance running. In: Lamb DR, Knuttgen HG, Murray R, eds. *Perspectives in Exercise Science and Sports Medicine*. Vol. 7. *Physiology and Nutrition for Competitive Sport*. Carmel, IN: Cooper Publishing, 1994: 329–72.

Maughan RJ. Sports drinks before, during and after running. In: Tunstall Pedoe D, ed. *Marathon Medicine*. London: Royal Society of Medicine Press, 2001: 147–58.

Maughan RJ, Bethell LR, Leiper JB. Effects of ingested fluids on exercise capacity and on cardiovascular and metabolic responses to prolonged exercise in man. *Exp Physiol* 1996;81:847–59.

Maughan RJ, Fenn CE, Leiper JB. Effects of fluid, electrolyte and substrate ingestion on endurance capacity. *Eur J Appl Physiol* 1989;58:481–6.

Maughan RJ, Leiper JB. Effects of sodium content of ingested fluids on post-exercise rehydration in man. *Eur J Appl Physiol* 1995;71:311–19.

Maughan RJ, Leiper JB, Shirreffs SM. Restoration of fluid balance after exercise-induced dehydration: effects of food and fluid intake. *Eur J Appl Physiol* 1996;73: 317–25.

Maughan RJ, Leiper JB, Thompson J. Rectal temperature after marathon running. *Br J Sports Med* 1985;19:192–6.

Maughan RJ, Owen JH, Shirreffs SM, Leiper JB. Post-exercise rehydration in man: effects of electrolyte addition to ingested fluids. *Eur J Appl Physiol* 1994;69: 209–15.

McConell G, Fabris S, Proietto J, Hargreaves M. Effect of carbohydrate ingestion on glucose kinetics during exercise. *J Appl Physiol* 1994;77:1537–41.

Merson SJ, Shirreffs SM, Leiper JB, Maughan RJ. Changes in blood, plasma and red cell volume after ingestion of hypotonic and hypertonic solutions. *Proc Nutr Soc* 2002 (in press).

Miller JM, Coyle EF, Sherman WM, Hagberg JM, Costill DL, Fink WJ, Terblanche SE, Holloszy JO. Effect of glycerol feeding on endurance and metabolism during prolonged exercise in man. *Med Sci Sports Exerc* 1983;15:237–42.

Mitchell JW, Nadel ER, Stolwijk JAJ. Respiratory weight losses during exercise. *J Appl Physiol* 1972;34:474–6.

Montain SJ, Coyle EF. Influence of graded dehydration on hyperthermia and cardiovascular drift during exercise. *J Appl Physiol* 1992a;73:1340–50.

Montain SJ, Coyle EF. Fluid ingestion during exercise increases skin blood flow independent of increases in blood volume. *J Appl Physiol* 1992b;73:903–10.

Montner P, Stark DM, Riedesel ML, Murata G, Robergs R, Timms M, Chick TW. Pre-exercise glycerol hydration improves cycling endurance time. *Int J Sports Med* 1996;17:27–33.

Nadel ER. Circulatory and thermal regulations during exercise. *Fed Proc* 1980;39:1491–7.

Nadel ER, Mack GW, Nose H. Influence of fluid replacement beverages on body fluid homeostasis during exercise and recovery. In: Gisolfi CV, Lamb DR, eds. *Perspectives in Exercise Science and Sports Medicine.* Vol. 3. *Fluid Homeostasis During Exercise.* Carmel, IN: Cooper Publishing, 1990: 181–205.

Nielsen B, Kubica R, Bonnesen A, Rasmussen IB, Stoklosa J, Wilk B. Physical work capacity after dehydration and hyperthermia. *Scand J Sports Sci* 1981;3:2–10.

Noakes TD, Goodwin N, Rayner BL, Branken T, Taylor RKN. Water intoxication: a possible complication during endurance exercise. *Med Sci Sports Exerc* 1985;17:370–5.

Noakes TD, Myburgh KH, du Plessis J, Lang L, Lambert M, van der Riet C, Schall R. Metabolic rate, not percent dehydration, predicts rectal temperature in marathon runners. *Med Sci Sports Exerc* 1991;23:443–9.

Nose H, Mack GW, Shi X, Nadel ER. Role of osmolality and plasma volume during rehydration in humans. *J Appl Physiol* 1988;65:325–31.

Ramsay DJ. The importance of thirst in the maintenance of fluid balance. In: Bayliss PH, ed. *Clinical Endocrinology and Metabolism.* Vol. 3. No. 2. *Water and Salt Homeostasis in Health and Disease.* London: Baillière Tindall, 1989: 371–91.

Riedesel ML, Allen DL, Peake GT, Al-Qattan K. Hyperhydration with glycerol solutions. *J Appl Physiol* 1987;63:2262–8.

Rolls BJ, Wood RJ, Rolls ET, Lind W, Ledingham JGG. Thirst following water deprivation in humans. *Am J Physiol* 1980;239:R476–R482.

Roth RN, Verdile VP, Grollman LJ, Stone DA. Agreement between rectal and tympanic membrane temperatures in marathon runners. *Ann Emerg Med* 1996;28:414–17.

Rowell LB. *Human Circulation.* New York: Oxford University Press, 1986.

Shirreffs SM. Post-exercise rehydration and recovery. In: Maughan RJ, Murray R, eds. *Sports Drinks.* Boca Raton, FL: CRC Press, 2001.

Shirreffs SM, Maughan RJ. Whole body sweat collection in man: an improved method with some preliminary data on electrolyte composition. *J Appl Physiol* 1997;82:336–41.

Sutton JR. Clinical implications of fluid imbalance. In: Gisolfi CV, Lamb DR, eds. *Perspectives in Exercise Science and Sports Medicine.* Vol. 3. *Fluid Homeostasis during Exercise.* Indianapolis, IN: Benchmark Press, 1990: 425–48.

Thecomata A, Nagashima K, Nose H, Morimoto T. Osmoregulatory inhibition of thermally induced cutaneous vasodilation in passively heated humans. *Am J Physiol* 1997;273:R197–R204.

Verbalis JG. Inhibitory controls of drinking: satiation of thirst. In: Ramsay DJ, Booth DA, eds. *Thirst: Physiological and Psychological Aspects. ILSI Human Nutrition Reviews.* London: Springer-Verlag, 1990: 313–34.

Vist GE, Maughan RJ. The effect of osmolality and carbohydrate content on the rate of gastric emptying of liquids in man. *J Physiol* 1995;486:523–31.

Walsh RM, Noakes TD, Hawley JA, Dennis SC. Impaired high-intensity cycling performance time at low levels of dehydration. *Int J Sports Med* 1994;15:392–8.

Wilmore JH, DL Costill. *Physiology of Sport and Exercise*. Champaign, IL: Human Kinetics, 1999.

CHAPTER 5

Mechanisms of muscle fatigue

Michael J. MCKENNA

Introduction

Muscle fatigue affects us throughout our daily lives but influences our activities at different stages. Fatigue is especially important in a sporting context, reducing muscular performance and having a major effect on sporting outcomes. Differences in levels of fatigue in individuals in a team game may determine which player gets to the ball first, thereby dictating subsequent play and possibly the final result of a match. In an individual sport, fatigue may determine the difference between just beating an opponent, and thus a gold or silver medal performance, or winning the vital final set in a tennis match.

Fatigue also affects people from all ages in recreational activities, limiting our capacity to perform routine tasks of daily living. Fatigue is emerging as a major factor responsible for reducing exercise capacity and, thus, quality of life, in many chronic diseases, including heart failure, kidney failure and severe respiratory disease.

There is a tendency to describe muscle fatigue as a single entity or process. Rather, it is a highly complex phenomenon comprising numerous different components and acting at multiple sites within both the central nervous system (CNS) and the muscle itself. The mechanisms of fatigue appear to be highly specific during muscular exercise of different intensities and durations and are likely to be very different in a 200-m sprint, a game of soccer and a marathon. Therefore, in this chapter it is specified, where possible, the type of muscular activity where a particular mechanism of fatigue has been shown or is likely to be active.

It is important to appreciate that our understanding of what causes muscle fatigue comes from many different experimental sources. Much research investigating mechanisms of fatigue uses laboratory animals, such as rats, in experiments that might involve whole-body exercise, contractions of whole (intact) muscles, or even of a single muscle cell (fibre). We often have difficulty understanding whether experiments using animal models are applicable to muscle fatigue in exercising humans. It is often assumed that this will be so, although this is not the case as pointed out in several important examples. Some researchers ignore work not done in humans. This is a mistake since the complexity of experiments that can be undertaken in an animal model often far exceeds our capabilities to study these processes in an exercising human. This chapter focuses on causes of muscle fatigue in humans but is based on essential information from a number of animal studies.

Finally, how should we view fatigue from a physiological and teleological perspective? In many contexts, muscle fatigue is often viewed as 'the bad guy'. From a sports science perspective this is reasonable since delaying or minimising fatigue will be performance enhancing. However, scientists increasingly view muscle fatigue not as an inadvertent failure of the system but, rather, as a well-regulated process that is a normal occurrence. Muscle fatigue has an important outcome: to preserve the integrity and (once recovered) subsequent function of skeletal muscle and survival of the organism. This is particularly true in the context of protection against complete adenosine triphosphate (ATP) loss, substantial lactic-acid-induced acidosis and calcium-induced cellular damage. In this context, muscle fatigue can then be viewed as an important survival strategy for the muscle—a 'good guy'.

Definitions and manifestations of fatigue

All athletes are aware of the feelings associated with muscle fatigue: the muscles feel tired, slow, weak and sometimes painful. We must firstly define fatigue so that we can then determine how to quantify it. Only then can we really understand what fatigue and its effects are and investigate means of delaying or attenuating the processes. For example, if we can quantify the magnitude of fatigue in reducing muscle performance, then we can rigorously test whether an ergogenic aid truly works in delaying the fatigue process (see Chapter 9).

Earlier definitions of fatigue focused on the loss of the force-producing capacity of muscle (e.g. Edwards 1981; Vøllestad & Sejersted 1988). These definitions were logical since many experiments at that time investigated fatigue in isometric muscle contractions, where force is produced without any external muscle shortening. In that context, muscle force development was the major variable of importance. In an isometric contraction, the physical manifestations of fatigue include a decrease not only in the maximum force output but also in the maximum rates of force development and relaxation. Hence with fatigue, force develops more slowly and to a lesser amount, and then the muscles relax more slowly.

Recent definitions focus on the importance of fatigue during dynamic contractions, involving force production and shortening/lengthening cycles. In dynamic contractions, the most important outcome of muscle contraction is the power output, defined as the product of force by velocity. The importance of muscle power can be seen in kicking a soccer ball. To achieve a maximum velocity of the ball, both muscle force and muscle shortening velocity must be high. A very large force production would not impact much speed to the ball if the leg muscles contracted only slowly. Thus, the effects of muscle fatigue on both muscle force and shortening velocity must be considered. If these are each reduced by fatigue, then the impairment in muscle power output will be even more dramatic. This is well illustrated in a classic study in rat gastrocnemius muscles stimulated until fatigue (de Haan et al. 1989). With fatigue the maximal isometric force declined by 52%, but since maximal velocity of shortening also declined by 66%, power output declined to a greater extent, falling by 75% (de Haan et al. 1989).

Muscle fatigue also occurs during prolonged submaximal exercise (e.g. Coyle et al. 1986), where maximal contractions are not required. This reflects the progressive decline in maximal force production of the muscle

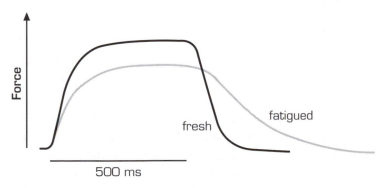

FIG. 5.1 Manifestations of fatigue during an isometric muscle contraction (from Cady et al. 1989a)

(Bigland-Ritchie et al. 1978) such that submaximal muscle contractions become progressively more stressful. The decline in muscle force, velocity of shortening and power accurately describe what is happening to the contractile performance of muscle during exercise, but on their own do not definitively prove fatigue, as they may also be a consequence of muscle damage. Thus, these impairments in contractile function must also be reversible during a recovery period. In conclusion, we can define muscle fatigue in exercising humans as a reduction in muscle power output during exercise, which is reversible during recovery.

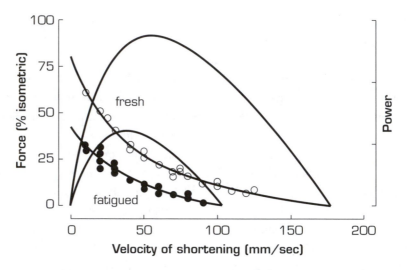

FIG. 5.2 Fatigue depresses both maximum force and velocity of shortening, with a large resultant decrease in maximal muscle power output (from de Haan et al. 1989)

Existence of both central and peripheral fatigue

What are the origins of fatigue? Does fatigue arise within the muscle itself or does this occur even before the muscle is activated? This is an important concept and is referred to as 'central' versus 'peripheral' muscle fatigue (Fig. 5.3). Peripheral muscle fatigue has been defined as any fatigue arising from the failure of mechanisms at or beyond (i.e. downstream of) the neuromuscular junction. Central fatigue can be defined as any fatigue originating before this point (upstream) in the neural pathways responsible for activation of muscle (Bigland-Ritchie 1981). Therefore, central fatigue could include processes such as the initiation of motor patterns in the motor

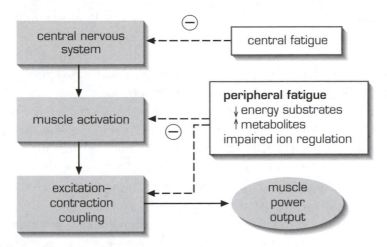

FIG. 5.3 Diagrammatic representation of central and peripheral sites of muscle fatigue, each manifested by a reduction in muscle power output

cortex, propagation of impulses down descending motor pathways, and excitation of alpha motor neurons and action potential (AP) propagation along the motor nerve, ultimately resulting in the recruitment of the muscle fibre. Central fatigue does occur during muscle contractions, as recently reviewed (Gandevia 2001).

Central fatigue occurs during isometric exercise

Bigland-Ritchie and colleagues (1978) were one of the first group of scientists to demonstrate convincingly that central fatigue could indeed occur in repeated contractions of large muscle groups in humans. They contrasted the force produced during maximal voluntary contractions with electrically stimulated maximal contractions during repeated fatiguing isometric contractions of the quadriceps muscles. Some individuals were unable to achieve maximal voluntary force equal to the maximal electrically stimulated force during repeated fatiguing contractions. These individuals were, therefore, unable to recruit all motor units fully and demonstrated central fatigue (Bigland-Ritchie et al. 1978).

The interpolated twitch technique has been extensively utilised to demonstrate the occurrence of central fatigue during repeated isometric contractions (McKenzie et al. 1992; Gandevia 2001). While performing a maximal muscle contraction, a brief electrical stimulation is superimposed to induce a muscle twitch contraction. If the electrical stimulation fails to produce any additional force above that produced by the voluntary contraction, then the muscle is fully activated (all motor units fully recruited). If, however, some additional force is produced with electrical stimulation, then motor unit recruitment is submaximal and activation is incomplete. If such incomplete activation develops during the presence of muscle fatigue, then central fatigue is evident. Central fatigue indicates that central drive to the muscles has diminished and accounts for some of the loss of force with fatigue. In simple terms, this means that the central nervous system is not 'driving' the muscles as hard as it needs to in order to maintain muscle force. This might be due to local reflex effects on the motor neuron or higher centres, reduced cortical drive or reduced drive through descending spinal pathways (Gandevia 2001).

Higher brain centres are involved in central fatigue, as transcranial magnetic stimulation of the cortex can increase muscle force during fatigue (Taylor et al. 2000; Gandevia 2001). A reflex inhibition of the alpha motor neuron has also been shown with fatiguing isometric muscle contractions, resulting in a reduced motor neuron firing rate and muscle excitation. However, this reflex preserves muscle force since relaxation also slows (Dawson et al. 1980). This is referred to as 'muscle wisdom', although this may be fortuitous rather than a coupled phenomenon (Gandevia 2001) and may not always be present (Garland & Gossen 2002).

The presence of central fatigue has been demonstrated on numerous occasions during isometric muscle contractions (McKenzie et al. 1992; Taylor et al. 2000; Fowles et al. 2002). Central fatigue typically accounts for a small proportion (10–20%) of the decline in muscle force with fatigue but can be more substantial in some individuals. This is emphasised by a recent study where central fatigue accounted for up to one-half of the overall force loss with fatigue after repeated isometric contractions of the quadriceps muscles (Fowles et al. 2002).

Central fatigue occurs during dynamic exercise

Few studies have convincingly demonstrated central fatigue during dynamic exercise but this appears to be mainly due to the complexity of undertaking these studies. Recent studies have increasingly used the twitch interpolation technique to study central fatigue during dynamic contractions. Central fatigue was found during repeated, fatiguing isokinetic quadriceps muscle contractions but could only account for 20% of the decline in power with fatigue (James et al. 1995). Conversely, no evidence of central fatigue was found during brief isokinetic cycle sprinting bouts (Beelen et al. 1995) or during repeated dynamic contractions of the elbow flexors (Gandevia et al. 1998). Central fatigue has recently been demonstrated following very prolonged exercise. After 5 hours of submaximal cycling at 55% of maximal oxygen uptake (VO_{2max}), maximal activation of the quadriceps muscles declined by 8%, representing about one-half of the 18% decline in maximal voluntary force (Lepers et al. 2002). Following a 65-km ultramarathon, this effect was even more marked, where almost all of the decline in maximal voluntary contraction (30%) could be explained by the decline (27%) in maximal activation (Millet et al. 2002). Thus, central fatigue may occur during isometric and dynamic contractions, although in most cases fatigue predominantly occurs in the periphery (Fig. 5.3).

Why would central fatigue exist? One possible and important advantage of central fatigue is that muscle power is allowed to fall to prevent the muscles from being driven progressively into more marked fatigue, with potentially catastrophic metabolic (e.g. ATP loss), ionic (e.g. Ca^{2+} overload or K^+ depletion), structural (e.g. muscle damage) and thermal (hyperthermia) consequences.

Impaired muscle membrane excitability and ionic disturbances

Excitation overview

The next major potential site of fatigue in the muscle activation pathway is membrane excitation, including both the sarcolemma and the transverse tubular membranes (Fig. 5.4). It is clear that transport of sodium (Na^+) and potassium (K^+) ions across the sarcolemmal and transverse tubular membranes is critical to maintain their large concentration gradients, which ensure cell excitability.

Disturbances in muscle ionic concentrations in fatigue

Many textbooks indicate that ion movements across the sarcolemma during an AP are minimal. This is true for a single AP, which induces very minor increases in Na^+ concentration (0.008 mM) and reductions in K^+ concentration of 0.005 mM within the cell (Hodgkin & Horowitz 1959). However, it is important to appreciate that in contracting skeletal muscle, the AP frequency may be as high as 50 Hz (i.e. 50 AP/s) in burst contractions and 10–30 Hz in more sustained contractions. Therefore, the extent of Na^+

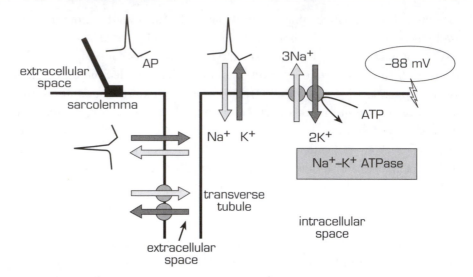

FIG. 5.4 Overview of the processes involved in membrane excitation, including action potential (AP) propagation along the sarcolemma and into the transverse tubular system. Interrelationships between AP, sodium (Na+) and potassium (K+) ion movements and the counteractive effects of the Na+–K+ ATPase enzyme (Na+–K+ pump) are shown. Dark arrows indicate Na+ ion movements and light arrows K+ ion movements. Note that outside the sarcolemma and within the transverse tubular system is an extracellular space

entry into and K+ loss from muscle are greatly magnified. In human muscles during exercise, muscle intracellular Na+ concentrations may double, rising from about 13 mM at rest to 24 mM at fatigue, while muscle intracellular K+ concentrations may decline by about 20%, from approximately 160 mM at rest to about 130 mM at fatigue (Sjøgaard et al. 1985). In electrically stimulated single muscle fibres from animal studies, even larger changes are found, with Na+ concentrations tripling and K+ concentrations falling by one-third (Balog & Fitts 1996).

Recent studies using the microdialysis technique have demonstrated remarkable increases in the muscle extracellular (interstitial) K+ concentration from 4–5 mM at rest to values as high as 10–15 mM during heavy muscle contractions (Green et al. 2000; Juel et al. 2000). As a consequence, the intracellular-to-extracellular K+ concentration ratio may decline by more than 50%, with a consequent decrease (depolarisation) in the muscle membrane potential of 8–10 mM from resting levels in human muscles (Sjøgaard et al. 1985) and in animal muscles (Balog et al. 1994). This results in the inactivation of fast Na+ channels, which are responsible for Na+ entry into the cell during the AP, with the consequent development of membrane inexcitability. The marked intramuscular water influx during heavy contractions will also affect these ion concentrations (see McKenna 1992).

Incubation of muscle in high K^+ concentrations typical of interstitial concentrations depresses force once the K^+ concentration exceeds about 8 mM, but this reduction in force is magnified when the extracellular Na^+ concentration also declines (Renaud et al. 1996). The rise in K^+ concentration and decline in Na^+ concentration could be marked within the transverse tubules due to their small local distribution volume, the circuitous network by which transverse tubules are connected to the sarcolemma (Fig. 5.5) and the lower concentration of Na^+–K^+ pumps in the transverse tubules (McKenna 1998). The extensive nature of the transverse tubular system is shown in Figure 5.5. This indicates the circuitous route by which K^+ ions released in the interior of the fibre and accumulating in the transverse tubules must travel before entering the interstitial space surrounding the fibre. Thus, it is possible that this localised K^+ accumulation may be more pronounced in the interior of the fibre and cause fatigue via impairment of membrane excitation.

A consequence of muscle membrane activation processes is a marked K^+ release from contracting muscle cells into the interstitium and then the blood. During maximal sprinting on a treadmill or cycle ergometer, arterial plasma K^+ concentrations may reach a peak of 7–8 mM and femoral venous

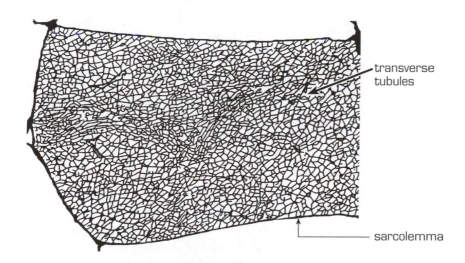

FIG. 5.5 Cross-section of a single frog muscle fibre, detailing the extensive and circuitous network of the t-tubular system (modified from Peachey and Eisenberg 1978). This should be contrasted to the commonly used stylised approach in Figure 5.4, which incorrectly suggests a 1:1 sarcolemmal–tubular membrane ratio.

plasma K^+ concentrations to 8 mM (Fig. 5.6; Hallen 1996; McKenna et al. 1997; Medbø & Sejersted 1990; Sejersted & Sjøgaard 2000). Since venous K^+ concentrations may exceed muscle interstitial K^+ concentrations by as much as 6 mM (Green et al. 2000), this indicates that muscle interstitial K^+ concentrations must be very high during heavy sprinting exercise in humans. However, this does not necessarily indicate that fatigue due to K^+ inactivation of membrane excitability must occur. A recent study has found that increased activity of the Na^+-K^+ ATPase enzyme that normally occurs during muscle contraction can also protect against muscle inactivation caused by a high-concentration K^+ solution (Nielsen et al. 2001).

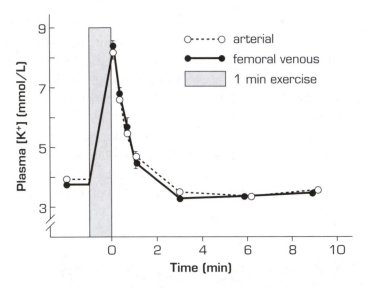

FIG. 5.6 Rise in arterial and femoral venous plasma K^+ concentrations after vigorous sprinting exercise (from Medbo & Sejersted 1990, reproduced with permission)

Impaired Na^+-K^+ ATPase activity with fatigue

The Na^+-K^+ ATPase enzyme (Na^+-K^+ pump) is mainly located in the sarcolemma and transports three Na^+ ions out of and two K^+ ions into the cell. These ions are transported against very large concentration gradients and the energy for this process comes from the hydrolysis of one ATP molecule (hence its name). The significance of this enzyme for cell function is indicated by the awarding of the Nobel Prize to its discoverer, Professor Jens Skou from Denmark, in 1997. In muscle cells undergoing contractions, Na^+-K^+ ATPase activity is rapidly increased to counteract the gain of Na^+

ions and the loss of K^+ ions associated with each AP. This activity exerts an electrogenic effect, which hyperpolarises the membrane. Recent research, mainly conducted in isolated rat muscles, has demonstrated an important role of Na^+–K^+ ATPase in muscle fatigue (see Nielsen & Clausen 2000 for review). When the Na^+–K^+ ATPase enzyme was inhibited (by the specific inhibitor ouabain), muscle fatigued more rapidly and recovered more slowly; when the enzyme activity was augmented, the muscle fatigued more slowly and recovered more rapidly. These experiments have not yet been performed in humans, so it is not yet possible to determine whether these findings can be extrapolated to contracting muscles in human exercise.

The Na^+–K^+ ATPase enzyme may also be directly adversely affected by fatigue. Following repeated isometric quadriceps contractions, the maximal Na^+–K^+ ATPase enzyme activity was reduced (Fowles et al. 2002). This was confirmed following dynamic exercise in untrained, endurance and resistance-trained athletes, suggesting that this was an obligatory change with fatigue (Fraser et al. 2002; Fig. 5.7). Since Na^+–K^+ ATPase activity counteracts muscle cellular K^+ loss and Na^+ gain, and thereby contributes to membrane depolarisation, these findings suggest that depression in the maximal Na^+–K^+ ATPase activity may result in worse regulation of cation movements and membrane potential, and thus directly contribute to muscle fatigue. An increase in K^+ release from muscle at fatigue is also consistent with this (Verburg et al. 1999).

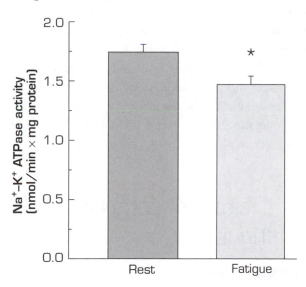

FIG. 5.7 Depressed maximal Na^+–K^+ ATPase enzyme activity in muscle with fatigue (modified from Fraser et al. 2002)

Membrane potential and M-waves: impaired excitation in fatigue

When human muscles undergo extremely high-frequency electrical stimulation (e.g. 100 Hz), muscle excitability is rapidly reduced, with smaller amplitude and widening of the AP, along with slowed conduction velocity (Jones 1996). Under these conditions force drops rapidly, a condition known as high-frequency fatigue. With more physiological, low-frequency stimulation, such extreme changes are not found (Jones 1996). Under these conditions muscle force declines, in particular during low-frequency stimulation, suggesting that fatigue is related to impairments in muscle calcium (Ca^{2+}) regulation (see p. 96).

To measure muscle excitability, many investigations have measured the area and amplitude of the M-wave, reflecting the muscle compound AP. This is the summation of many individual APs, usually from muscle fibres close to the muscle surface. Close relationships have been demonstrated between muscle force and M-wave area in isolated muscles incubated in high K^+ solutions to simulate high-intensity contractions (see Nielsen & Clausen 2000). It is not known whether similar changes occur in human muscles during sprinting-type contractions. Motor neuron activation rates of up to 50 Hz in contractions suggest that membrane excitation could be impaired under these conditions. A recent study demonstrated a 25% reduction in M-wave area after repeated isometric contractions of the quadriceps muscles (Fowles et al. 2002). Impairment of excitability is much more likely to occur in transverse tubular membranes rather than in the sarcolemma (Nielsen & Clausen 2000).

An involvement of membrane inexcitability in fatigue makes sense since this represents an early stage in muscle activation, and failure at one or more of these sites would be energetically economic. Failure could occur prior to exhaustion of metabolic fuels, thus preserving muscle ATP, preventing muscle rigour and ensuring cell survival.

Failure of excitation–contraction coupling (ECC) in fatigue

Overview of muscle ECC

The coupling between membrane excitation and the sarcoplasmic reticulum (SR) in the development of force is the next possible link affected in muscle fatigue. To understand fatigue effects it is firstly necessary to briefly review some of the structures and proteins linking membrane excitation to Ca^{2+} release from the SR.

Two vital proteins are involved in the link between membrane excitation and the increase in Ca^{2+} concentration within the cell cytosol, which then enables muscle contraction (Fig. 5.8a). The dihydropyridine receptor (DHPR) is located in the transverse tubular membrane and acts as a 'voltage sensor', detecting the change in voltage as the AP propagates along the transverse tubular membrane. The ryanodine receptor (RyR) is located in the terminal cisternae of the SR and is the physiological Ca^{2+}-release channel in the SR (Lamb 2000). The RyR is also in contact with numerous other proteins that exert modulatory effects on RyR function. The DHPR and RyR are located directly opposite each other in the membrane, but in an alternating fashion (i.e. at a DHPR:RyR ratio of about 2:1). The DHPR are thought to communicate mechanically with the opposing RyR. Therefore, some RyR cannot be activated mechanically by an opposing DHPR but are probably activated by Ca^{2+} released from an adjacent RyR. Activation of the RyR (i.e. opening the Ca^{2+}-release channel) results in Ca^{2+} being released from the SR lumen, where it is bound to calsequestrin, with Ca^{2+} then flooding out into the cell cytoplasm (Fig. 5.8b). In resting muscle cells, the Ca^{2+} concentration is tightly regulated at an extremely low concentration of 50–100 nM (about one-millionth the concentration of resting blood lactate concentration, which is about 1 mM). In contracting muscle cells, the Ca^{2+} concentration rises by between 10- and 100-fold, to 1–10 µmol/L (1000 nmol/L) (Westerblad et al. 1998).

Normal intracellular ATP in resting muscle is about 6 mM, which would open the RyR, but this effect is overwhelmed by the inhibitory effect of magnesium (Mg^{2+}) at the normal resting concentration of about 1 mM. In the intact cell the mechanical link between the DHPR and the RyR is essential for RyR opening. However, many other factors also regulate opening/closure of the RyR and many of these are important in muscle fatigue. These include Ca^{2+} ions; the metabolic fuels ATP, phosphocreatine (PCr) and glycogen; metabolites such as inorganic phosphate (P_i) and lactate; and drugs such as caffeine (see Stephenson et al. 1998).

Fatigue impairs SR Ca^{2+} release: techniques and major findings

A growing number of scientific studies provide evidence that the SR RyR is a major site of peripheral muscle fatigue, if not the most important (see reviews: Fitts 1994; Allen et al. 1995; Favero 1999; Westerblad et al. 1998;

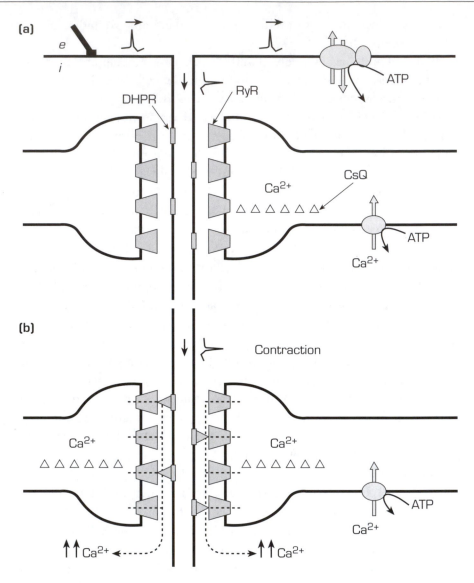

FIG. 5.8 Schematic representation of structures and proteins involved in excitation–contraction coupling. The dihydropyridine receptor (DHPR), or voltage sensors, are indicated by rectangular boxes in transverse tubules and the ryanodine receptor (RyR) by cone-shaped proteins on the sarcoplasmic reticulum (SR). Note that these are located opposite each other in an alternate fashion. Calsequestrin (CsQ), indicated by triangular shapes, binds Ca^{2+} within the SR.
(a) Resting muscle. (b) Contracting muscle

Lamb 2000). Four important techniques have been used to examine the effects of intense muscle contractions on SR Ca^{2+} release and its role in muscle fatigue.

The first technique involves the microinjection of ion-selective fluorescent dyes (e.g. Indo, Fura, which bind Ca^{2+}) into a single intact fibre, allowing determination of the intracellular ion concentration (Fig. 5.9). A landmark study by Allen et al. (1989) demonstrated that muscle intracellular Ca^{2+} concentration declined markedly during fatiguing contractions, combined with a decline in muscle force. When caffeine, the RyR opener, was applied to the fatigued muscle fibre, both muscle intracellular Ca^{2+} concentration and force were restored to resting levels! This suggested that a failure of the RyR opening was directly responsible for muscle fatigue in that preparation (Fig. 5.9).

A similar outcome from a different study is shown in Figure 5.10.

A limitation of this technique is that it can only be performed on a single intact cell. It is therefore impossible to employ in human single muscle fibres, since these are cut during the biopsy process. So the important question arises: does impairment of SR Ca^{2+} release also occur in human muscles in fatigue? Based on studies using vesicle preparations and Ca^{2+}-sensitive dyes in human muscles, it would appear so (Hill et al. 2001; Li et al. 2002). Using this technique, the muscle biopsy sample is homogenised, causing formation of membrane vesicles (spheres of membranes) to study Ca^{2+} release from the RyR (Fig. 5.11). Results from these studies have confirmed that SR Ca^{2+} release is reduced following intense dynamic muscle contractions (Hill et al. 2001; Li et al. 2002), consistent with data from investigations in isolated muscle fibres (Allen et al. 1995). This depression appears to reflect structural changes in the RyR, rather than ionic or metabolic perturbations (Li et al. 2002). Thus, impaired SR Ca^{2+} release also plays a major role in fatigue in

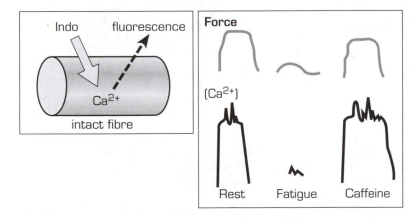

FIG. 5.9 Microinjection of the fluorescent dye Indo into a single intact fibre to determine muscle intracellular Ca^{2+} concentration during fatigue

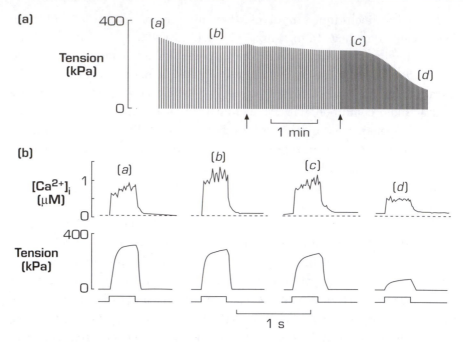

FIG. 5.10 Fatigue effects on muscle force and intracellular Ca^{2+} concentration in a single muscle fibre. The individual intracellular Ca^{2+} concentration and force records at each of the time points labelled (a)–(d) on the upper trace are magnified in the two lower records. Note the marked decline in intracellular Ca^{2+} concentration from traces (a) to (d), when muscle force (tension) is also severely depressed (from Westerblad et al. 1998)

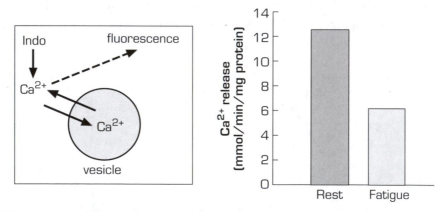

FIG. 5.11 Use of dyes in human muscle vesicle preparations to determine muscle SR RyR function with fatigue. SR Ca^{2+} release was depressed after 50 maximal isokinetic quadriceps contractions (modified from Li et al. 2002)

human muscles. SR Ca^{2+} release was also depressed in fatigue induced by prolonged exercise in rat soleus muscle (Favero et al. 1993) and it is highly likely that similar depression will be found in human muscles.

This vesicle technique has also been employed in human muscle to demonstrate that Ca^{2+} uptake into the SR by the Ca^{2+} ATPase enzyme is reduced in fatigue (Fig. 5.11). This effect occurs after brief intense exercise (Li et al. 2002), high-intensity intermittent exercise bouts (Hargreaves et al. 1998), isometric contractions (Gollnick et al. 1991) and prolonged exhaustive exercise (Booth et al. 1997). Similarly, depressed SR Ca^{2+} uptake has been observed in vesicle preparations after brief and prolonged fatiguing exercise in rats and in horses (Byrd et al. 1989 a, b). Depressed SR Ca^{2+} uptake would reduce SR loading, potentially reducing releasable Ca^{2+}, as well as exposing the muscle to higher Ca^{2+} concentrations, which might lead to activation of proteases and membranous damage (Clarkson 1992). Thus, it is likely that depressed SR Ca^{2+} uptake plays an important role in muscle fatigue.

RyR channel function has been studied directly, using RyR proteins embedded in a lipid bilayer, thus allowing the effect of specific ions (e.g. lactate, H^+, Mg^{2+}) on RyR function to be determined (Favero 1999; Laver et al. 2001). While this technique has been extremely useful in understanding RyR function, it has led to some erroneous claims about muscle fatigue. For example, increased lactate and H^+, both of which accompany intense muscle contractions, inhibit RyR opening in this preparation (Favero et al. 1995) but not in single fibres (Dutka & Lamb 2000; Lamb et al. 1992). The fourth technique is the mechanically skinned muscle fibre, which exposes the interior of the fibre to easily controlled external solutions (e.g. low pH, low PCr, high lactate), yet also allows activation of the muscle fibre via the normal voltage activation (i.e. DHPR–RyR) pathway (Stephenson et al. 1998). These techniques have allowed scientists to determine the effects of many substrates and metabolites on the muscle fibre, under conditions mimicking muscle fatigue.

Mechanisms of SR dysfunction in muscle fatigue

The major factor thought to be responsible for the depressed SR Ca^{2+} release in fatigue is the increase in muscle P_i as a result of PCr depletion (Fryer et al. 1995; Posterino & Fryer 1998; Allen & Westerblad 2001). P_i is thought to enter the SR and bind with Ca^{2+} ions therein, thus reducing the Ca^{2+} available for release. This is consistent with a decline in the rapidly releasable pool of Ca^{2+} with fatigue (Kabbara & Allen 1999). This is supported by evidence from mice lacking creatine kinase in their muscles: PCr cannot be broken down in these muscles and no decline in muscle intracellular Ca^{2+} concentration is seen with fatigue (Dahlstedt & Westerblad 2001). Other metabolic factors are also important. Glycogen is associated with the SR and low muscle glycogen levels impair muscle ECC (Stephenson et al. 1999). Creatine kinase is closely associated with the SR; localised depletion of PCr also impairs muscle Ca^{2+} release. This strongly suggests that a local supply of ATP is critical for RyR function (Duke & Steele 1998). Therefore, any adverse impact of exercise on muscle energy status will also directly affect SR Ca^{2+} release.

Some ionic factors are also thought to contribute to impaired ECC. In an intact muscle fibre, even transient increases in Ca^{2+} concentration can impair muscle ECC (Lamb et al. 1995), but lactate nor acidosis do not. Finally, the rate of Ca^{2+} transport from the cytoplasm back into the SR is reduced with fatigue (Westerblad & Allen 1993). This is not the cause of the reduced muscle relaxation time with fatigue, which appears to be due to slowed detachment of cross bridges (Westerblad & Allen 1993; Booth et al. 1997). Rather, reduced Ca^{2+} transport into the SR may reduce loading of the SR for subsequent Ca^{2+} release and thus also contribute to decreased muscle force with fatigue.

Accumulation of free radicals in fatigue has also been shown to exert important adverse effects on SR function, although these are not yet well understood (Reid 2001). The sensitivity of the muscle to Ca^{2+} is reduced with fatigue (Westerblad et al. 1998). This means that a higher intracellular Ca^{2+} concentration is required to achieve the same muscle force output in fatigued muscle. Since intracellular Ca^{2+} concentration in fact falls with fatigue, a reduced Ca^{2+} sensitivity therefore exacerbates the decline in force in fatigue. Accumulation of P_i also directly affects force produced by the cross bridges.

The failure of Ca^{2+} release from the SR in muscle fatigue appears to result from numerous causes of metabolic and ionic origins. Depletion of localised substrates ATP, PCr and glycogen and accumulation of P_i, Mg^{2+} and Ca^{2+} all affect RyR opening and Ca^{2+} release. The consequent decline in intracellular Ca^{2+} concentration, together with a reduced Ca^{2+} sensitivity of the myofibrils, directly results in reduced muscle force and power. This makes excellent energetic sense from the muscle's perspective since failure occurs at this site before the metabolic fuel supplies become exhausted, thus preserving muscle ATP, preventing muscle rigour and ensuring cell survival. Impaired SR Ca^{2+} release is a major factor in fatigue in isolated muscle fibres, in contractions lasting only a few minutes in duration. Depressed Ca^{2+} release has also been demonstrated in intense contractions in humans and seems highly probable in intermittent and prolonged contractions as well.

Metabolism is intricately involved in muscle fatigue

Metabolism and fatigue in intense, brief muscle contractions

Is metabolism important in muscle fatigue during high-intensity sprinting exercise? The answer is yes and links several mechanisms already discussed in this chapter. High-intensity exercise lasting several minutes and continued until exhaustion results in almost total depletion of muscle PCr (Hultman et al. 1967). The depletion of muscle phosphagens (ATP and PCr) was therefore regarded as the source of muscular fatigue during heavy exercise (Hultman et al. 1967). Almost total depletion of muscle PCr has been confirmed following repeated bouts of intense cycling exercise (McCartney et al. 1986), isometric knee extensor contractions held to fatigue (Sahlin & Henriksson 1984) and electrical stimulation of human quadriceps muscle under anaerobic conditions (Spriet et al. 1987). Under these conditions, the maximum rate of ATP resynthesis must be reduced, making PCr unavailability an important factor in muscle fatigue. However, muscle PCr is usually not fully depleted during most exercise conditions and thus fatigue cannot be simply attributed to the complete depletion of PCr. What appears to be more important is the rate of PCr hydrolysis, since this will indicate the rate of ATP resynthesis via the creatine kinase reaction.

It is apparent that the *rate* of PCr hydrolysis declines rapidly during brief, high-intensity exercise. During a 6-s sprint, muscle PCr and ATP contents decreased by 57% and 13%, respectively (Gaitanos et al. 1993). If these hydrolytic rates could continue, PCr and ATP would be completely depleted within 10 and 46 seconds, respectively. This would be disastrous for muscle! It would mean that an elite 400-m sprinter would have to go into muscle rigour to gain a place in an Olympic final. Following a 30-s maximal sprint, muscle ATP and PCr contents had decreased by 40% and 70% (Cheetham et al. 1986), which are well below changes predicted at rates observed in the first 6 seconds. Such dramatic metabolic rates simply cannot be sustained (Bogdanis et al. 1998). This is likely due not only to limited availability of these stores, but also to the fact that other peripheral (and possibly central) factors intervene to down-regulate contractile performance.

Interestingly, elite sprinters have shown a decline in muscle PCr of 75% and ATP of 40% within only 10 seconds (Hirvonen et al. 1987). This might reflect the greater initial decline in muscle PCr in type II rather than type I fibres (Casey et al. 1996). A recent study has demonstrated that depletion of ATP and PCr may be 75% and 89% in some type II fibres following an exhaustive 25-s sprint bout (Karatzaferi et al. 2001). Finally, important evidence in support of a key role for PCr in muscle fatigue during brief, intense exercise is that recovery of muscle power after exercise is closely correlated with muscle PCr resynthesis (Bogdanis et al. 1995).

Muscle glycogen is also an important energy source during intense exercise, for both anaerobic and aerobic pathways. During a 6-s 'all out' sprint, muscle glycogen decreases by 14%, while after a 30-s sprint glycogen levels had decreased by 25% (Cheetham et al. 1986). At the highest glycogenolytic rate, muscle glycogen would be totally depleted within 43 seconds. Reduced glycogen availability would restrict the rate of anaerobic ATP production from glycolysis and thus contribute further to the decline in ATP turnover and decline in muscle power.

Taken collectively, the results from these investigations indicate that muscle ATP is not depleted by intense exercise. However, one important limitation in interpreting results from these studies is that ATP and PCr contents were average measurements over the whole muscle sample. Since the ATP hydrolysing enzymes (Na^+–K^+ ATPase, Ca^{2+} ATPase and myosin ATPase) are located at specific sites, then it is highly likely that regions exist within the contracting muscle where even more dramatic reductions in muscle PCr and ATP occur. Localised ATP depletion could thus affect each of membrane excitation, intracellular Ca^{2+} concentrations and force development (Green 1998). The case for this possibility is even stronger with recent findings that muscle ATP in single fibres may fall to extremely low values in some fibres (Karatzaferi et al. 2001). A reduced rate of ATP resynthesis relative to hydrolysis is indicated by the massive rise in muscle inosine monophosphate (IMP) after intense fatiguing exercise (Stathis et al. 1994).

By-products of such high rates of energy metabolism include lactate, ADP, IMP, H^+ ions and P_i. Although muscle lactate content rose by 28-fold after a 30-s sprint (Cheetham et al. 1986), there does not appear to be an important mechanism whereby this might contribute to fatigue. The obvious candidate is acidosis. Intense muscle contractions may reduce muscle pH from 7.1 at rest to 6.5 at fatigue (Hermansen & Osnes 1972). This acidosis has long been thought to be an important mechanism in muscle fatigue (Hermansen 1981). However, in many of the early studies demonstrating depressive effects of acidosis on muscle force, the experiments were conducted on muscle fibres at room temperature. Under these conditions, both muscle force and shortening velocity were impressively reduced by acidosis. However, at more physiological temperatures (35°C), acidosis had only a very minor effect on muscle force and shortening velocity (Westerblad et al. 1997). Thus, acidosis is not an important factor in muscle fatigue.

This raises two interesting and unresolved questions. Firstly, why does intensive training (Sharp et al. 1986) or hypoxia (Gore et al. 2001) induce an increase in muscle buffering capacity? Secondly, why does alkalosis induce enhanced muscular performance (Sutton et al. 1976)? Other mechanisms must clearly be involved.

Muscle P_i rises dramatically following exhaustive exercise (Sahlin 1978). After maximal forearm exercise, phosphorus-31 labelled nuclear magnetic resonance (NMR) analyses show a fourfold to fivefold rise in total muscle P_i (Cady et al. 1989b; Wilson et al. 1988). Increased P_i has a marked inhibitory effect on force development (Cooke et al. 1988) and is related to the decline in force output reported in animal single fibres (Dawson et al. 1980), as well as in fatigued human forearm muscle (Wilson et al. 1988). This inhibitory effect of P_i is likely to be exerted on the cross bridges, although P_i may also precipitate Ca^{2+} within the SR and reduce Ca^{2+} release for exercise lasting more than several minutes (Allen & Westerblad 2001).

Another important metabolic by-product is the production of oxygen free radicals. There are many different radicals and several have been linked with fatigue in isolated animal muscle experiments (Barclay & Hansel 1991; Reid 2001). However, the link with fatigue in human muscles is not yet well established. An intriguing study demonstrated that infusion of the antioxidant compound *N*-acetyl cysteine reduced muscular fatigability during low-frequency stimulation, suggesting that free radicals do induce fatigue in human muscles (Reid et al. 1994).

In summary, reductions in the rate of ATP resynthesis due to falling rates of ATP resynthesis from PCr and, to a lesser extent, glycogen breakdown appear to be of vital importance in fatigue occurring during brief, high-intensity exercise bouts. This is most likely mediated at the sites of ATP breakdown, with loss of excitability (within the transverse tubules), impaired rate of Ca^{2+} release and reduced cross bridge force development.

Metabolism and fatigue in intermittent sports

Relatively little is known about muscle metabolism and fatigue during team sports that are typically characterised by a large number of brief, high-intensity bouts of exercise, separated by a variable recovery interval undertaken for 1–3 hours. For example, during a competition match, soccer players on average may cover a total distance of 9–10 km by running and walking, perform 60–80 sprints or high-intensity runs, 10–16 jumps,

13 tackles and 50 turns (Tumilty 1993). There are few studies of muscle metabolism during such activities, making it difficult to determine their relevance in muscle fatigue. However, it is clear that muscle glycogen availability is critically important.

Muscle glycogen content fell by 94% at the end of an exhibition match in Scandinavian soccer players (Saltin 1973). In a subgroup of players who commenced the match with approximately half-normal resting glycogen content, muscle glycogen was extremely low by half-time and completely exhausted by the end of the match, in which they also exhibited a large reduction in time running at maximum speed (Saltin 1973). Muscle glycogen depletion after a game in elite Swedish soccer players was approximately equal in type I and II muscle fibres (Jacobs et al. 1982). Blood lactate concentrations in elite soccer players at half-time were in the range of 7–10 mM, and at the end of the match of 4–11 mM (Ekblom 1986). This strongly suggests high muscle lactate content, which together with the nature of the match, implies that muscle PCr would also be heavily utilised. Therefore, a reduced ATP resynthesis rate is likely to be a major factor in fatigue during intermittent sports.

Metabolism and fatigue during prolonged exercise

The most important variable linked with fatigue in prolonged exercise is muscle glycogen depletion. This was largely determined more than three decades ago by a group of Scandinavian researchers, who reported during prolonged exercise that muscle glycogen content may fall to nearly zero at exhaustion (Hermansen et al. 1967; Bergstrom et al. 1967). Increased dietary carbohydrate intake could enhance muscle glycogen content and prolong performance, while a reduction of dietary carbohydrate intake had the reverse effect. Many studies have subsequently investigated the role of carbohydrate ingestion before and during exercise upon muscle glycogen utilisation and performance (see Chapter 2).

The possible link between lowered glycogen and impaired performance was suggested by the finding of a sharp rise in muscle IMP at fatigue, indicating a reduced rate of ATP resynthesis relative to hydrolysis with falling carbohydrate oxidation rates (Sahlin 1992). Consistent with this, carbohydrate supplements also reduce muscle IMP accumulation and enhance prolonged exercise performance (McConell et al. 1999). However, increased IMP did not occur at fatigue in trained athletes despite low muscle glycogen levels (Baldwin et al. 1999) and was also unrelated to muscle glycogen content or performance at fatigue (Febbraio & Dancey

1999). Further, numerous studies have found that individuals have fatigued while still retaining considerable amounts of muscle glycogen. There may be several reasons for these inconsistencies.

Muscle glycogen utilisation occurs primarily in type I fibres, which are heavily recruited during prolonged exercise (Vøllestad et al. 1984). Reductions in glycogen would be expected to be greater around the SR, since glycogen is preferentially used to fuel Ca^{2+} uptake and most likely also Ca^{2+} release. This suggests even more severe localised depletion of ATP resynthesis rates, thereby severely compromising SR Ca^{2+} release (see p. 96). SR uptake rates in human muscle are depressed with prolonged exercise (Booth et al. 1997). Muscle glycogen has also been shown to have an important stabilising role in muscle ECC (Stephenson et al. 1999). Finally, prolonged exercise performance may be affected by central fatigue (Lepers et al. 2002; Millet et al. 2002). This may be a factor in the observation that muscle fatigue also coincides with body core temperature reaching a critical level of 40°C (Nybo & Nielsen 2001). Temperature-dependent cessation of exercise during prolonged exercise might occur to prevent further hyperthermia and dehydration, and the associated deterioration in major organs.

Conclusion

Muscle fatigue is a highly complex phenomenon with multifactorial causes. Many sites in the muscle force development pathway appear to be affected by fatigue under some exercise conditions. Central fatigue certainly occurs, although most fatigue resides within the peripheral muscles themselves. Membrane excitability appears to be susceptible to fatigue under conditions of very high-intensity, brief contractions. Impairment of muscle SR Ca^{2+} release may be a major factor in many forms of fatigue, although the mechanisms may differ and its application to human muscles in exercise is only just beginning. Metabolism also plays a clear role in fatigue, through diminished rates of ATP supply and via interactions with each of the ATP-consuming processes in membrane excitability, ECC and cross bridge detachment and cycling. Finally, muscle fatigue should be viewed as an evolved protective strategy. The numerous fatigue factors act in concert to reduce muscle contractile performance and protect the muscle cell against the associated harsh metabolic, ionic, fluid and thermal disturbances. This explains why ergogenic aids can delay or reduce fatigue but can never completely prevent it.

References

Allen DG, Lannergren J, Westerblad H. Muscle cell function during prolonged activity: cellular mechanisms of fatigue. *Exp Physiol* 1995;80(4):497–527.

Allen DG, Lee JA, Westerblad H. Intracellular calcium and tension during fatigue in isolated single muscle fibres from *Xenopus laevis. J Physiol* 1989;415:433–58.

Allen DG, Westerblad H. Role of phosphate and calcium stores in muscle fatigue. *J Physiol* 2001;536(Pt 3):657–65.

Baldwin J, Snow RJ, Carey MF, Febbraio MA. Muscle IMP accumulation during fatiguing submaximal exercise in endurance trained and untrained men. *Am J Physiol Regul Integr Comp Physiol* 1999;277(1):R295–R300.

Balog EM, Fitts RH. Effects of fatiguing stimulation on intracellular Na^+ and K^+ in frog skeletal muscle. *J Appl Physiol* 1996;81(2):679–85.

Balog EM, Thompson LV, Fitts RH. Role of sarcolemma action potentials and excitability in muscle fatigue. *J Appl Physiol* 1994;76(5):2157–62.

Barclay JK, Hansel M. Free radicals may contribute to oxidative skeletal muscle fatigue. *Can J Physiol Pharmacol* 1991;69(2):279–84.

Beelen A, Sargeant AJ, Jones DA, de Ruiter CJ. Fatigue and recovery of voluntary and electrically elicited dynamic force in humans. *J Physiol* 1995;484(Pt 1):227–35.

Bergstrom J, Hermansen L, Hultman E, Saltin B. Diet, muscle glycogen and physical performance. *Acta Physiol Scand* 1967;71(2):140–50.

Bigland-Ritchie B, Jones DA, Hosking GP, Edwards RH. Central and peripheral fatigue in sustained maximum voluntary contractions of human quadriceps muscle. *Clin Sci Mol Med* 1978;54(6):609–14.

Bigland-Ritchie B. EMG and fatigue of human voluntary and stimulated contractions. *Ciba Found Symp* 1981;82:130–56.

Bogdanis GC, Nevill ME, Boobis LH, Lakomy HK, Nevill AM. Recovery of power output and muscle metabolites following 30 s of maximal sprint cycling in man. *J Physiol* 1995;482(Pt 2):467–80.

Bogdanis GC, Nevill ME, Lakomy HK, Boobis LH. Power output and muscle metabolism during and following recovery from 10 and 20 s of maximal sprint exercise in humans. *Acta Physiol Scand* 1998;163(3):261–72.

Booth J, McKenna MJ, Ruell PA, Gwinn TH, Davis GM, Thompson MW, Harmer AR, Hunter SK, Sutton JR. Impaired calcium pump function does not slow relaxation in human skeletal muscle after prolonged exercise. *J Appl Physiol* 1997;83(2):511–21.

Byrd SK, Bode AK, Klug GA. Effects of exercise of varying duration on sarcoplasmic reticulum function. *J Appl Physiol* 1989a;66(3):1383–9.

Byrd SK, McCutcheon LJ, Hodgson DR, Gollnick PD. Altered sarcoplasmic reticulum function after high-intensity exercise. *J Appl Physiol* 1989b;67(5):2072–7.

Cady EB, Elshove H, Jones DA, Moll A. The metabolic causes of slow relaxation in fatigued human skeletal muscle. *J Physiol* 1989a;418:327–37.

Cady EB, Jones DA, Lynn J, Newham DJ. Changes in force and intracellular metabolites during fatigue of human skeletal muscle. *J Physiol* 1989b;418:311–25.

Casey A, Constantin-Teodosiu D, Howell S, Hultman E, Greenhaff PL. Creatine ingestion favorably affects performance and muscle metabolism during maximal exercise in humans. *Am J Physiol* 1996;271(1 Pt 1):E31–E37.

Cheetham ME, Boobis LH, Brooks S, Williams C. Human muscle metabolism during sprint running. *J Appl Physiol* 1986;61(1):54–60.

Clarkson PM. Exercise-induced muscle damage—animal and human models. *Med Sci Sports Exerc* 1992;24(5):510–11.

Clausen T. The Na+–K+ pump in skeletal muscle: quantification, regulation and functional significance. *Acta Physiol Scand* 1996;156(3):227–35.

Cooke R, Franks K, Luciani GB, Pate E. The inhibition of rabbit skeletal muscle contraction by hydrogen ions and phosphate. *J Physiol* 1988;395:77–97.

Coyle EF, Coggan AR, Hemmert MK, Ivy JL. Muscle glycogen utilization during prolonged strenuous exercise when fed carbohydrate. *J Appl Physiol* 1986;61(1): 165–72.

Dahlstedt AJ, Westerblad H. Inhibition of creatine kinase reduces the rate of fatigue-induced decrease in tetanic [Ca2+]$_i$ in mouse skeletal muscle. *J Physiol (Lond)* 2001;533(3):639–49.

Dawson MJ, Gadian DG, Wilkie DR. Mechanical relaxation rate and metabolism studied in fatiguing muscle by phosphorus nuclear magnetic resonance. *J Physiol* 1980;299:465–84.

de Haan A, Jones DA, Sargeant AJ. Changes in velocity of shortening, power output and relaxation rate during fatigue of rat medial gastrocnemius muscle. *Pfluegers Arch* 1989;413(4):422–8.

Duke AM, Steele DS. Effects of caffeine and adenine nucleotides on Ca^{2+} release by the sarcoplasmic reticulum in saponin-permeabilized frog skeletal muscle fibres. *J Physiol (Lond)* 1998;513(1):43–53.

Dutka TL, Lamb GD. Effect of lactate on depolarization-induced Ca(2+) release in mechanically skinned skeletal muscle fibers. *Am J Physiol Cell Physiol* 2000;278(3):C517–C525.

Edwards RH. Human muscle function and fatigue. *Ciba Found Symp* 1981;82:1–18.

Ekblom B. Applied physiology of soccer. *Sports Med* 1986;3(1):50–60.

Favero TG. Sarcoplasmic reticulum Ca(2+) release and muscle fatigue. *J Appl Physiol* 1999;87(2):471–83.

Favero TG, Pessah IN, Klug GA. Prolonged exercise reduces Ca^{2+} release in rat skeletal muscle sarcoplasmic reticulum. *Pfluegers Arch* 1993;422(5):472–5.

Favero TG, Zable AC, Bowman MB, Thompson A, Abramson JJ. Metabolic end products inhibit sarcoplasmic reticulum Ca^{2+} release and [3H]ryanodine binding. *J Appl Physiol* 1995;78(5):1665–72.

Febbraio MA, Dancey J. Skeletal muscle energy metabolism during prolonged, fatiguing exercise. *J Appl Physiol* 1999;87(6):2341–7.

Fitts RH. Cellular mechanisms of muscle fatigue. *Physiol Rev* 1994;74(1):49–94.

Fowles JR, Green HJ, Tupling R, O'Brien S, Roy BD. Human neuromuscular fatigue is associated with altered Na+–K+-ATPase activity following isometric exercise. *J Appl Physiol* 2002;92(4):1585–93.

Fraser S, Li JL, Carey MF, Wang XN, Sangkabutra T, Sostaric S, Selig SE. Fatigue depresses maximal in vitro skeletal muscle Na+–K+ ATPase activity in untrained and trained individuals. *J Appl Physiol* 2002; 93:1650–9.

Fryer MW, Owen VJ, Lamb GD, Stephenson DG. Effects of creatine phosphate and P(i) on Ca^{2+} movements and tension development in rat skinned skeletal muscle fibres. *J Physiol* 1995;482(Pt 1):123–40.

Gaitanos GC, Williams C, Boobis LH, Brooks S. Human muscle metabolism during intermittent maximal exercise. *J Appl Physiol* 1993;75(2):712–9.

Gandevia SC. Spinal and supraspinal factors in human muscle fatigue. *Physiol Rev* 2001;81(4):1725–89.

Gandevia SC, Herbert RD, Leeper JB. Voluntary activation of human elbow flexor muscles during maximal concentric contractions. *J Physiol* 1998;512(Pt 2):595–602.

Garland SJ, Gossen ER. The muscular wisdom hypothesis in human muscle fatigue. *Exerc Sport Sci Rev* 2002;30(1):45–9.

Gollnick PD, Korge P, Karpakka J, Saltin B. Elongation of skeletal muscle relaxation during exercise is linked to reduced calcium uptake by the sarcoplasmic reticulum in man. *Acta Physiol Scand* 1991;142(1):135–6.

Gore CJ, Hahn AG, Aughey RJ, Martin DT, Ashenden MJ, Clark SA, Garnham AP, Roberts AD, Slater GJ, McKenna MJ. Live high:train low increases muscle buffer capacity and submaximal cycling efficiency. *Acta Physiol Scand* 2001;173(3): 275–86.

Green HJ. Cation pumps in skeletal muscle: potential role in muscle fatigue. *Acta Physiol Scand* 1998;162(3):201–13.

Green S, Langberg H, Skovgaard D, Bulow J, Kjaer M. Interstitial and arterial–venous [K+] in human calf muscle during dynamic exercise: effect of ischaemia and relation to muscle pain. *J Physiol (Lond)* 2000;529(3):849–61.

Hallen J. K+ balance in humans during exercise. *Acta Physiol Scand* 1996;156(3): 279–86.

Hargreaves M, McKenna MJ, Jenkins DG, Warmington SA, Li JL, Snow RJ, Febbraio MA. Muscle metabolites and performance during high-intensity, intermittent exercise. *J Appl Physiol* 1998;84(5):1687–91.

Hermansen L. Effect of metabolic changes on force generation in skeletal muscle during maximal exercise. *Ciba Found Symp* 1981;82:75–88.

Hermansen L, Hultman E, Saltin B. Muscle glycogen during prolonged severe exercise. *Acta Physiol Scand* 1967;71(2):129–39.

Hermansen L, Osnes JB. Blood and muscle pH after maximal exercise in man. *J Appl Physiol* 1972;32(3):304–8.

Hill CA, Thompson MW, Ruell PA, Thom JM, White MJ. Sarcoplasmic reticulum function and muscle contractile character following fatiguing exercise in humans. *J Physiol* 2001;531(Pt 3):871–8.

Hirvonen J, Rehunen S, Rusko H, Harkonen M. Breakdown of high-energy phosphate compounds and lactate accumulation during short supramaximal exercise. *Eur J Appl Physiol Occup Physiol* 1987;56(3):253–9.

Hodgkin AL, Horowitz P. Movements of Na and K in single muscle fibres. *J Physiol* 1959;145:405–32.

Hultman E, Bergstrom J, Anderson NM. Breakdown and resynthesis of phosphorylcreatine and adenosine triphosphate in connection with muscular work in man. *Scand J Clin Lab Invest* 1967;19(1):56–66.

Jacobs I, Westlin N, Karlsson J, Rasmusson M, Houghton B. Muscle glycogen and diet in elite soccer players. *Eur J Appl Physiol Occup Physiol* 1982;48(3):297–302.

James C, Sacco P, Jones DA. Loss of power during fatigue of human leg muscles. *J Physiol* 1995;484(Pt 1):237–46.

Jones DA. High- and low-frequency fatigue revisited. *Acta Physiol Scand* 1996;156(3): 265–70.

Juel C, Pilegaard H, Nielsen JJ, Bangsbo J. Interstitial K(+) in human skeletal muscle during and after dynamic graded exercise determined by microdialysis. *Am J Physiol Regul Integr Comp Physiol* 2000;278(2):R400–R406.

Kabbara AA, Allen DG. The role of calcium stores in fatigue of isolated single muscle fibres from the cane toad. *J Physiol* 1999;519(Pt 1):169–76.

Karatzaferi C, de Haan A, Ferguson RA, van Mechelen W, Sargeant AJ. Phosphocreatine and ATP content in human single muscle fibres before and after maximum dynamic exercise. *Pfluegers Arch* 2001;442(3):467–74.

Lamb GD. Excitation-contraction coupling in skeletal muscle: comparisons with cardiac muscle. *Clin Exp Pharmacol Physiol* 2000;27(3):216–24.

Lamb GD, Junankar PR, Stephenson DG. Raised intracellular $[Ca^{2+}]$ abolishes excitation-contraction coupling in skeletal muscle fibres of rat and toad. *J Physiol* 1995;489(Pt 2):349–62.

Lamb GD, Recupero E, Stephenson DG. Effect of myoplasmic pH on excitation–contraction coupling in skeletal muscle fibres of the toad. *J Physiol* 1992;448: 211–24.

Laver DR, Lenz GK, Lamb GD. Regulation of the calcium release channel from rabbit skeletal muscle by the nucleotides ATP, AMP, IMP and adenosine. *J Physiol* 2001;537(Pt 3):763–78.

Lepers R, Maffiuletti NA, Rochette L, Brugniaux J and Millet GY. Neuromuscular fatigue during a long-duration cycling exercise. *J Appl Physiol* 2002;92(4):1487–93.

Li JL, Wang XN, Fraser SF, Carey MF, Wrigley TV, McKenna MJ. Effects of fatigue and training on sarcoplasmic reticulum Ca^{2+} regulation in human skeletal muscle. *J Appl Physiol* 2002;92(3):912–22.

McCartney N, Spriet LL, Heigenhauser GJ, Kowalchuk JM, Sutton JR, Jones NL. Muscle power and metabolism in maximal intermittent exercise. *J Appl Physiol* 1986;60(4):1164–9.

McConell G, Snow RJ, Proietto J, Hargreaves M. Muscle metabolism during prolonged exercise in humans: influence of carbohydrate availability. *J Appl Physiol* 1999;87(3):1083–6.

McKenna MJ. The roles of ionic processes in muscular fatigue during intense exercise. *Sports Med* 1992;13(2):134–45.

McKenna MJ. Role of the skeletal muscle Na^+–K^+ pump during exercise. In: Hargreaves M, Thomson M, eds. *Biochemistry of Exercise X*. Champaign, IL: Human Kinetics, 1998: 71–97.

McKenna MJ, Heigenhauser GJ, McKelvie RS, MacDougall JD, Jones NL. Sprint training enhances ionic regulation during intense exercise in men. *J Physiol* 1997;501(Pt 3):687–702.

McKenzie DK, Bigland-Ritchie B, Gorman RB, Gandevia SC. Central and peripheral fatigue of human diaphragm and limb muscles assessed by twitch interpolation. *J Physiol* 1992;454:643–56.

Medbø JI, Sejersted OM. Plasma potassium changes with high intensity exercise. *J Physiol* 1990;421:105–22.

Millet GY, Lepers R, Maffiuletti NA, Babault N, Martin V, Lattier G. Alterations of neuromuscular function after an ultramarathon. *J Appl Physiol* 2002;92(2): 486–92.

Nielsen OB, Clausen T. The Na(+)/K(+)-pump protects muscle excitability and contractility during exercise. *Exerc Sport Sci Rev* 2000;28(4):159–64.

Nielsen OB, de Paoli F, Overgaard K. Protective effects of lactic acid on force production in rat skeletal muscle. *J Physiol (Lond)* 2001;536(1):161–6.

Nybo L, Nielsen B. Hyperthermia and central fatigue during prolonged exercise in humans. *J Appl Physiol* 2001;91(3):1055–60.

Peachey LD & Eisenberg BR, Helicoids in the T system and striation of frog skeletal muscle fibres seen by high voltage electron microscopy. *Biophys J* 1978;22:145–54.

Posterino GS, Fryer MW. Mechanisms underlying phosphate-induced failure of Ca^{2+} release in single skinned skeletal muscle fibres of the rat. *J Physiol* 1998;512 (Pt 1):97–108.

Reid MB. Invited review: redox modulation of skeletal muscle contraction: what we know and what we don't. *J Appl Physiol* 2001;90(2):724–31.

Reid MB, Stokic DS, Koch SM, Khawli FA, Leis AA. N-acetylcysteine inhibits muscle fatigue in humans. *J Clin Invest* 1994;94(6):2468–74.

Renaud JM, Gramolini A, Light P, Comtois A. Modulation of muscle contractility during fatigue and recovery by ATP sensitive potassium channel. *Acta Physiol Scand* 1996;156(3):203–12.

Sahlin K. Intracellular pH and energy metabolism in skeletal muscle of man. With special reference to exercise. *Acta Physiol Scand* 1978;455(Suppl.):1–56.

Sahlin K. Metabolic factors in fatigue. *Sports Med* 1992;13(2):99–107.

Sahlin K, Henriksson J. Buffer capacity and lactate accumulation in skeletal muscle of trained and untrained men. *Acta Physiol Scand* 1984;122(3):331–9.

Saltin B. Metabolic fundamentals in exercise. *Med Sci Sports* 1973;5(3):137–46.

Sejersted OM, Sjøgaard G. Dynamics and consequences of potassium shifts in skeletal muscle and heart during exercise. *Physiol Rev* 2000;80(4):1411–81.

Sharp RL, Costill DL, Fink WJ, King DS. Effects of eight weeks of bicycle ergometer sprint training on human muscle buffer capacity. *Int J Sports Med* 1986;7(1): 13–17.

Sjøgaard G, Adams RP, Saltin B. Water and ion shifts in skeletal muscle of humans with intense dynamic knee extension. *Am J Physiol* 1985;248(2 Pt 2):R190–R196.

Spriet LL, Soderlund K, Bergstrom M, Hultman E. Anaerobic energy release in skeletal muscle during electrical stimulation in men. *J Appl Physiol* 1987;62(2):611–15.

Stathis CG, Febbraio MA, Carey MF, Snow RJ. Influence of sprint training on human skeletal muscle purine nucleotide metabolism. *J Appl Physiol* 1994;76(4):1802–9.

Stephenson DG, Lamb GD, Stephenson GM. Events of the excitation-contraction-relaxation (E-C-R) cycle in fast- and slow-twitch mammalian muscle fibres relevant to muscle fatigue. *Acta Physiol Scand* 1998;162(3):229–45.

Stephenson DG, Nguyen LT, Stephenson GM. Glycogen content and excitation-contraction coupling in mechanically skinned muscle fibres of the cane toad. *J Physiol (Lond)* 1999;519(1):177–87.

Sutton JR, Jones NL, Toews CJ. Growth hormone secretion in acid-base alterations at rest and during exercise. *Clin Sci Mol Med* 1976;50(4):241–7.

Taylor JL, Allen GM, Butler JE, Gandevia SC. Supraspinal fatigue during intermittent maximal voluntary contractions of the human elbow flexors. *J Appl Physiol* 2000;89(1):305–13.

Tumilty D. Physiological characteristics of elite soccer players. *Sports Med* 1993;16(2): 80–96.

Verburg E, Hallen J, Sejersted OM, Vøllestad NK. Loss of potassium from muscle during moderate exercise in humans: a result of insufficient activation of the $Na^+–K^+$-pump? *Acta Physiol Scand* 1999;165(4):357–67.

Vøllestad NK, Sejersted OM. Biochemical correlates of fatigue. A brief review. *Eur J Appl Physiol Occup Physiol* 1988;57(3):336–47.

Vøllestad NK, Vaage O, Hermansen L. Muscle glycogen depletion patterns in type I and subgroups of type II fibres during prolonged severe exercise in man. *Acta Physiol Scand* 1984;122(4):433–41.

Westerblad H, Allen DG. The contribution of $[Ca^{2+}]_i$ to the slowing of relaxation in fatigued single fibres from mouse skeletal muscle. *J Physiol* 1993;468:729–40.

Westerblad H, Allen DG, Bruton JD, Andrade FH, Lannergren J. Mechanisms underlying the reduction of isometric force in skeletal muscle fatigue. *Acta Physiol Scand* 1998;162(3):253–60.

Westerblad H, Bruton JD, Lannergren J. The effect of intracellular pH on contractile function of intact, single fibres of mouse muscle declines with increasing temperature. *J Physiol* 1997;500(Pt 1):193–204.

Wilson JR, McCully KK, Mancini DM, Boden B, Chance B. Relationship of muscular fatigue to pH and diprotonated P_i in humans: a 31P-NMR study. *J Appl Physiol* 1988;64(6):2333–9.

CHAPTER 6

Overtraining

Harm **KUIPERS** and Eric **VAN BREDA**

Introduction

The primary goal of athletic training is to enhance performance outcomes (see Chapter 7). It is generally assumed that in order to extend performance capacity to its upper limit, a high volume of intensive training is necessary. Consequently, athletes are often balancing on a fine edge between the optimal amount of training to enhance performance and overtraining. Indeed, one of the most difficult parts of the training process is to find the correct balance between training and recovery. Such a balance is of utmost importance, since the difference between winning and losing is small. For example, Snyder and Foster (1994) reported that in the 1988 Olympic speed skating event in Calgary, the difference in average velocity between all gold and silver medal performances was approximately 0.3%, while the mean difference between all the gold medallists and the fourth placegetters was 1.3%. In professional cycling, stage-races such as the Tour de France are won and lost by even smaller margins: over the course of a 3-week race lasting about 300 000 seconds, the difference between first and second place is often 200–400 seconds, which represents 0.07–0.13% of the total race time (Jeukendrup et al. 2000).

Unfortunately, little scientific data currently exists about the optimal amount of training for peak performance. However, there does appear to be an inverted U-shaped relationship between training volume (load) and subsequent performance (see Fig. 6.1). Although it is assumed that there is an optimal training impulse that will result in the best performance outcome, this training load is poorly defined.

The overtraining syndrome

From a practical point of view overtraining can be defined as a loss of performance despite the maintenance of or an increase in training effort. However, a decrease in performance is often viewed as the result of too little training. As a consequence, training volume and/or intensity is often increased, resulting in a downward spiral effect that may eventually end in the full-blown overtraining syndrome (see Fig. 6.1). The incidence of the full-blown syndrome in athletes is relatively rare and other environmental factors besides physical exercise, such as work-related, financial, travel for international competitions, psychological and social factors, often play an underlying role in the development and incidence of the overtraining syndrome in athletes.

As previously noted, few scientific data exist about the optimal training regimen(s) to attain peak performance (see Chapter 7). Noakes (1991) documented the case of former long-distance runner Ron Hill, who kept meticulous records of his daily training over his competitive career. From these data Noakes (1991) observed that Hill's best (marathon) performances

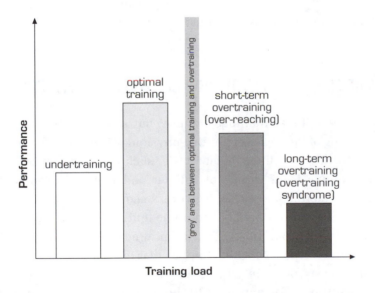

FIG. 6.1 Performance is directly linked to the amount of training. Too little training results in poor performance, while too much training also results in suboptimal performance. Too much training in combination with psychological, social and economical factors may result in the full-blown overtraining syndrome, which results in a decrement in performance. The 'grey' area indicates the area between balanced training and overtraining

coincided with training volumes around 150–170 km/week. Both a lesser and a greater training load resulted in a decrement in performance.

In support of the classic relationship observed between training load and performance (Fig. 6.1), our own personal experience during training supervision reveals trends similar to that noted by Noakes (1991). We have kept daily training logs and competition results for athletes from a number of different sports over several years. The training can be classified as a mix of endurance workouts and intermittent exercise at or near to competitive race intensity. When the total training duration exceeded 15 h/week, there was a consistent decrement in competitive performance independent of the athlete's race duration. Overtraining syndrome or staleness was more likely to occur when the training load was more than 20 h/week (Kuipers, unpublished observations).

In this regard, Costill and co-workers (1991) studied the effect of increasing the training volume on performance in well-trained collegiate swimmers. They found that a doubling of the training volume from 1.5 h/day to 3 h/day for 6 weeks failed to induce a further increase in any of the performance indices under investigation. Interpretation of these results suggests that overtraining can not only be diagnosed by a reduction in performance but also when performance fails to improve in the face of an increase in training load, as previously noted.

Training and recovery to avoid overtraining

To obtain the optimal training 'impulse' but avoid overtraining, a good understanding of the basics of training physiology is needed. Exercise leads to a disturbance in cellular homeostasis: such exercise-induced changes are the stimulus for a variety of cellular and morphological responses initiated to restore homeostasis. However, recovery processes do not stop when homeostasis is restored but continue until a small overcompensation is attained (Viru 1984, 1994). The training adaptations are specific and reversible (see Chapter 7), which implies that the training stimulus should be as specific as possible and should be repeated on a regular basis. The optimal timing for transition to the next training phase is when the overcompensation (read 'supercompensation') is at its highest level (Fig. 6.2). However, relatively little is known about the recovery process and no simple and easily measurable variables are available to afford insight into this phenomenon.

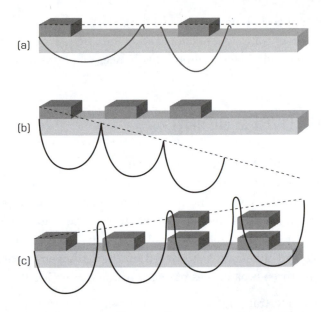

FIG. 6.2 Different methods of training. (a) The training stimulus (load) is either too low or applied too late after the first stimulus; thus no training adaptation or improvement in performance will occur. (b) Training is too heavy or applied too early. A downward spiral in performance will occur that may eventually lead to overtraining. (c) The right training stimulus is applied. The next training occurs at the optimum moment and will lead to an increase in performance. Training adaptation takes place during the upward part of the curve (recovery)

As noted, the actual adaptation to training takes place in the recovery phase, so recovery is an essential component of the overall training process. In this regard many athletes and coaches probably place too much emphasis on training per se and pay too little attention to recovery processes. Although little is known about recovery, it appears that the duration of the recovery phase is not always consistent and depends, among other things, on the training history and ability level of the athlete, the prevailing volume and intensity of training, and other (non-training related) factors affecting the individual athlete. In addition, the recovery rate is different in different organ systems (McArdle et al. 1991).

As discussed previously, recovery is initiated by disturbance of homeostasis. Viru and co-workers (1985) found evidence that recovery processes are modulated by the endocrine environment. During exercise the neuroendocrine system supports catabolic processes. During the recovery phase anabolic processes are most important. The endocrine environment can modify and amplify the recovery and adaptation process. There is not one single hormone which modifies recovery but the hormonal system working in a concerted manner (Viru 1985). Cortisol seems to have a dual role: in low concentrations it enhances the effect of anabolic hormones but when present in high concentrations it enhances catabolism (Viru 1985).

Types of overtraining

When exercise and the concomitant disturbance in homeostasis are not compensated for by adequate recovery, at the time of the next training, the athlete is, in effect, overtraining. For optimal results it is important that the sports practitioner is able to detect when the athlete is undertaking too much training or is not completely recovering between training sessions in the early stages of this condition. Based on the pathogenesis and affected organ systems, three broad types of overtraining can be identified:

- mechanical overtraining
- metabolic overtraining or over-reaching
- overtraining syndrome or staleness

Mechanical overtraining

Mechanical overload involves the locomotor system. Connective tissue and connective tissue-derived tissues, such as cartilage and bone, have a relatively poor blood supply and consequently a low metabolic rate and slow recovery (Puddu et al. 1994). The balance between exercise and recovery is a fragile one and can easily be disturbed. Too much training, too rapid an increase in training loads, and inappropriate equipment (such as footwear) may tip the balance towards overtraining (Kilber et al. 1992; Kuipers & Keizer 1988). An imbalance between exercise and recovery is usually local and often manifests itself as an overuse sport injury.

Metabolic overtraining or over-reaching

Intensive training relies predominantly on carbohydrate (CHO) to supply energy for non-oxidative and oxidative metabolism. As such, endogenous muscle (and liver) glycogen stores are of prime importance for muscular contraction. When high intensity exercise is commenced with low muscle (and liver) glycogen levels, this may lead to an imbalance between energy supply processes and the metabolic demand for ATP. This, in turn, leads to an accumulation of ADP. In order to restore the ADP/ATP ratio, 2 ADP form 1 ATP and 1 AMP, which is further broken down to IMP and eventually to uric acid. Ammonia is also formed in this process (De Haan 1993; Sahlin et al. 1989; Sahlin & Katz 1993).

When insufficient time for recovery is allowed, there may be decline of the resting energy-rich phosphate pool up to 24 hours after the last exercise bout, as has been found in overtrained race horses (Bruin et al. 1994). This metabolic type of overtraining is probably associated with over-reaching (Lehmann et al. 1993; Stone et al. 1991).

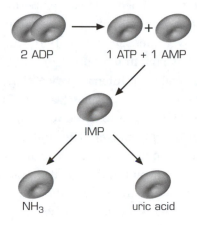

FIG. 6.3 Metabolic overtraining. An accumulation of ADP through an imbalance between ATP splitting and ATP generation may eventually lead to depletion of the energy-rich phosphate pool

Carbohydrates and overtraining

During their daily high-intensity exercise athletes uses CHO as the primary energy source. As a result, glycogen stores become depleted and acute fatigue can occur (Karlsson & Saltin 1971). From these and later findings, scientists have put forward the 'glycogen depletion hypothesis' to explain the overtraining syndrome. Costill et al. (1988) reported that swimmers who consumed less than the recommended proportion of CHO, based on total energy expenditure, were susceptible to over-reaching and/or overtraining, detected by early fatigue in daily training sessions. In contrast, the findings from our own laboratory (Snyder 1998) revealed that athletes undergoing 2 weeks of intense training in combination with a CHO intake sufficient to maintain the level of intra-muscular glycogen concentrations still met some of the generally accepted criteria for short-term over-reaching. Few long-term human training studies have been conducted, making it difficult to postulate a mechanism to explain these findings.

Indeed, few studies have linked reductions in CHO intake to over-reaching and/or overtraining. The recommended intake of CHO for athletes is approximately 70% of the daily total energy intake, which is better expressed as an absolute intake based on the athlete's body mass (i.e. 7 g CHO/kg BM/day). It is generally recognised, however, that in daily practice athletes usually consume less energy from carbohydrates than is typically recommended by sports nutritionists and exercise physiologists. From these findings we can draw the hypothesis that, in the long-term, this reduction in CHO intake could lead to detrimental effects on performance and may even lead to over-reaching or the development of the overtraining syndrome.

An elegant study by Simonsen et al. (1991) revealed that collegiate rowers consuming a diet containing 10 g CHO/kg BM/day (70% of total energy intake) for 4 weeks of intense, twice daily training showed a significant improvement in performance (as measured by an enhanced time trial performance) in contrast to those who ingested only 5 g CHO/kg BM/day (42% of total energy intake). The findings, however, cannot be related to over-reaching or overtraining, since rowers consuming both the high- and low-CHO diet showed improvements in performance (increase in power output and time trial). Furthermore, the athletes who consumed the low-CHO diet showed little decrement in muscle glycogen content over the period of the investigation. Similar results have been published by Sherman et al. (1993), who reported significant reductions in muscle glycogen content in a group of athletes consuming 5 g CHO/kg/day but could not find any relation between CHO intake, glycogen content and performance parameters. Finally, Lamb et al. (1990) reported that collegiate swimmers undertaking double workouts each day for 9 days while consuming either a high (83% of total energy intake) or low-CHO diet (43% of total energy intake) had similar swim-training velocities and no differences in a number of major physiological parameters (heart rates, blood glucose level, perceived exertion).

There are two plausible explanations for the absence of the hypothesised effect of changed CHO intake on performance:

- there might be a rapid physiological adaptation to a changed diet

- training volume and intensity are hard to preserve in elite athletes since yet-unknown mechanisms prevent our body from excessive overload

Overtraining syndrome or staleness

When the hypothalamus is unable to cope with the total amount of stress, a dysfunction of the neuroendocrine system and changes in behaviour may occur (Barron et al. 1985). This general form of overstress in athletes is generally referred to as overtraining syndrome or staleness (Fry et al. 1991; Kuipers & Keizer 1988). The overtraining syndrome is marked by premature fatigue during exercise, a decline in performance, mood changes, emotional instability and decreased motivation (Stone et al. 1991). In addition, overtraining and staleness may be associated with changes in immune function (Fry et al. 1992) and increased risk of injury (Keizer & Kuipers 1993). The propensity for infections has been attributed to changes in glutamine metabolism (Newsholme et al. 1991). These workers suggested that intensive exercise may cause a decrease in plasma glutamine levels. As glutamine is thought to be essential for immune cell functioning, decreased plasma glutamine levels could lead to decreased immune function. This, in turn, would lead to an increased uptake of tryptophan in the brain and increased production of the neurotransmitter 5-hydroxytryptamine (5-HT). This is supposed to be associated with central fatigue and symptoms of overtraining syndrome. However, there is no solid scientific evidence supporting this hypothesis (Lehmann et al. 1992, 1994; Rowbottom et al. 1995).

Indeed, a recent study by Mackinnon and Hooper (1996) showed that in swimmers with symptoms of staleness, plasma glutamine levels may not necessarily be lowered. This suggests that the decline in plasma glutamine is not proportionally related to the severity of staleness. Paradoxically, during starvation lymphocytic glutamine uptake increases in spite of low plasma levels. So, it is unlikely that decreased glutamine levels lead to decreased immune function.

There is a gradual transition from adequate recovery via short-term overstress to an overtraining syndrome. When overtraining syndrome or staleness presents, the training alone is seldom the primary cause. Rather, it is that the total amount of stress exceeds the organism's capacity to cope. Contributing factors for an overtraining syndrome are: too many competitions, too much training, infectious diseases, allergic reactions, mental stress, nutritional deficiencies and jet lag (Kuipers & Keizer 1988). From German literature on clinical symptoms, two types of overtraining can be distinguished: the sympathetic type and the parasympathetic type (Israel 1958). The sympathetic or Basedowian type is characterised by increased sympathetic tone in the resting state, while in the parasympathetic or

Addisonoid type the parasympathetic tone dominates in the resting state as well as during exercise. The main characteristics of both types of overtraining are summarised in Table 6.1.

Sympathetic overtraining syndrome is most often observed in team sports and sprint events, while parasympathetic overtraining is preferentially observed in endurance athletes (Lehmann et al. 1993). The characteristics of the parasympathetic type of the overtraining syndrome are misleading to the athlete and the coach because the symptoms suggest excellent health. Although the pathophysiological mechanism of both types of overtraining is virtually unknown, it is hypothesised that both types reflect different stages of the overtraining syndrome. During the early stage of the overtraining syndrome, the sympathetic system is supposed to be continuously on alert, while during advanced overtraining the activity of the sympathetic system is inhibited, resulting in a dominance of the parasympathetic system. This would also explain the increased proneness for hypoglycaemia during exercise because the glucose counter-regulation is mediated via the sympathetic system.

Table 6.1 The main symptoms of the sympathetic and parasympathetic type of staleness or overtraining syndrome

SYMPATHETIC TYPE OF OVERTRAINING	PARASYMPATHETIC TYPE OF OVERTRAINING
Increased heart rate at rest and during exercise	Low or normal resting pulse rate
Slow recovery after exercise	Relatively low exercise heart rate
Poor appetite, weight loss	Fast recovery of heart rate after exercise
Mental instability and irritability	Hypoglycaemia during exercise, good appetite
Increased blood pressure in the resting state	Normal sleep, lethargy, depression
Menstrual irregularities, oligomenorrhoea or amenorrhoea in females	Low resting blood pressure
Disturbed sleep: difficulties in falling asleep and early wakening	Low plasma lactate levels during submaximal and maximal exercise (lactate paradox)

Diagnosis of overtraining

Because the transition from adequate training to overtraining is a gradual one, it is rather difficult to diagnose the overtraining syndrome in its earliest stage. Several attempts have been made to establish parameters that can be easily measured during the daily routines of training, especially parameters that indicate early signs of over-reaching. Besides the many blood chemical variables that have been suggested as indicators (Bruin et al. 1994; Rowbottom et al. 1995), heart rate measurements at rest are a practical indicator of overtraining or over-reaching. Although increments in resting heart rate have been reported in a number of investigations, other investigators have been unable to detect such changes (Urhausen 2002).

Another tool used to detect overtraining is the Profile of Mood State (POMS) inventory (Morgan et al. 1987; Urhausen et al. 1998). The POMS scale yields information about the global measure of mood, tension, depression, anger, vigour, fatigue and confusion. By monitoring the mood state by the POMS scale, signs of overtraining can be hopefully detected in an early stage. Another approach is to have the athletes complete a self-designed questionnaire on a visual analogue scale containing questions about fatigue, recovery, motivation, irritability and sleep. The disadvantage of self-designed questionnaires is that they lack validation.

Other subjective scales that might be useful include sleep disturbances, feelings of anxiety and other subjective parameters. It has to be kept in mind, however, that the outcome is dependent on the individual and can easily be manipulated by the athlete.

Since staleness is also associated with hormonal changes, hormones have also been suggested as early markers for the detection of over-reaching. Adlercreutz and co-workers (1986) have suggested that the ratio of free testosterone and cortisol would be indicative of the balance between anabolic and catabolic processes. Other investigators, however, have found evidence that the free testosterone/cortisol ratio is not a reliable marker for early staleness (Lehmann et al. 1992; Urhausen et al. 1995; Vermulst et al. 1991). Some studies suggest that behavioural changes are the first signs of an imminent overtraining syndrome (Bruin et al. 1994; Urhausen et al. 1998).

Usually, overtraining syndrome is diagnosed by excluding other causes for underperformance. The first step should be to use the athlete's training log to identify possible factors that could explain the increased fatigue. If this does not lead to a clear explanation for decreased performance, routine blood tests such as haemoglobin concentration, haematocrit, ferritin concentration, red blood cell sedimentation rate, white blood cell count, white blood cell differentiation, liver and kidney functions can be undertaken.

If these tests show no abnormal findings, the next step is laboratory exercise testing. In the overtrained state the maximal workload attained in an incremental test is decreased, while at submaximal exercise intensity the lactate concentration is also decreased. In addition to a lower peak power output, peak lactate levels are also decreased. This 'lactate paradox' has been reported by several independent investigators (Foster et al. 1988; Jeukendrup et al. 1992; Jeukendrup & Hesselink 1994). Because overtraining is difficult to diagnose it is most important to try to prevent it. The following guidelines are helpful:

- develop a well-balanced training program, with individual adjustment
- have field or laboratory performance tests at regular intervals
- emphasise proper diet (> 6 g CHO/kg BM/day)
- have the athletes keep a training log in which resting heart rate and body weight are recorded

Can recovery be accelerated?

Recovery consists basically of two components: a fast component including restoration of energy substrates, and a slow component which includes training adaptations. It has been suggested that supplementing testosterone in individuals who have low testosterone levels after exercise should enhance recovery. Although direct evidence is lacking, it has been shown that the application of androgenic anabolic steroids enhances muscle protein synthesis (Griggs et al. 1989; Salmons 1992).

Treatment of overtraining

The treatment of overtraining depends on its type and cause. In the case of mechanical overtraining a number of measures need to be considered. Wearing proper clothing, especially proper footwear, is important. Very often a rapid increase in training loads is the cause of mechanical overtraining. Gradual increases should prevent this from happening. With metabolic overtraining, a decrease in training volume is the most important indicator that can be measured. Emphasis should be placed on sufficient rest, recovery and a diet sufficiently high in CHO (Kuipers & Keizer 1988). Usually metabolic overtraining is reversible within a few days. Systemic overtraining usually requires one to several weeks for recovery. The contributing factors must be identified and sometimes counselling is necessary. There are no specific known drugs or treatments. Because it is so difficult to detect, it is important to try to prevent overtraining from occurring in the first place, and here nutritional factors may play a role.

Final considerations

Sports science continues its search for the responsible mechanisms that underlie the development of the overtraining syndrome. Scientifically based, systematic increases in training, and a long-term approach to competition, combined with optimal nutrition, avoidance of non-athletic stressors such as sleep loss and time differences due to international competitions, seem to be the best way of preventing overtraining. In conclusion, we suggest that adjustment of training regimens, inclusion of complete rest days and prevention of general life stressors are the best ways we have today of preventing an athlete from developing the full-blown overtraining syndrome. It has been frequently stated that choosing your parents wisely is the best guarantee of becoming an elite athlete. However, in light of the subjective life stress parameters that only the athlete's trainers and coaches can observe and monitor, it would seem that choosing your coach wisely is of equal importance in whether athletes optimise their genetic potential or become overtrained.

This chapter is dedicated to the memory of Professor Manfred Lehmann.

References

Adlercreutz H, Harkonen M, Kuoppasalmi K, Naveri H, Huhtaniemi I, Tikkanen H, Remes K, Dessypris A, Karvonen J. Effect of training on plasma anabolic and catabolic steroid hormones and their response during physical exercise. *Int J Sports Med* 1986;7(Suppl. 1):27–8.

Barron GL, Noakes TD, Levy W, Smith C, Millar RP. Hypothalamic dysfunction in overtrained athletes. *J Clin Endocrinol Metab* 1985;60(4):803–6.

Bruin G, Kuipers H, Keizer HA, VanderVusse GJ. Adaptation and overtraining in horses subjected to increased training loads. *J Appl Physiol* 1994;76(5):1908–13.

Costill DL, Flynn MG, Kirwan JP, Houmard JA, Mitchell JB, Thomas R, Park SH. Effects of repeated days of intensified swimming on muscle glycogen and swimming performance. *Med Sci Sports Exerc* 1988;20:249–54.

Costill DL, Thomas R, Robergs RA, Pascoe DA, Lambert C, Fink WJ. Adaptations to swimming training: influence of training volume. *Med Sci Sports Exerc* 1991:23:371–7.

Foster C, Snyder AC, Thompson NN, Kuettel K. Normalization of the blood lactate profile. *Int J Sports Med* 1988;9:198–200.

Fry RW, Morton AW, Garcia-Webb P, Crawford GPM, Keast D. Biological responses to overload training in endurance sports. *Eur J Appl Physiol* 1992;64:335–44.

Fry RW, Morton AW, Keast D. Overtraining in athletes: an update. *Sports Med* 1991: 63:228–34.

Griggs RC, Kingston W, Jozefowicz RF, Herr BE, Forbes G, Halliday D. Effect of testosterone on muscle mass and muscle protein synthesis. *J Appl Physiol* 1989;66: 498–503.

Haan de A. Muscle metabolism during fatiguing exercise. In: Sargeant T & Kernell D (eds). *Neuromuscular Fatigue.* Amsterdam: North Holland, 1993: 16–23.

Hooper SL, Mackinnon LT, Howard A, Gordon RD, Bachmann AW. Markers for monitoring overtraining and recovery. *Med Sci Sports Exerc* 1995;27:106–12.

Israel S. Die Erscheinungsformen des Uebertrainings. *Sportmedizin* 1958;9:207–9.

Jeukendrup AE, Craig NP, Hawley JA. The bioenergetics of world class cycling. *J Sci Med Sport* 2000;3:414–33.

Jeukendrup AE, Hesselink MKC. Overtraining, what do lactate curves tell us? *Br J Sports Med* 1994;28:239–40.

Jeukendrup AE, Hesselink MKC, Snyder AC, Kuipers H, Keizer HA. Physiological changes in male competitive cyclists after two weeks of intensified training. *Int J Sports Med* 1992;13(7):534–41.

Karlsson J, Saltin B. Diet, muscle glycogen and endurance performance. *J Appl Physiol* 1971;31:203–6.

Keizer HA, Kuipers H. Endocrinological deregulation and musculoskeletal injuries. In: Renström PA (ed). *Sports Injuries.* London: Blackwell Scientific, 1993: 87–95.

Kilber WB, Chandler TJ, Straceber ES. Musculoskeletal adaptations and injuries to overtraining. In: Holloszy JO (ed). *Exercise and Sport Sciences Reviews.* Vol. 20. Baltimore, MA: Williams & Wilkins, 1992: 99–126.

Kuipers H, Keizer HA. Overtraining in elite athletes; review and directions for the future. *Sports Med* 1988;6:79–92.

Lamb DR, Rinehardt KF, Bartels RL, Sherman WM, Snook JT. Dietary carbohydrate and intensity of interval swim training. *Am J Clin Nutr* 1990;52(6):1058–63.

Lehmann M, Foster C, Keul J. Overtraining in endurance athletes: a brief review. *Med Sci Sports Exerc* 1993;25(7):854–62.

Lehmann M, Gastmann U, Petersen KG, Bachl N, Seidel A, Khalaf AN, Fischer S, Keul J. Training–overtraining: influence of a defined increase in training volume versus training intensity on performance, catecholamines and some metabolic parameters in experienced middle- and long-distance runners. *Eur J Appl Physiol* 1992;64: 169–77.

Lehmann M, Schiestl G, Schmidt K, Bauer S, Wieland H, Keul J. BCAA supplementation related performances in cyclists. *Eur J Appl Physiol* 1994;69(Suppl.):36.

Mackinnon LT, Hooper SL. Plasma glutamine and upper respiratory infection during intensified training in swimmers. *Med Sci Sports Exerc* 1996;28:285–90.

McArdle WD, Katch FI, Katch VL. *Exercise Physiology.* Philadelphia: Lea & Febiger, 1991: 136–41.

Morgan WP, Brown DR, Raglin JS, O'Connor PJ, Ellickson KA. Psychological monitoring of overtraining and staleness. *Br J Sports Med* 1987;21:107–14.

Newsholme EA, Parry-Billings M, McAndrew N, Budgett R. A biochemical mechanism to explain some characteristics of overtraining. In: Brouns F (ed). *Advances in Nutrition and Top Sport.* Basel: Karger, *Med Sport Sci*, 1991;32:79–93.

Noakes TD. *Lore of Running*. Champaign, IL: Human Kinetics Press, 1991: 263–361.

Puddu G, Scala A, Cerullo G, Franco V, de Paulis F, Michelini O. Achilles tendon injuries. In: Renström PA (ed). *Clinical Practice of Sports Injury Prevention and Care*. London: Blackwell Scientific, 1994: 188–216.

Rowbottom DG, Keast D, Goodman C, Morton AR. The haematological, biochemical and immunological profile of athletes suffering from the overtraining syndrome. *Eur J Appl Physiol* 1995;70:502–9.

Sahlin K, Broberg S, Ren JM. Formation of inosine monophosphate (IMP) in human skeletal muscle during incremental dynamic exercise. *Acta Physiol Scand* 1989;136:193–8.

Sahlin K, Katz A. Adenine nucleotide metabolism. In: Poortmans JR (ed). *Principles of Exercise Biochemistry*. Basel: Karger, 1993: 137–57.

Salmons S. Myotrophic effects of an anabolic steroid in rabbit limb muscle. *Muscle Nerve* 1992;15:806–12.

Sherman WM, Doyle JA, Lamb DR, Strauss RH. Dietary carbohydrate, muscle glycogen, and exercise performance during 7 d of training. *Am J Clin Nutr* 1993;57(1):27–31.

Simonsen JC, Sherman WM, Lamb DR, Dernbach AR, Doyle JA, Strauss R. Dietary carbohydrate, muscle glycogen, and power output during rowing training. *J Appl Physiol* 1991;70(4):1500–5.

Snyder AC, Foster C. Physiology and nutrition for skating. In: Lamb DR, Knuttgen HG, Murray R, eds. *Perspectives in Exercise Science and Sports Medicine*. Carmel, IN: Cooper Publishing Group, 1994: 181–219.

Stone MH, Keith RE, Kearny JT, Fleck SJ, Wilson GD, Triplett NT. Overtraining: a review of the signs, symptoms and possible causes. *J Appl Sport Sci Res* 1991;5: 35–50.

Urhausen A, Gabriel H, Kindermann W. Blood hormones as markers of training stress and overtraining. *Sports Med* 1995;20:251–76.

Urhausen A, Gabriel HHW, Weiler B, Kindermann W. Ergometric and psychological findings during overtraining: a long term follow-up study in endurance athletes. *Int J Sports Med* 1998;19:114–20.

Urhausen A, Kinderman W. Diagnosis of overtraining: what tools do we have? *Sports Med* 2002;32:95–102.

Vermulst LJM, Vervoorn C, Boelens-Quist AM, Koppeschaar HPF, Erich WBM. Analysis of seasonal training volume and working capacity in elite female rowers. *Int J Sports Med* 1991;12(6):567–72.

Viru A. *Hormones in Muscular Activity*. Vol. 1. Florida: CRC Press, 1985: 25–114.

Viru A. Molecular cellular mechanisms of training effects. *J Sports Med Phys Fitness* 1994;34:309–14.

Viru A. The mechanism of training effects: a hypothesis. *Int J Sports Med* 1984;5: 219–27.

CHAPTER 7

Training for enhancement of sports performance

John A. HAWLEY

Introduction and historical development of training practices

Physical training in preparation for competitive sport is not, and likely never will be, a purely scientific pursuit. Our contemporary knowledge of the optimal training practices for enhancing performance in a wide variety of sports has evolved during the past century from the trial-and-error methods and field-based observations of a few innovative and risk-taking coaches working with a limited number of athletes and teams, rather than innovations arising from modern-day, laboratory-based studies. For the most part, science has played a post-hoc role, determining some of the physiological mechanisms that help explain why already accepted training practices result in enhanced athletic performance. As such, it must be recognised that the present scientific knowledge of the effects of specific training interventions undertaken by competitive athletes on selected adaptive responses and their consequences for improving performance is severely limited.

Part of the reason for this lack of knowledge is because it has proved difficult for sport scientists to persuade athletes in general, and elite athletes in particular, to experiment with their existing training regimens. Furthermore, access to samples of blood and muscle from athletes for biochemical analyses (to elucidate possible training-induced mechanisms underlying performance changes) is difficult. Therefore, most investigations of the effect of various training programs on performance typically include only a few highly trained athletes in a study population. More often than not, healthy, moderately trained, predominantly male volunteers are studied before and after short-term (8–12 week) exercise-training interventions. The results obtained from these studies are not likely to be relevant, or directly applicable to the training practices of genetically endowed competitive athletes who have engaged in intense training for many years. Finally, the large variety of different training techniques currently practised by athletes and the possible combinations of these make it very difficult for scientists to evaluate the benefits of any single regimen on performance changes effectively.

In the past decade, however, science has started to make a valuable contribution to assist coaches in the preparation of athletes. There are several possible reasons for this recent progress, including:

■ substantial government funding to establish National Sports Institutes in various countries around the world, which provide the infrastructure and expertise required to provide a closer working relationship between scientists, coaches and athletes (e.g. Australian Institute of Sport)

■ talent identification programs aimed at early discovery of potential medal-winning athletes

■ improvements in athlete testing and monitoring along with the early detection of symptoms of 'overtraining' and associated immune-system suppression

■ the publication and dissemination in scientific journals and the popular press of the results from a large number of well-controlled studies of the effect of a multitude of nutrition and ergogenic aids on training and athletic performance

■ the application of several 'cutting-edge', industry-based techniques to science in general and sport science in particular (e.g. aerospace engineering and the development and testing of aerodynamic equipment and associated micro technologies).

While it is appropriate to acknowledge the gaps in our current knowledge with regard to the precise effect of various training techniques on athletic performance, advances are being made in several areas to assist the coach and athlete in their preparation for competition. This chapter focuses on the science of physical training and, in particular, on those training strategies currently undertaken by competitive athletes that have been shown to enhance performance.

The objectives of physical training

The ability of multiple human organ systems, particularly skeletal muscle, to adapt to repeated bouts of physical activity over time so that exercise capacity is improved is termed physical training (Booth & Thomason 1991). For the competitive endurance athlete, the primary objective of such training is to increase the ability to sustain the highest *average* power output or speed of movement to overcome resistance (air or water) or drag (friction) for a predetermined distance or time such that performance will be enhanced (Coyle et al. 1994; Hawley 2002a). In the case of an athlete whose event depends on exerting maximal power/force, then the primary objective of training is to increase the *peak* power output or speed of movement to overcome gravitational resistance (or an opponent) and delay the onset of muscle fatigue (i.e. delay a significant decline in power output).

All movement (or work) ultimately depends on the rate and efficiency at which chemical energy can be converted into mechanical energy for skeletal muscle contraction. Accordingly, it has been proposed (Coyle et al. 1994; Hawley 2002a) that training for enhancement of athletic performance should aim to induce multiple physiological and metabolic adaptations that enable an athlete to:

- increase the rate of energy production and force capability from both aerobic (endurance and ultra-endurance events) and oxygen-independent (power/speed events) adenosine triphosphate (ATP)-generating pathways
- maintain tighter metabolic control (i.e. match ATP production with ATP hydrolysis)
- minimise cellular disturbances
- increase economy of motion
- improve the resistance of the working muscles to fatigue during exercise.

The general physiological responses to short-term (12 week) training programs undertaken by previously sedentary (but healthy) individuals have been well documented (Clausen 1977; Saltin 1991). Of specific interest in this chapter are the adaptations and responses arising from the high-volume, high-intensity training undertaken by well-trained competitive athletes which subsequently result in enhanced performance.

The scientific principles of training

Performance outcomes in many athletic events can, to some extent, be largely predicted if a scientist or coach has a thorough knowledge of the training history of an individual athlete. This is because the human body responds in a relatively predictable and uniform manner to the scientific principles of training. The most widely accepted general training principles include the principle of overload, specificity, reversibility and individuality. For a comprehensive synopsis of these fundamental training concepts, the reader is referred to several reviews (Coyle et al. 1994; Hawley 2002b; Hawley & Burke 1998; Maughan et al. 1997).

Although the general principles of training are similar for all athletes, the *rate* and *magnitude* of adaptation varies greatly from one individual to another, presumably due to differences in genetic endowment (Bouchard et al. 1992). It would appear that athletes capable of superior performances are not only genetically endowed with the necessary physical attributes for success but are also fortunate enough to have the potential to optimise these factors to the greatest possible extent through training (Hawley & Burke 1998). In this regard, Lortie et al. (1984) reported that following a 20-week endurance-training program, previously untrained subjects improved their endurance capacity (determined by the work subjects could complete during a 90-minute maximal cycle ergometer test) by, on *average*, 50%. However, the *range* of improvement in performance output was as low as 16% in some individuals and as high as 97% in others (Lortie et al. 1984). Human variation in trainability is also observed for short-duration (< 90 s), high-intensity performance measures. Simoneau et al. (1986) reported that after 15 weeks of sprint cycle training, previously untrained volunteers significantly improved 10-s and 90-s sprint performance. However, individual differences in the training response were large, with a five- to ninefold range between the low and high responders.

The concept of genetic endowment can be further highlighted by the information in Table 7.1, which lists the recommended criteria for classifying endurance-trained cyclists (Jeukendrup et al. 2000). Based exclusively on physiological criteria, it is clear that certain individuals can be classified as 'well-trained' or even 'elite'. However, these same individuals lack the genetic endowment necessary for superior performance capabilities. On the other hand, those athletes with excellent genetic endowment may attain superior physiological ratings without (much) training. In this context, a world class cyclist may be described as 'untrained' if he/she has not performed any training for a long period of time.

TABLE 7.1 Criteria for classification of trained, well-trained, elite and world class road cyclists

CATEGORY	TRAINED	WELL-TRAINED	ELITE	WORLD CLASS/ PROFESSIONAL
Training and race status				
Training frequency (times/week)	2–3	3–7	5–8	5–8
Training duration (min)	30–60	60–240	60–360	60–360
Training background (year)	1	3–5	5–15	5–30
Racing status (days/year)	0–10	0–20	50–100	90–110
International Cycling Union (ICU) ranking	–	–	First 2000	First 200
Physiological variables				
VO_{2max} (L/min)[a]	4.0–4.5	5.0–5.3	5.3–6.0	5.4–7.0
VO_{2max} (mL/kg/min)	60–64	65–70	70–75	75–90
PPO (W)[b]	240–400	300–450	350–500	400–600
Economy (W/L/min)	72–74	74–75	76–77	>78

[a] VO_{2max}: maximal aerobic power.
[b]   PPO: peak sustained power output attained during a maximal test.
    Adapted from Jeukendrup et al. (2000)

Because of individual variability in response to a training regimen, the objective of any training program should be to maximise each athlete's unique phenotypic potential: training should be viewed as a means by which an individual ultimately determines how close he/she comes to reaching his/her genetic limits. As athletic training is undertaken for the sole intent of enhancing performance, it is well to remember that its purpose is very different from participation in regular exercise for health-related benefits: training is planned, systematic and goal orientated.

The training stimulus and the training response

The key components of any training program aimed to enhance athletic performance are volume, intensity and frequency (Hawley 2002b; Hawley & Burke 1998; Hawley & Stepto 2001; Maughan et al. 1997) with the sum of these inputs termed the training impulse (Bannister 1991). Adaptations to both endurance and strength/power training are related to the volume and intensity of work performed (Brooks & Fahey 1984). For endurance athletes (runners), several studies have reported a strong positive relationship between training volume (km/week) and subsequent race performance (Hagan et al. 1981; Sjödin & Svedenhag 1985).

However, as noted (Maughan 1994), the association between training volume and performance, while statistically significant, does not always imply a cause-and-effect relationship. Indeed, there is obviously a maximal duration beyond which additional volume stimulus does not induce further increases in functional capacity and may lead to injury, illness and the overtraining syndrome (see Chapter 6). As the relationship between training volume and subsequent performance enhancement is not linear, this implies that the control mechanisms signalling adaptive responses are eventually titrated by exercise duration (Booth & Watson 1985). Such a plateau in adaptive response is of practical significance because many runners (Hawley 2000; Wells & Pate 1988), swimmers (Pyne et al. 2001), cyclists (Jeukendrup et al. 2000) and rowers (Hagerman 1994) undertake prodigious volumes of training in the strong belief of a direct relationship between the amount of work performed in training and subsequent performance.

Irrespective of whether endurance or power/speed training is performed, subsequent training adaptations are highly specific to the mode of exercise undertaken and the corresponding patterns of muscle recruitment. The greatest adaptations in skeletal muscle are observed in those muscles involved directly in the training activity with little or no adaptation in untrained limbs (Gollnick et al. 1971). This implies that the signals for adaptation are local (within the muscle) rather than systemic.

Different training impulses give rise to different adaptive responses. Training to optimise performance in power/speed events principally involves intermittent bouts of low-frequency repetition with high workloads and extended recoveries between work bouts (for review see Kraemer et al. 1996). The adaptive responses to such stimuli rely initially on altered neural activation of the trained musculature to mediate a large portion of the strength increases attributable to such training, in the absence of large increases in cross-sectional area (Ploutz et al. 1994). The ability to activate all (available) motor units in a muscle (or muscle group) may also be a large part of the strength gains seen in the early phases of resistance training. This neural adaptation is followed by muscle hypertrophy in which the myofibres increase in size and cross-sectional area but otherwise retain their initial ultrastructural and biochemical properties (Hakkinen & Komi 1983; Moritani & de Vries 1979; Sale 1992). Typically, muscle hypertrophy requires more than 16 workouts to produce significant gains in muscle cross-sectional area (Staron et al. 1994). When hypertrophy of skeletal muscle fibres can no longer explain improvements in maximal force and power (as during an advanced stage of training), neural alterations may, again, assume the predominant role on the adaptation response (Sale 1992). For example, Häkkinen et al. (1988) reported minimal changes in muscle fibre size in competitive Olympic weight-lifters during a 2-year training period, although strength and power were markedly improved.

Training for endurance sports, on the other hand, requires high-frequency repetition workouts with low workloads, performed continuously for prolonged periods. The response to such loading is markedly enhanced enzymatic and structural characteristics often accompanied by changes in microvasculature, but little or no skeletal muscle hypertrophy (Booth & Thomason 1991). The differential molecular, cellular and functional response to endurance and power/speed training has practical significance: if well-trained competitive athletes attempt to combine heavy resistance training (to enhance power/speed) with aerobic training (to enhance endurance), then strength/power development by skeletal muscle is less rapid than with resistance training only and vice versa (Dudley & Djamil 1985; Hickson 1980; Kraemer et al. 1995; Sale et al. 1990). This is probably because endurance training interferes with the ability of the neuromuscular system to generate maximal force (Kraemer et al. 1995; Leveritt et al. 1999; McCarthy et al. 2002).

There is currently much controversy as to whether endurance performance is enhanced in highly trained athletes who undergo resistance training (discussed subsequently). However, concurrent strength/endurance workouts in recreational athletes training only three days/week does not appear to interfere with either strength development (McCarthy et al. 1995, 2002) or endurance capacity (Hickson 1980; Kraemer et al. 1995; McCarthy et al. 1995, 2002; Sale et al. 1990), at least in the short-term (up to 12 weeks). There is also debate as to whether males and females respond in a similar fashion to a training stimulus (Ivey et al. 2000; O'Hagan et al. 1995). This latter issue is discussed in detail in Chapter 12.

Finally, the processes by which stable, long-term (chronic) adaptations occur are distinct from the immediate or short-term (acute) physiological responses that provide energy for muscle during contraction and recovery, or modulate contractile force during a single bout of exercise. Chronic adaptations require changes in gene expression mediated by changes in the rate of transcription of specific target genes and in the rate of synthesis of specific proteins (Booth & Thomason 1991; Williams & Neufer 1996). While the major disruptions to cellular homeostasis occur *during* a training bout, the time-course responses of several of the intracellular signalling pathways are up-regulated *post exercise* and may be the stimulus for chronic intracellular adaptations (Widegren et al. 2001: Yu et al. 2003).

Classification of different sport activities

Based largely on the characteristics of movement patterns and the duration of competition, athletic events can be broadly classified into four main categories:

1 Power events: typically involving one or several maximal contractions lasting < 10 s and sometimes repeated after moderate (5–10 min) recoveries (e.g. throwing, jumping, lifting).

2 Speed events: typically involving continuous movement for < 60 s (e.g. running, swimming, cycling).

3 Endurance events: lasting > 10 min but < 4 h (including team sports).

4 Ultra-endurance events lasting > 4 h.

The power systems used to supply energy for muscle contraction for these distinct events have been detailed in Chapter 2. It is only during the past 20 years that our knowledge of the physiology and biochemistry of sprint exercise has come close to matching our understanding of the energetics of prolonged, submaximal aerobic exercise (see Nevill et al. 1994 for a comprehensive review of muscle metabolism during sprinting). It should be noted that sprint exercise is synonymous with sport events that require the athlete to generate the *maximal* rate of energy production from the onset of exercise. Accordingly, the average power output during a sprint lasting approximately 30 seconds is often three to four ti\mes higher than that required to elicit the 'maximum' oxygen uptake (VO_{2max}).

Although the energetics of continuous (sprint and endurance) events in which an athlete has to cover a predetermined distance in the minimum time possible are now reasonably well characterised (Bangsbo et al. 1990; Brandon 1995; Costill et al. 1973; Conley & Krahenbuhl 1980; Coyle et al. 1994; Farrell et al. 1979; Hagerman 1994; Lakomy 2000; Nevill et al. 1994), far less is known about the energy demands of intermittent, stochastic exercise undertaken for prolonged periods (60–90 min). The scarcity of scientific studies dedicated to the activity patterns typical of most team sports is surprising given that such sports have, by far, the greatest number of worldwide participants.

Current training practices of athletes

There is currently much debate among scientists and athletes as to what constitutes the 'optimal' training program that best promotes the necessary physiological attributes for successful performance in a given event. Such discussion is likely to continue until sport scientists conduct well-controlled studies using competitive athletes under 'real life' conditions (i.e. typical training and nutritional practices) such that their results are meaningful to coaches. In the meantime, it seems intuitive to suggest that the 'perfect' training regimen for performance enhancement in a sport should incorporate most of the training techniques and methods currently practised by the top athletes in that discipline. Although such an approach does not take into account differences in genetic endowment (discussed previously) that make it impossible to predict the rate at which an individual adapts to a specified training load, it does provide a 'state-of-the-art' impression of modern-day training practices.

Power/speed events

The current training methods practised by athletes competing in events that predominantly require strength or power/speed can be summarised as follows:

- prolonged involvement in sport since early age
- year-round training (2–3 h/day), often with double periodisation of training during the competitive year
- emphasis on aerobic training during general conditioning phase, with the inclusion of alternative modes of activity to an athlete's primary event
- extensive use of resistance/strength training, starting with a phase of high-volume, low-intensity work and moving towards lower volumes of training with maximal or supramaximal intensities
- plyometric training and bounding exercises to develop explosive muscle power
- circuit training
- use of drills and technique work to develop mechanical and neuromuscular skills required for the sport/event
- stretching and use of active recovery processes such as massage
- extensive use of specialised dietary (and other) supplements during extensive periods of training to augment muscle growth and recovery
- peaking or tapering before major competitions.

Endurance events

The current training methods practised by athletes competing in events that predominantly rely on endurance can be summarised as follows:

■ prolonged involvement in sport since early age

■ year-round training (3–4 h/day) and competition with only short (2–4 week) breaks for active recovery between seasons

■ a high volume of aerobic conditioning throughout the year

■ prolonged (>2 h) steady-state aerobic workouts performed as a single, continuous training session

■ speed work, performed at velocities or power outputs that are faster than planned competition pace/effort

■ a 'hard–easy' pattern to the overall organisation of daily training

■ high-volume, low-intensity resistance training in the non-competitive phase

■ sustained race-pace workouts or pace training (i.e. interval training)

■ use of time trials over intermediate distances to assess fitness and pace judgment

■ stretching and mobility exercises

■ special dietary practices before, during and after training

■ peaking or tapering before major competitions

■ special dietary practices before major competitions ('dietary periodisation').

Importance of practice training

Several issues are worthy of mention with regard to the current training practices of athletes competing in either strength/power events or endurance sports. Firstly, there is likely to be a link between the number of years of prior training and current performance capacity: regardless of event speciality, successful athletes have a longstanding history of training in their chosen sport. In this regard, Coyle et al. (1991) have hypothesised that the superior performance capacity of endurance cyclists that allows them to develop greater forces during the down stroke of the pedalling action is directly related to the number of years spent cycling. It may well be that an important component of sustained, intense training over a period of many seasons is a direct alteration in skeletal muscle contractility: improved patterns of neuromuscular recruitment in response to sport-specific overload patterns would explain why performances of highly trained athletes continue to improve independently of little or no measurable changes in many of the most common laboratory-determined physiological variables, such as VO_{2max} (Daniels et al. 1978).

Secondly, the influx of sponsorship into professional sport has dramatically raised the level of competitiveness required for success. As a direct result of this increased competitiveness, the 'entry' point for athletes in all sports has been raised. This, in turn, necessitates that modern-day athletes undertake a training load greater than that of their predecessors. While it is widely accepted that heavy training doses are required to optimise performance (Brooks & Fahey 1994), the extension of the competition year means that it is now commonplace for athletes to maintain intense training all year round. Chronic exposure to such training is not without its pitfalls, however (see Chapter 6).

Planning a training program

Wells and Pate (1988) have suggested that, prior to planning any training program, several questions need to be addressed by the sport scientist and coach:

- What are the physiological demands of the sport?
- What is the athlete's (or team's) ability to meet these demands?
- What is the magnitude of improvement required by the athlete to be successful in the sport? Is this realistic?
- What type of movements are required for this sport (e.g. eccentric contractions, concentric contractions, sustained, intermittent)?
- What are the training demands for this sport?
- Are these demands realistic for this athlete?
- What environmental stresses will be encountered during training?
- What are the athlete's strengths and weaknesses in his/her sport?
- Should the training program aim to enhance the athlete's particular strengths further, or counteract and reduce the athlete's weaknesses?

Answers to these questions should provide the coach with a starting point on which to base a training plan constructed according to the scientific principles of training. The organisation of that plan is referred to as the 'periodisation of training'.

Constructing a training program: the periodisation of training

The development of the training concept, now referred to as 'periodisation' (Martveyev 1972), probably represents one of the most significant advances in training program development. This training approach originally detailed a theoretical framework in the development of training programs used by weight-lifters in the then Soviet Union and Eastern bloc countries (Martveyev 1972).

Periodisation involves the manipulation of the intensity and volume of exercise performed within a training cycle. Although periodisation was not a totally innovative way to compartmentalise training, it was the first formal approach to scientific training organisation. Periodisation of training is now commonly used by athletes in both power/speed sports and endurance events, and has been reported to be superior to a wide variety of programs that do not provide variation in training stimulus (Stone et al. 1981; Stowers et al. 1983; Willoughby 1993).

It is beyond the scope of this chapter to provide the reader with comprehensive training programs for a multitude of different sports. This is because even within a discipline (e.g. track and field, swimming, cycling, rowing) numerous separate and physiologically distinct events exist that cover a wide range of performance distances and durations. Furthermore, it seems possible to achieve success at the highest level by employing a variety of different training methods (Maughan 1994). However, a comprehensive review of the scientific training literature reveals that for the vast majority of sports, the core components that constitute a year-round training program are strikingly similar and can be divided into several distinct phases:

- the general preparatory phase, often referred to as general conditioning or base training
- the transition or competition preparation phase
- the taper and competition phase
- the recovery phase.

During each of these distinct phases of physical preparation, primary emphasis is placed on the development and enhancement of one or more specific physiological objectives. As an athlete progresses from general to more specific training, the overall volume of training decreases, while the specificity of training routines along with the intensity of exercise increase.

The general preparatory, conditioning phase of training

For most athletes, general preparatory training will be performed during the non-competitive period of a macro-cycle, typically during the winter. As a general rule, the longer the duration of an athlete's event, the greater the time that will be spent in this phase of the cycle. However, in sports with a high technique component requiring power/speed (such as Olympic weight-lifting and power-lifting), the duration of the general conditioning phase is largely a function of the skill level of an athlete. Accordingly, for a new lifter, the preparatory or conditioning phase may last as long as 8–10 months to allow an athlete to gain the necessary motor skills and techniques to perform lifts satisfactorily (Kraemer & Koziris 1994). For an endurance athlete, such as an international marathon runner, the general preparatory phase may last up to 6 months, whereas a high school or Masters runner might devote as little as 8–10 weeks for general conditioning (Hawley 2000). In the case of a double-periodised year in which an athlete may be competing throughout a 12-month period (such as summer seasons in both Northern and Southern Hemispheres), the general preparatory/conditioning phase will have to be reduced accordingly.

During the general conditioning phase the volume and frequency of training is high (Wells & Pate 1988) and the magnitude of adaptation is likely to be greatest when the athlete's training load is just below the threshold that would eventually lead to staleness and fatigue (Hawley 2000). The primary physiological adaptations to this type of training for athletes competing in both power/speed events and endurance sports have been detailed elsewhere (Hagerman 1994; Hawley & Burke 1998; Maughan et al. 1997; Snyder & Foster 1994; Wells & Pate 1988; Williams & Gandy 1994).

It has been suggested that athletes should continue general conditioning until such a time when performance of their specialist event (as determined by time trials or other performance related benchmarks) fails to improve (Hawley & Burke 1998). Although such a hypothesis has not been scientifically validated, it does provide a definitive time point at which an individual should shift the focus of attention to more specific competition preparation.

As noted previously, controversy exists as to potential benefits of resistance training for enhancing endurance performance in well-trained athletes. Weight-training programs along with many forms of resistance training are regularly used by endurance athletes, and while these training techniques *probably* contribute to improved endurance performance, there is little scientific documentation of such a benefit (Wells & Pate 1988). In this regard, Hagerman (1994) compared the effects of weight training versus no weight training during the general preparatory phase on muscular strength and power, maximal aerobic power (endurance), and rowing ergometer performance in elite male and female rowers. Rowers who performed off-season weight training experienced a significant *reduction* in maximal aerobic power and failed to improve their rowing ergometer performance compared to the rowers who did not participate in weight training. Perhaps more importantly, the off-season weight training detracted from in-season rowing on-water performance. Accordingly, it was concluded 'elite rowers benefit more from performing only simulated or actual rowing training during the off-season rather than including resistance training' (Hagerman 1994).

In support of these findings, Bell et al. (1989) studied 18 well-trained rowers who undertook two different resistance-training programs during their general conditioning phase. In addition to their on-water endurance training, one group added high-volume (~20 repetitions), low-resistance, high-velocity resistance training, while another group added low-volume (6–8 repetitions), high resistance, low-velocity training. All resistance training was rowing specific (i.e. used the same musculature employed in the rowing movement), and was undertaken on variable-resistance hydraulic equipment four times per week for 5 weeks. A third group of rowers acted as controls and followed the same general conditioning program, without any resistance training. After the 5-week intervention, the high-volume, low-resistance group performed better in high-velocity movements, while those rowers who performed low-volume, high-resistance training were better at low-velocity actions. However, when tested under controlled laboratory conditions on a rowing ergometer, there were no differences between peak power output and rowing performance for either of the two resistance-trained groups when compared to the control group.

Although 5 weeks of resistance training is unlikely to elicit the changes in muscle morphology that might ultimately underlie performance enhancements (for review see Kraemer et al. 1996), the results of that study (Bell et al. 1989) highlight the concept of the specificity of training adaptation, and demonstrate that even 'sport-specific' resistance training effects do not transfer to the coordinated whole-body rowing action. From a practical perspective, coaches often stress that resistance (or other) supplementary training regimens may actually restrict the volume of sport-specific training that an (endurance) athlete can perform and may result in a decrement in performance. It is clear that more applied research is needed to address this important issue.

The transition or competition preparation phase

Unlike general preparatory conditioning, which can last many months, the transition or competition preparation phase typically lasts 3–6 weeks depending on the length of the subsequent competition period. The primary goal of this phase of training is to provide athletes with workouts that closely match their planned competition intensity. The shift from general conditioning to the transition or competition preparation phase signifies that training becomes more event specific.

During this phase of training, athletes whose event requires strength/power emphasise very high-intensity workouts (e.g. heavy weights, low volume, extended recovery) that stress technique. The transition from general conditioning to competition preparation for an athlete whose event largely requires endurance is facilitated by the introduction of 'simulated competitions'. For most endurance athletes, these 'simulated competitions' typically take the form of time trials over a variety of intermediate distances, usually less than the planned race distance. In addition to the physiological demands, which closely replicate the anticipated race demands, the use of time trials helps to develop an athlete's pace judgment and the necessary skills and techniques likely to be encountered at race speed.

The effects of transition training (or intensified training) on the performances of already well-trained endurance athletes are summarised in Table 7.2. Although the vast majority of studies described in Table 7.2 have been undertaken using well-trained endurance cyclists, the findings from these investigations are likely to be applicable across a number of endurance sports.

In the vast majority of studies, transition training was undertaken on two occasions per week for a period of approximately 3–4 weeks, although in one investigation (Acevedo & Goldfarb 1989) an 8-week intervention was employed. However, increasing this phase of training beyond 3–4 weeks does not result in further performance enhancement (Hawley et al. 1997). Indeed, independent of the period of intervention, performance of events lasting 30–60 minutes is typically improved by approximately 2.5% after intensified training. Such an improvement in performance is substantial and much greater than the smallest worthwhile enhancement of performance for an athlete in an international event, which is usually in the order of 0.4–0.7% of the typical within-athlete variation in performance (see Hopkins et al. 1999 for discussion). The mechanisms underlying such a performance enhancement after transition training include less reliance on carbohydrate as a fuel for muscular contraction, improved muscle buffering, decreased

TABLE 7.2 Effects of intensified training in well-trained athletes on endurance performance and selected physiological markers

SUBJECTS/TRAINING STATUS	TRAINING INTERVENTION	PERFORMANCE MEASURE	PHYSIOLOGICAL OUTCOMES	REFERENCE
8 ET[a] runners VO_{2peak} 65.3 ± 2.3 mL/kg/min[b]	8 weeks of 3 sessions/week of: interval workouts, fartlek and race-pace training	10 km TT[c] ↓ 2.9% 35:27 vs 34:24 min:s ($P< 0.05$)	Decreases in plasma [lactate] at 85% and 90% of VO_{2peak} after intensified training	Acevedo & Goldfarb (1989)
8 ET cyclists 305 ± 38 km/week VO_{2peak} 65.7 ± 0.05 mL/kg/min	3 weeks of 2 sessions/week of: 6–8 × 5 min repetitions @ 85% VO_{2peak} with 60 s recovery	40 km TT ↓ 3.5% 56:24 ± 3:36 vs 54.24 ± 3:12 min:s ($P< 0.001$)	No physiological measures taken	Lindsay et al. (1996)
8 ET cyclists 294 ±65 km/week VO_{2peak} 66.2 ± 2.6 mL/kg/min	3 weeks of 2 sessions/week of: 6–8 × 5 min repetitions @ 85% VO_{2peak} with 60 s recovery	40 km TT ↓ 3.5% 56.24 ± 3.36 vs 54.24 ± 3:12 min:s ($P< 0.001$)	βm[d] ↑ 16% Citrate synthase, PFK[e] and HK[f], NS	Weston et al. (1977)
4 ET cyclists VO_{2peak} 60.3 ± 0.05 mL/kg/min	3 weeks of 2 sessions/week of: 12 × 30 s repetitions @ 175% PPO with 4.5 min recovery	40 km TT ↓ 2.4%	No differences in CHO[g] oxidation, plasma [lactate] or heart rate during submaximal cycling after training	Stepto et al. (1999)
3 ET cyclists VO_{2peak} 62.8 ± 0.17 mL/kg/min	3 weeks of 2 sessions/week of: 12 × 60 s repetitions @ 100% PPO with 4 min recovery	40 km TT: NS	No differences in CHO oxidation, plasma [lactate] or heart rate during submaximal cycling after training	Stepto et al. (1999)
4 ET cyclists VO_{2peak} 69.8 ± 0.01 mL/kg/min	3 weeks of 2 sessions/week of: 12 × 2 min repetitions @ 90% PPO with 3 min recovery	40 km TT: NS	No differences in CHO oxidation, plasma [lactate] or heart rate during submaximal cycling after training	Stepto et al. (1999)
4 ET cyclists VO_{2peak} 61.2 ± 0.01 mL/kg/min	3 weeks of 2 sessions/week of: 8 × 4 min repetitions @ 85% PPO with 90 s recovery	40 km TT ↓ 2.8%	No differences in CHO oxidation, plasma [lactate] or heart rate during submaximal cycling after training	Stepto et al. (1999)

(continues)

TABLE 7.2 Effects of intensified training in well-trained athletes on endurance performance and selected physiological markers (*continued*)

SUBJECTS/TRAINING STATUS	TRAINING INTERVENTION	PERFORMANCE MEASURE	PHYSIOLOGICAL OUTCOMES	REFERENCE
4 ET cyclists VO_{2peak} 61.5 ± 0.04 mL/kg/min	3 weeks of 2 sessions/week of: 4 × 8 min repetitions @ 80% PPO with 1 min recovery	140 km TT: NS	No differences in CHO oxidation, plasma [lactate] or heart rate during submaximal cycling after training	Stepto et al. (1999)
8 ET cyclists 300 ± 86 km/wk VO_{2peak} 65.3 ± 2.35 mL/kg/min	3 weeks of 2 sessions/week of: 6–9 × 5 min repetitions @ 85% VO_{2peak} with 60 s recovery	40 km TT ↓ 2.3%	↑ absolute (291 ± 43 vs 327 ± 51 W) and relative (72.6 ± 5.3 vs 78.1 ± 2.8%; $P < 0.05$) work rates after intensified training ↓ CHO oxidation, plasma [lactate] and ventilation during submaximal cycling ($P < 0.05$)	Westgarth-Taylor et al. (1977)

(a) ET: endurance trained.
(b) VO_{2peak}: peak oxygen uptake.
(c) TT: time trial.
(d) βm: skeletal muscle buffering capacity.
(e) PFK: phosphofructokinase.
(f) HK: hexokinase.
(g) CHO: carbohydrate.
All values are mean ± SD.

plasma lactate accumulation, and an increase in fractional utilisation of aerobic capacity (Table 7.2).

Of particular interest to both scientists and coaches are the findings of Stepto et al. (1999), who systematically determined the effects of a diverse range of different interval-training programs on cycling time-trial performance (Table 7.2). These workers showed that six sessions of the shortest, most intense sessions (12 repetitions 30 s at maximal aerobic power output with 4–5 min recovery) were just as effective at improving 40-km time-trial performance (lasting ~55 min) as were longer interval sets (8 repetitions 4 min at 85% VO_{2max} with 1 min recovery). The nadir in performance enhancement after 'supramaximal' versus more 'event specific' aerobic interval training sets suggests that there may be more than one mechanism by which interval training enhances endurance performance. In this regard, intensified training is known to up-regulate the proton-linked monocarboxylate transporters that function to transport lactate across the sarcolemma in skeletal muscle (Brooks et al. 1999; Juel & Pilegaard 1999; Pilegaard et al. 1999). An increased lactate transport capacity is likely to be an important training-induced adaptation that might explain the improvement in performance observed after high-intensity sprint-type training. Whatever the precise mechanism underlying performance enhancement, it has been recommended that supramaximal repeated sprint workouts be incorporated into the competition preparation of all endurance athletes (Hawley & Stepto 2001).

The taper and competition phase

For athletes competing in either explosive events necessitating bouts of maximal strength/power, or endurance sports requiring sustained, submaximal power outputs for prolonged periods, tapering of training has become a widely accepted component of preparation for a major competition (Wells & Pate 1988). During taper, several variables can be manipulated to reduce the training impulse and maximise subsequent performance. These include the *duration* of the taper, the *intensity* of training undertaken during the taper and the *frequency* of training sessions throughout the taper. Several investigations have been undertaken with athletes from a variety of sports to determine the optimal taper that results in the best performance. While tapers vary between sports, several common features emerge as being essential to a successful taper (Houmard 1991; Mujika 1998).

Firstly, training *volume* is reduced in an incremental or stepwise fashion for 1–2 weeks so that in the days immediately prior to a major competition it is almost zero. A prolonged (~21 day) taper is common in sports such as swimming (Costill et al. 1985; Houmard & Johns 1994; Mujika et al. 1996; Neufer et al. 1987) and is also likely to be undertaken by athletes aiming for a single major competitive peak in a meso-cycle (i.e. the Olympic Games) that requires multiple qualifying rounds. However, a taper undertaken for longer than 21 days maintains rather than improves performance.

Despite a marked reduction in training volume, the *intensity* of training is maintained, or even slightly increased during a taper. In one of the most frequently cited studies of taper, Shepley et al. (1992) reported that competitive college cross-country runners training 80 km per week showed greater improvements in performance after a 7-day low-volume, high-intensity taper compared to a low-volume (30 km per week), low-intensity regimen or no training at all. Similarly, Gibala et al. (1994) reported that resistance-trained athletes improved concentric strength for at least 8 days following a 10-day taper in which training volume was reduced by 50% but training intensity was maintained.

Finally, the reduction in training volume should not be achieved at the expense of a drastic decline in the number of training sessions undertaken by an athlete. In the only study to systematically manipulate training *frequency* during a taper, Mujika et al. (2002) determined the effects of reduced training rate in two groups of well-trained middle-distance runners who performed a 6-day taper consisting of an 80% non-linear progressive reduction in high-intensity interval training. One group of runners trained daily during the taper (high frequency) whereas the other group rested every third day (low frequency). Performance (800-m time), assessed during competitions before and after the taper, improved significantly after the high-frequency taper (121.8 s vs 124.2 s), but not after the low-frequency taper (126.6 s vs 127.1 s). The improvement in 800-m race time with the high-frequency taper could not be explained by differences in any of the physiological indices measured by the investigators (Mujika et al. 2002), leading them to speculate that 'a potential loss of "feel" may have taken place for the runners who undertook the low-frequency taper group, despite only a moderate (33%) reduction in training frequency'.

On a practical note, many endurance athletes commonly complain that they lose 'feel' for their activity if forced to reduce the frequency of training sessions by more than 30%. Such a complaint is often voiced by swimmers when they are forced to miss a pool session for more than 24 hours. Although not scientifically proven, the body of anecdotal evidence for a loss of sensory feel with a significant reduction in training frequency is likely to be accompanied by changes in gross mechanical efficiency and economy of movement. In strength/power events, particularly those involving a high technique component, frequent training sessions are a necessity for maintaining acquired and skilled motor patterns (Kraemer et al. 1994). Although many athletes fear a loss of training adaptation (detraining) in the taper, such an apprehension appears unwarranted: provided the training frequency is not reduced by more than 20–25%, markers of training status (VO_{2max}, maximal heart rate, maximal speed or workload) are well maintained for 10–21 days after reductions in training volume of up to 70% (for review see Houmard 1991).

With regard to the likely performance enhancement after a taper, the results from a large number of studies indicate that, independent of event duration, competitive athletes typically improve performance by approximately 2.5% (Houmard 1991; Houmard & Johns 1994; Houmard et al. 1994; Mujika 1998; Mujika et al. 2000). The mechanisms underlying endurance performance enhancement include elevations in resting muscle and liver glycogen stores, increased total blood volume and associated haematological changes, and improvements in economy of movement. For the strength/power trained athletes, a taper may induce physiologically important changes in muscle contractile function that allow the individual to generate greater peak forces and sustain faster maximal contraction velocities, possibly by greater motor unit activation (Hawley 2000).

Regardless of the precise mechanisms, when the effect of a taper is added to the improvement in performance attributable to transition training, the combined outcome is an enhancement in the order of approximately 5% compared to the performance an athlete might attain after a period of general conditioning. When viewed against the extremes of training undertaken by the modern-day athlete, such improvements in performance capacity seem, at first sight, rather modest. However, the difference between winning and losing in many professional sports is small (see Hopkins et al. 1999). For example, the winning margin in the Tour de France is in the order of 200–400 s over the course of a 3-week race lasting about 300 000 s. Such a margin represents just 0.07–0.13% of total race time (Jeukendrup et al. 2000). Paradoxically, in events requiring speed/power, the margin of victory, while small, is slightly greater: in the men's 100-m and 200-m sprint finals at the 2000 Sydney Olympic Games, the difference between winning the gold medal and last place was 2.46%.

The recovery phase

Depending on the periodisation of the athlete's year and his/her ability level, the recovery phase may last anywhere between 2 and 6 weeks. The primary aim of this phase is to allow the athlete an extended period of recuperation from the preceding season. Depending on the presence of chronic injuries or other maladies, the athlete may need a period of complete inactivity before embarking on a regimen of alternative activity where training is gradually resumed. Nowadays, most competitive athletes will only take a limited time off from their primary activity and even then usually undertake some form of alternative training to maintain a degree of general fitness. If technical aspects of an athlete's discipline need to be made, such adjustments should be made before the commencement of the general conditioning phase. For both the coach and athlete, the recovery phase allows for an objective appraisal of the previous season's training and, if necessary, the revision of future goals based on the athlete's progress (or lack of) to that point.

Evaluation of training methods

The final result of any training program is an athlete's or team's performance in a given competition. As such, training methods can be objectively evaluated because the outcome measures (e.g. time taken, distance covered, position, ranking) are easily observed and quantified. Although frequent competitions are the best way to evaluate the efficacy of different training methods, such an approach is not practical in events where athletes only compete once or twice a year (such as marathon and ultra-marathon races). In these situations an alternative option would be to simulate competition demands (i.e. speed of motion, power output) in a controlled environment (laboratory or field) and have the athlete complete a reduced portion of his/ her race distance/duration. Guidelines for the construction of an effective athlete-testing program have been reviewed elsewhere (Hawley 1999). The most important criterion of such an evaluation is that it provide useful information to the coach and scientist concerning the development and effects of a specific training intervention.

Table 7.3 provides physiological test data from elite American rowers over an 8-month period. The individual lactate threshold was determined during

TABLE 7.3 Physiological responses of elite American rowers during 2000-m simulated competitions undertaken on a Concept II ergometer

VARIABLE	DECEMBER	FEBRUARY	MAY	JULY
Peak power (W)	345 ± 19	380 ± 17	393 ± 17[c]	457 ± 18
Peak VO$_2$ (L/min)[a]	5.61 ± 0.59	5.65 ± 0.63	6.16 ± 0.36[c]	6.35 ± 0.29[c]
Peak VO$_2$ (mL/kg/min)	61.4 ± 2.1	62.0 ± 1.9	68.4 ± 1.9[c]	71.3 ± 1.9[c][d]
VO$_2$ @ LT[b] (L/min)	4.04 ± 0.73	4.26 ± 0.69	5.14 ± 0.81[d]	5.46 ± 0.77[d]
LT (% of peak VO$_2$)	72.0 ± 1.0	75.0 ± 1.3	83.0 ± 1.1[c]	86 ± 1.2[c]

(a) VO$_2$: oxygen uptake.
(b) LT: lactate threshold. Values are mean ± SD.
(c) Significantly different to December ($P < 0.05$).
(d) Significantly different to December ($P < 0.01$).
Data from Hagerman (1994)

an incremental rowing ergometer test commencing at a power output of 100 W and increasing in power by 50 W every 2 minutes until exhaustion.

Over the period of monitoring (from the onset of general conditioning in December through to the competition phase in July) there were impressive overall gains in peak power (~25%), peak VO$_2$ (~13%) and VO$_2$ at the individual lactate threshold (~26%). Of particular interest is the time course of adaptation of these variables. As might be expected with the general conditioning phase (from December through February), there are modest (statistically non-significant) increases in most of the parameters under investigation (Table 7.3). However, with the onset of more intense transition/competition preparation (May through July), all parameters improve so that, by July, all maximal and submaximal values are significantly different from the data collected in December (Table 7.3). It is of note that improvements in laboratory indices (13–26%) always exceed subsequent performance enhancement in competitions (~5%).

While acknowledging the value of laboratory testing as a useful adjunct to the field-based observations of coaches, the ultimate test of any athlete's ability will always be his/her competitive performance. Evaluation of training should, therefore, be viewed as a process that aids the coach in assessing an athlete's strengths and weaknesses and in monitoring progress in response to a specified training program. Testing and monitoring should be viewed as an ongoing, long-term process that incorporates regular revision of plans within all phases of training. In the final analysis, effective training requires that the coach, sport scientist and athlete work jointly to continually modify training plans on the basis of laboratory data, practical experience and the results of performance in competition.

References

Acevedo EO, Goldfarb AH. Increased training intensity effects on plasma lactate, ventilatory threshold, and endurance. *Med Sci Sports Exerc* 1989;21:563–8.

Bangsbo J, Gollnick PD, Graham TE, Juel C, Kiens B, Mizuno M, Saltin B. Anaerobic energy production and O_2 deficit-debt relationship during exhaustive exercise in humans. *J Physiol (Lond.)* 1990;422:539–59.

Bannister EW. Modeling elite athletic performance. In: Green HJ, McDougall JD, Wenger H, eds. *Physiological Testing of Elite Athletes*. Champaign, IL: Human Kinetics, 1991:403–24.

Bell GJ, Petersen SR, Quinney AH, Wenger HA. The effect of velocity-specific strength training on peak torque and anaerobic rowing power. *J Sports Sci* 1989;7:205–14.

Booth FW, Thomason DR. Molecular and cellular adaptation of muscle in response to exercise: Perspectives of various models. *Physiol Rev* 1991;71:541–85.

Booth FW, Watson PS. Control of adaptations in protein levels in response to exercise. *Fed Proc* 1985;44:2293–300.

Bouchard C, Dionne FT, Simoneau JA, Boulay MR. Genetics of aerobic and anaerobic performances. In: Holloszy JO, ed. *Exercise and Sport Sciences Reviews*. Vol. 20. Baltimore: Williams & Wilkins, 1992: 27–58.

Brandon LJ. Physiological factors associated with middle distance running performance. *Sports Med* 1995;19:268–77.

Brooks GA, Dubouchard H, Brown M, Sicurello JP, Butz CE. Role of mitochondrial lactate dehydrogenase and lactate oxidation in the intracellular lactate shuttle. *Proc Natl Acad Sci* 1999;96:1129–34.

Brooks GA, Fahey TD. Exercise Physiology. *Human Bioenergetics and its Applications*. New York: Macmillan Publishing Company, 1984: 429.

Clausen JP. Effect of physical training on cardiovascular adjustments to exercise. *Physiol Rev* 1977;57:779–815.

Costill DL, King DS, Thomas R, Hargreaves M. Effects of reduced training on muscular power in swimmers. *Physician Sportsmed* 1985;13:94–101.

Costill DL, Thomason H, Roberts E. Fractional utilization of the aerobic capacity during distance running. *Med Sci Sports* 1973;5:246–52.

Conley DL, Krahenbuhl GS. Running economy and distance running performance of highly trained athletes. *Med Sci Sports Exerc* 1980;12:357–60.

Coyle EF, Feltner ME, Kautz SA, Hamilton MT, Montain SJ, Baylor AM, Abraham LD, Petrek GW. Physiological and biomechanical factors associated with elite endurance cycling performance. *Med Sci Sports Exerc* 1991;23:93–107.

Coyle EF, Spriet L, Gregg S, Clarkson P. Introduction to physiology and nutrition for competitive sport. In: Lamb DR, Knuttgen HG, Murray R, eds. *Perspectives in Exercise Science and Sports Medicine*. Vol. 7. *Physiology and Nutrition for Competitive Sport*. Carmel, IN: Cooper Publishing Group, 1994: xv–xxix.

Daniels JT, Yarborough RA, Foster C. Changes in VO_{2max} and running performance with training. *Eur J Appl Physiol* 1978;39:249–54.

Dudley GA, Djamil R. Incompatibility of endurance- and strength-training modes of exercise. *J Appl Physiol* 1985;59:1446–51.

Farrell PA, Wilmore JH, Coyle EF, Billing JE, Costill DL. Plasma lactate accumulation and distance running performance. *Med Sci Sports Exerc* 1979;11:338–44.

Gibala MJ, MacDougall JD, Sale DG. The effects of tapering on strength performance in trained athletes. *Int J Sports Med* 1994;15:492–7.

Gollnick PD, Armstrong RB, Saubert CW 4th, Piehl K, Saltin B. Enzyme activity and fiber composition in skeletal muscle of untrained and trained men. *J Appl Physiol* 1971;33:312–19.

Hagan RD, Smith MG, Gettman LR. Marathon performance in relation to maximal aerobic power and training indices. *Med Sci Sports Exerc* 1981;13:185–9.

Hagerman FC. Physiology and nutrition for rowers. In: Lamb DR, Knuttgen HG, Murray R, eds. *Perspectives in Exercise Science and Sports Medicine.* Vol. 7. *Physiology and Nutrition for Competitive Sport.* Carmel, IN: Cooper Publishing Group, 1994: 221–99.

Häkkinen K, Komi PV. Electromyographic changes during strength training and detraining. *Med Sci Sports Exerc* 1983;15:455–60.

Häkkinen K, Pakarinen A, Alen M, Kauhanen H, Komi PV. Neuromuscular and hormonal adaptations in athletes to strength training in two years. *J Appl Physiol* 1988:65:2406–12.

Hawley JA. Guidelines for laboratory and field testing of athletic potential and performance. In: Maughan RJ, ed. *Basic and Applied Sciences for Sports Medicine.* Oxford: Butterworth-Heinemann, 1999: 312–35.

Hawley JA. Training for successful running performance. In: Hawley JA, ed. *Handbook of Sports Medicine and Science. Running.* Oxford: Blackwell Science, 2000: 44–57.

Hawley JA. Adaptations of skeletal muscle to prolonged, intense endurance training. *Clin Exp Pharmacol Physiol* 2002a;29:218–22.

Hawley JA. Physiological preparation for high-performance cycling: Designing a training program. In: Jeukendrup AE, ed. *High Performance Cycling.* Champaign, IL: Human Kinetics, 2002b: 3–12.

Hawley JA, Burke LM. *Peak Performance: Training and Nutritional Strategies for Sport.* Sydney: Allen & Unwin, 1998.

Hawley JA, Myburgh KH, Noakes TD, Dennis SC. Training techniques to improve fatigue resistance and endurance performance. *J Sports Sci* 1997;15:325–33.

Hawley JA, Stepto NK. Adaptation to training in endurance-trained cyclists. Implications for performance. *Sports Med* 2001;31:511–20.

Hickson RC. Interference of strength development by simultaneously training for strength and endurance. *Eur J Appl Physiol* 1980;45:255–63.

Hopkins WG, Hawley JA, Burke LM. Design and analysis of research on sport performance enhancement. *Med Sci Sports Exerc* 1999;31:472–85.

Houmard JA. Impact of reduced training on performance in endurance athletes. *Sports Med* 1991;12:380–93.

Houmard JA, Johns RA. Effects of taper on swim performance. Practical implications. *Sports Med* 1994;17:224–32.

Houmard JA, Scott BK, Justice CL, Chenier TC. The effects of taper on performance in distance runners. *Med Sci Sports Exerc* 1994;26:624–31.

Ivey FM, Roth SM, Ferrell RE, Tracy BL, Lemmer JT, Hurlbut DE, Martel GF, Siegel EL, Fozard JL, Metter EJ, Fleg JL, Hurley BF. Effects of age, gender, and myostatin genotype on the hypertrophic response to heavy resistance strength training. *J Gerentol* 2000;55A:M641–M648.

Jeukendrup AE, Craig NP, Hawley JA. The bioenergetics of world class cycling. *J Sci Med Sport* 2000;3:414–33.

Juel C, Pilegaard H. Lactate exchange and pH regulation in skeletal muscle. In: Hargreaves M, Thompson M, eds. *Biochemistry of Exercise*. Vol. X. Champaign, IL: Human Kinetics, 1999: 185–200.

Kraemer WJ, Fleck SJ, Evans WJ. Strength and power training: Physiological mechanisms of adaptation. In: Holloszy JO, ed. *Exercise and Sport Sciences Reviews*. Vol. 24. Baltimore: Williams & Wilkins, 1996: 363–97.

Kraemer WJ, Koziris LP. Olympic weightlifting and power lifting. In: Lamb DR, Knuttgen HG, Murray R, eds. *Perspectives in Exercise Science and Sports Medicine*. Vol. 7. *Physiology and Nutrition for Competitive Sport*. Carmel, IN: Cooper Publishing Group, 1994: 1–46.

Kraemer WJ, Patton JF, Gordon SE, Harman EA, Deschenes MR, Reynolds K, Newton RU, Triplett NT, Dziados JE. Compatibility of high-intensity strength and endurance training on hormonal and skeletal muscle adaptations. *J Appl Physiol* 1995;78:976–89.

Lakomy HKA. Physiology and biochemistry of sprinting. In: Hawley JA, ed. *Handbook of Sports Medicine and Science. Running*. Oxford: Blackwell Science, 2000: 1–13.

Leveritt M, Abernethy PJ, Barry BK, Logan PA. Concurrent strength and endurance training: A review. *Sports Med* 1999;28:413–27.

Lindsay FH, Hawley JA, Myburgh KH, Schomer HH, Noakes TD, Dennis SC. Improved athletic performance in highly trained cyclists after interval training. *Med Sci Sports Exerc* 1996;28:1427–34.

Lortie G, Simoneau JA, Hamel P, Boulay MR, Landry F, Bouchard C. Responses of maximal aerobic power and capacity to aerobic training. *Int J Sports Med* 1984;5: 232–6.

Maughan RJ. Physiology and nutrition for middle distance and long distance running. In: Lamb DR, Knuttgen HG, Murray R, eds. *Perspectives in Exercise Science and Sports Medicine*. Vol. 7. *Physiology and Nutrition for Competitive Sport*. Carmel, IN: Cooper Publishing Group, 1994: 329–64.

Maughan RJ, Gleeson M, Greenhaff PL. *Biochemistry of Exercise and Training*. Oxford: Oxford University Press, 1997.

Martveyev LP. *Periodisienang das Sportlichen Training*. Berlin: Beles & Wernitz, 1972.

McCarthy JP, Agre JC, Graf BK, Pozniak MA, Vailas AC. Compatibility of adaptive responses with combining strength and endurance training. *Med Sci Sports Exerc* 1995;27:429–36.

McCarthy JP, Pozniak MA, Agre JC. Neuromuscular adaptations to concurrent strength and endurance training. *Med Sci Sports Exerc* 2002;34:511–19.

Moritani T, de Vries HA. Neural factors versus hypertrophy in the time course of muscle strength gain. *Am J Phys Med* 1979;58:115–30.

Mujika I. The influence of training characteristics and tapering on the adaptation in highly trained individuals: A review. *Int J Sports Med* 1998;19:439–46.

Mujika I, Busso T, Lacoste L, Barale F, Geyssant A, Chatard JC. Modelled responses to training and taper in competitive swimmers. *Med Sci Sports Exerc* 1996;28: 251–8.

Mujika I, Goya A, Padilla S, Grijalba A, Gorostiaga E, Ibanez J. Physiological responses to a 6-day taper in middle-distance runners: influence of training intensity and volume. *Med Sci Sports Exerc* 2000;32:511–17.

Mujika I, Goya A, Ruiz E, Grijalba A, Santisteban J, Padilla S. Physiological and performance responses to a 6-day taper in middle-distance runners: influence of training frequency. *Int J Sports Med* 2002 23:367–73.

Neufer PD, Costill DL, Fielding RA, Flynn MG, Kirwan JP. Effect of reduced training on muscular strength and endurance in competitive swimmers. *Med Sci Sports Exerc* 1987;19:486–90.

Nevill ME, Bogdanis GC, Boobis LH, Lakomy HKA, Williams C. Muscle metabolism and performance during sprinting. In: Maughan RJ, Shirreffs SM, eds. *Biochemistry of Exercise IX*. Champaign, IL: Human Kinetics, 1994: 243–59.

O'Hagan FT, Sale DG, MacDougall JD, Garner SH. Response to resistance training in young women and men. *Int J Sports Med* 1995;16:314–21.

Pilegaard H, Terzis G, Halestrap A, Juel C. Distribution of the lactate/H^+ transporter isoforms MCT1 and MCT4 in human skeletal muscle. *Am J Physiol* 1999;276: E843–E848.

Ploutz LL, Tesch PA, Biro RL, Dudley GA. Effect of resistance training on muscle use during exercise. *J Appl Physiol* 1994;76:1675–81.

Pyne DB, Lee H, Swanick KM. Monitoring the lactate threshold in world-ranked swimmers. *Med Sci Sports Exerc* 2001;33:291–7.

Sale DG. Neural adaptation to strength training. In: Komi PV, ed. *Strength and Power in Sports*. Oxford: Blackwell Scientific Publications, 1992: 249–65.

Sale DG, MacDougall JD, Jacobs I, Garner S. Interaction between concurrent strength and endurance training. *J Appl Physiol* 1990;68:260–70.

Saltin B. Physiological effects of physical conditioning. *Med Sci Sport* 1991:1:50–6.

Shepley B, MacDougall JD, Cipriano N, Sutton JR, Tarnopolsky MA, Coates G. Physiological effects of tapering in highly trained athletes. *J Appl Physiol* 1992;72: 706–11.

Simoneau JA, Lortie G, Boulay MR, Marcotte M, Thibault MC, Bouchard C. Inheritance of human skeletal muscle and anaerobic capacity adaptation to high-intensity intermittent training. *Int J Sports Med* 1986;7:167–71.

Sjödin B, Svedenhag J. Applied physiology of marathon running. *Sports Med* 1985;2: 83–99.

Snyder AC, Foster C. Physiology and nutrition for skating. In: Lamb DR, Knuttgen HG, Murray R, eds. *Perspectives in Exercise Science and Sports Medicine*. Vol. 7. *Physiology and Nutrition for Competitive Sport*. Carmel, IN: Cooper Publishing Group, 1994:181–215.

Staron RS, Karapondo DL, Kraemer WJ, Fry AC, Gordon SE, Falkel JE, Hagerman FC, Hikida RS. Skeletal muscle adaptations during the early phase of heavy resistance training in men and women. *J Appl Physiol* 1994;76:1247–55.

Stepto NK, Hawley JA, Dennis SC, Hopkins WG. Effects of different interval-training programs on cycling time-trial performance. *Med Sci Sports Exerc* 1999;31: 736–41.

Stone MH, O'Bryant HS, Garnhammer J. A hypothetical model for strength training. *J Sports Med Phys Fitness* 1981;21:342–51.

Stowers TJ, McMillan D, Scala D, Davis V, Wilson D, Stone M. The short-term effects of three different strength-power training methods. *National Strength Cond Assoc J* 1983;5:24–7.

Wells CL, Pate RR. Training for performance of prolonged exercise. In: Lamb DR, Murray R, eds. *Perspectives in Exercise Science and Sports Medicine*. Vol. 1. *Prolonged Exercise*. Indianapolis, IN: Benchmark Press, 1988: 357–88.

Westgarth-Taylor C, Hawley JA, Rickard S, Myburgh KH, Noakes TD, Dennis SC. Metabolic and performance adaptations to interval training in endurance-trained cyclists. *Eur J Appl Physiol* 1997;75:298–304.

Weston AR, Myburgh KH, Lindsay FH, Dennis SC, Noakes TD, Hawley JA. Skeletal muscle buffering capacity and endurance performance after high-intensity training by well-trained cyclists. *Eur J Appl Physiol* 1997;75:7–13.

Widegren U, Ryder JW, Zierath JR. Mitogen-activated protein kinase signal transduction in skeletal muscle: effects of exercise and muscle contraction. *Acta Physiol Scand* 2001;172:227–38.

Williams C, Gandy G. Physiology and nutrition for sprinting. In: Lamb DR, Knuttgen HG, Murray R, eds. *Perspectives in Exercise Science and Sports Medicine*. Vol. 7. *Physiology and Nutrition for Competitive Sport*. Carmel, IN: Cooper Publishing Group, 1994: 55–98.

Williams RS, Neufer PD. Regulation of gene expression in skeletal muscle by contractile activity. In: Rowell LB, Shepherd JT, eds. *Handbook of Physiology*. Section 12. *Exercise: Regulation and Integration of Multiple Systems*. New York: Oxford, 1996: 1124–50.

Willoughby DS. The effects of meso-cycle length weight training programs involving periodization and partially equated volumes on upper body strength. *J Strength Cond Res* 1993;7:2–8.

Yu M, Stepto NK, Chibalin AV, Fryer LGD, Carling D, Krook A, Hawley JA, Zierath JR. Metabolic and mitogenic signal transduction in human skeletal muscle after intense cycling exercise. *J Physiol* 2003 (in press).

CHAPTER 8

Nutrition for training and competition

Louise M. BURKE

Introduction

In the past few decades we have seen an increased awareness in the relationship between nutrition and athletic performance, and the sophistication of both the advice that can be offered to athletes and the scientific evidence that underpins such advice. The benefits of a sound nutrition plan are most immediate and obvious in the area of competition performance, where strategies of food or fluid intake before and during the event reduce or delay the onset of factors that would otherwise cause fatigue. Recovery after the event will determine the athlete's ability to maintain performance over a tournament or from heats to the final. However, everyday eating patterns are just as important, supplying the athlete with the fuel and nutrients needed to optimise the adaptations achieved during training sessions and to recover quickly between workouts. The athlete must also eat to stay in good health and to achieve and maintain an optimal physique. A summary of the goals of sports nutrition is provided in Table 8.1.

Despite the knowledge that is available, sports nutritionists observe that many athletes do not achieve sound dietary practices for either optimal health or sports performance. Factors that prevent good eating practices include poor knowledge of food composition and the practical skills needed to choose and prepare meals, dietary extremism, and reduced access to food due to the busy lifestyle and frequent travel that are typical of high-level athletes. This chapter addresses the major issues in sports nutrition, including issues of the everyday or training diet (energy balance, achieving protein and micronutrient needs) as well as nutrition strategies for competition (e.g. carbohydrate [CHO] and fluid intake before, during and after an event). Of course, acute strategies of rehydration and refuelling are also important for optimal performance in training sessions and should be incorporated into everyday eating.

TABLE 8.1 The goals of sports nutrition

During training, athletes should aim to:

1 meet the energy and fuel requirements needed to support their training program

2 achieve and maintain an ideal physique for their event; manipulate training and nutrition to achieve a level of body mass, body fat and muscle mass that is consistent with good health and good performance

3 refuel and rehydrate well during each training session so that they perform at their best at each session

4 practise any intended competition nutrition strategies so that beneficial practices can be identified and fine-tuned

5 enhance adaptation and recovery between training sessions by providing all the nutrients associated with these processes

6 maintain optimal health and function, especially by achieving the increased needs for some nutrients resulting from a heavy training program

7 reduce the risk of sickness during heavy training periods by maintaining a healthy physique and energy balance, and by supplying nutrients believed to assist immune function (e.g. consume CHO during prolonged exercise sessions)

8 make use of supplements and specialised sports foods which have been shown to enhance training performance or meet training nutrition needs

9 eat for long-term health by paying attention to community nutrition guidelines

10 continue to enjoy food and the pleasure of sharing meals.

For competition athletes should:

1 in weight-division sports, achieve the competition weight division with minimal harm to health or performance

2 'fuel up' adequately prior to an event; consume CHO and achieve exercise taper during the day(s) prior to the event according to the importance and duration of the event; utilise CHO loading strategies when appropriate before events of greater than 90–120 min duration

3 minimise dehydration during the race by using opportunities to drink fluids before, during and after the event

4 consume CHO during events more than 1 h in duration or other events where body carbohydrate stores become depleted

5 achieve pre-event and during-event eating/drinking strategies without causing gastrointestinal discomfort or upsets

6 promote recovery after the event, particularly during multi-day competitions such as tournaments and stage races

7 during a prolonged competition program, not allow event nutrition to compromise overall energy and nutrient intake goals

8 make use of supplements and specialised sports foods which have been shown to enhance competition performance or meet competition nutrition goals.

Energy needs of the athlete

An athlete's energy intake is of interest for several reasons (Burke 2001):

1 It sets the potential for achieving the athlete's requirements for energy-containing macronutrients (especially protein and carbohydrate) and the food needed to provide vitamins, minerals and other non-energy containing dietary compounds required for optimal function and health.

2 It assists the manipulation of muscle mass and body fat levels to achieve the specific physique that is ideal for athletic performance.

3 It affects the function of hormonal and immune systems.

4 It challenges the practical limits to food intake set by issues such as food availability and gastrointestinal comfort.

The energy requirements of individual athletes vary markedly between and within sports and are influenced by body size, the need to lose or gain weight, growth and the training load (frequency, duration and intensity). The training programs of athletes vary according to their event, their level of competition and the time of the athletic season. Results from dietary surveys reveal that male athletes typically report energy intakes varying from 12–20 MJ/day over prolonged periods, with endurance-training athletes reporting higher energy intakes expressed per kilogram of body mass (BM) than those in non-endurance sports (Burke et al. 2001). The expected (absolute) energy requirements of female athletes should be 20–30% lower than their male counterparts, principally to take into account their smaller size. However, it is a common finding of dietary surveys that even when energy intake is expressed per kilogram BM, the reported energy intakes of females are still substantially lower than that reported by their male counterparts (Burke et al. 2000).

It should be remembered that the results of dietary surveys do not necessarily represent the *actual* and *usual* energy intakes of athletes. Rather, they present the results of what athletes *report* eating during a *particular* period of time. Experts in dietary survey methodology are keenly aware that such studies rely on athletes accurately reporting what they consumed, as well as the study period being a true representation of their usual eating patterns (Burke et al. 2001). Errors typically occur because athletes are not accurate and truthful about everything they eat and drink, or because they modify their intake during the period of the dietary survey. In general, dietary surveys underestimate the true intakes of most people because subjects under-eat or under-report their usual intake while they are being investigated. The energy requirements of athletes can be determined using techniques such as indirect calorimetry, doubly-labelled water tracer protocols and factorial prediction equations (Manore & Thompson 2000).

Although most individuals are able to achieve remarkable energy balance over long periods, the athlete is often faced with the challenge of managing energy intakes that are either extremely high or extremely low. High-energy intakes are expected of athletes who have a large body mass to support, extremely high training/exercise loads or the additional energy requirement for growth or purposeful increase in lean body mass. Such athletes are often recommended to consume extra energy, particularly in the form of CHO and/or protein, at special times or in greater quantities than that which would be provided in an everyday diet, or dictated by their appetite and hunger. These athletes may also need to consume energy during and after exercise when the availability of foods and fluids, or opportunities to consume them, are limited. Practical issues interfering with the achievement of energy-intake goals during post-exercise recovery include loss of appetite and fatigue, poor access to suitable foods, and distraction from other activities.

In contrast, other athletes need to restrict energy intake to reduce or maintain low body mass and body fat levels. This can be difficult to achieve in the face of hunger, customary eating patterns or the eating habits of peers. These athletes may also need to address their requirements for other nutrients within a reduced energy allowance. Specialised advice from a sports dietitian is often useful to assist in the achievement of the energy intake challenges faced by individual athletes. However, general principles that may assist in achieving such goals include being organised to have suitable foods on hand in a busy day, choosing foods that are either compact and easy to eat (for high-energy consumers) or high in satiety value (for those with low energy needs), and considering the micronutrient and macronutrient content of food within the framework of total energy allowances (for more information see Burke 2001).

Energy discrepancies in athletes: apparently low energy intakes

Dietary survey data shows that some athletes report large energy intakes commensurate with the energy requirements of prolonged daily training or competition sessions, or efforts to gain muscle size and strength. However, many endurance athletes, particularly females, appear to consume lower energy intakes than would be expected (Burke et al. 2001); in fact, these energy intakes often appear to be insufficient to support their training loads, let alone their basal energy requirements (Barr 1987). Several factors may explain apparently low energy intakes:

■ The athlete has been surveyed during a period of deliberate loss of body mass/body fat and is in a state of negative energy balance.

■ Energy efficiency.

■ Artefact of dietary survey methodology.

Although many athletes have a real requirement to undertake weight/fat loss to improve their health or performance (see section below), it is unlikely that all situations of apparently low energy intake by athletes arise from a deliberate and active phase of negative energy balance. As an alternative explanation, it has been suggested that some athletes are 'energy efficient'— that they can balance their basal metabolic needs and the energy cost of eating and exercise at a substantially lower than predicted energy intake (Manore & Thompson 2000). In addition to the dietary surveys of athletes that consistently report low energy intake, most dietary counsellors are familiar with challenging situations involving athletes who claim that they can't lose weight/body fat despite 'hardly eating anything'. The situation may be worse for female athletes, who already face strong societal pressure to be lean yet naturally carry higher levels of body fat despite undertaking similar training to their male counterparts. Some studies report that female distance runners with menstrual disturbances maintain energy balance on lower energy intakes than regularly menstruating runners who are matched for training volume (Barr 1987), although it is not clear whether menstrual dysfunction is the cause or effect of energy efficiencies.

There is research evidence both to support (Thompson et al. 1995) and to contradict (Edwards et al. 1993) the theory of energy efficiency. Athletes may have truly reduced energy requirements due to a reduction in resting metabolic rate, low activity levels outside the training program or an efficient exercise technique. Although these characteristics have been shown to exist in some individuals (Thompson et al. 1995), they are not as widespread as is commonly reported. In fact, in some studies of athletes whose apparent energy intakes were well below estimated energy requirements, there was convincing evidence of under-recording or under-eating during the period of investigation (Edwards et al. 1993; Schulz et al. 1992). It is suspected that athletes who are weight/physique conscious or dissatisfied with their body image are at highest risk of significant under-estimation errors when undertaking dietary surveys (Schulz et al. 1992; Edwards et al. 1993; Fogelholm et al. 1995). Reporting errors can be minimised when athletes are motivated to receive a true dietary assessment and when training to enhance record-keeping skills has been undertaken. Nevertheless, researchers and practitioners should be cautious in their interpretation of the results of self-reported assessments of dietary intake.

Achieving optimal physique

Physical characteristics, such as height, limb lengths, body mass, muscle mass and levels of body fat levels can all play a role in the performance of sport. An athlete's physique is determined by inherited characteristics, as well as the conditioning effects of his/her training program and diet.

There are several techniques that can be used to assess body fat levels or other aspects of physique, ranging from techniques that are best suited to the laboratory (e.g. underwater weighing, dual-energy X-ray absorptiometry [DEXA] scans) to protocols that are suited to the field. In practice, useful information about body composition can be collected from anthropometric data, such as skin-fold (subcutaneous) fat measurements, and various body girths and circumferences (Kerr 2000). Coaches or sports scientists who make these assessments on athletes should be well trained so that they have a small degree of error in repeating measurements. Often, coaches set rigid criteria for the 'ideal' physique of their athletes based on the characteristics of successful competitors. However, this process fails to take into account the considerable variability in the physical characteristics of athletes, even between individuals in the same sport. Therefore, it is dangerous to prescribe rigid targets for individuals, particularly with regard to body mass or body fat levels. The preferable strategy is to nominate a range of acceptable values for body fat and body mass within each sport, and then monitor the health and performance of individual athletes within this range. Sometimes it takes many years of training and maturation for an athlete to finally achieve his/her ideal shape and body composition.

Some athletes easily achieve the body composition that is best suited to their sport. However, others may need to manipulate characteristics such as muscle mass or body fat levels through changes in diet and training. Gain of muscle mass is desired by many athletes whose performance is linked to size, strength or power. In addition to the increase in muscle mass and strength that occurs during adolescence, particularly in males, many athletes pursue specific muscle hypertrophy gains through a program of progressive muscle overload. The chief nutritional requirement to support such a program is additional energy; this is required for the manufacture of new muscle tissue, as well as to provide fuel for the training program that supplied the stimulus for this muscle growth. Many athletes do not achieve a sufficiently positive energy balance to optimise muscle gains during a strength-training program; individual advice can help the athlete to improve this situation by making foods/drinks accessible and easy to consume (Burke 2001). It should be noted that there is little rigorous scientific study of the amount of energy required, the optimal ratio of macronutrients supplying this energy and the requirements for micronutrients to enhance muscle size.

Since protein forms the most significant structural component of muscle, it is tempting to conclude that additional protein intake will stimulate muscle gain. Many strength-trained athletes consume very high protein intakes (> 2–3 g/kg BM/day), two to three times the dietary reference intakes (DRIs) for protein in most countries, in the belief that this will enhance the gains from resistance training programs. However, the value of very high protein intakes per se in optimising muscle gains remains unsupported by the scientific literature (Lemon 1991; Lemon 2000). Instead, there is recent evidence that *timing* the intake of protein and *carbohydrate* immediately after, or even before, a resistance training session is a useful strategy to increase the muscle retention of protein and overall protein balance (Rasmussen et al. 2000; Tipton et al. 2001). Protein needs for athletes are discussed on page 160.

There are situations when athletes are clearly carrying excess body fat and will improve their health and performance by reducing body fat levels. This may occur due to heredity or lifestyle factors, or because the athlete has been in a situation of sudden energy imbalance; for example, failing to reduce energy intake while injured or taking a break from training. Loss of body fat should be achieved through a program based on a sustained and moderate energy deficit; that is, a decrease in dietary energy intake and, perhaps, an increase in energy expenditure through aerobic exercise or activity (O'Connor et al. 2000). In other sports, however, low body fat levels offer performance advantages in terms of the energy cost of movement (e.g. distance running, cycling, gymnastics) or aesthetics (e.g. gymnastics, body building). In many such weight/fat-conscious sports, athletes strive to achieve minimum body fat levels per se, or at least reduce body fat levels below what seems their 'natural' or 'healthy' level. In the short-term this may produce an improvement in performance. However, the long-term disadvantages include outcomes related to having very low body fat stores, as well as the problems associated with unsound weight loss methods. Excessive training, chronically low intakes of energy and nutrients, and psychological distress are often involved in fat loss strategies and may cause long-term damage to health, happiness or performance.

Some sports set competition goals of matching competitors of equal size and strength via the setting of weight divisions; these sports include combative sports (e.g. boxing, judo, wrestling), lightweight rowing and weight-lifting. Unfortunately, the culture and common practice in these sports is to try to compete in a weight division that is considerably lighter than normal training body mass (Brownell et al 1987; Steen & Brownell 1990). Athletes then 'make weight' over the days prior to competition by dehydrating (e.g. via saunas, exercising in 'sweat clothes', diuretics) and restricting food and fluid intake. There are a number of disadvantages arising from these practices: the short-term penalties include the effects of dehydration and inadequate fuel status on performance, while the long-term penalties include psychological stress, chronic inadequate nutrition and effects on hormone status (for review see Walberg-Rankin 2000). The potential problems associated with extreme weight-making practices should not be underestimated. The worst-case scenario is the death of the athlete, as occurred in 1997 in three separate situations involving college wrestlers in the United States. Athletes in these sports are guided to make better choice of the appropriate competition weight division and to achieve necessary weight loss by safe and long-term strategies to reduce body fat levels (Walberg-Rankin 2000).

'Ideal' weight and body fat targets should be set in terms of ranges and should consider measures of long-term health and performance, as well as the athlete's ability to eat a diet that is adequate in energy and nutrients, and free of unreasonable food-related stress. Some racial groups or individuals are naturally light and have low levels of body fat, or can achieve these without paying a substantial penalty. Furthermore, some athletes vary their body fat levels over a season so that very low levels are achieved only for a specific and short time. In general, however, athletes should not undertake strategies to minimise body fat levels unless they can be sure there are no side-effects or disadvantages. Compared to sedentary populations, there appears to be a higher risk of eating disorders or disordered eating behaviour and body perceptions among female athletes, and among athletes in sports in which success is associated with specific weight targets or low body fat levels. Even where clinical eating disorders do not exist, many athletes appear to be 'restrained eaters', reporting not only energy intakes that are considerably less than their expected energy requirements but considerable stress related to food intake. The 'female athlete triad'—the coexistence of disordered eating, disturbed menstrual function and suboptimal bone density—has received considerable publicity and will be discussed in greater detail on page 164. Expert advice from sports medicine professionals, including dietitians, psychologists and physicians, is important in the early detection and management of problems related to body composition and nutrition.

Meeting requirements for protein and micronutrients

Protein requirements for exercise

Prolonged daily training increases protein requirements, not only to support muscle gain and repair of damaged body tissues but to meet the small contribution of protein oxidation to the fuel requirements of prolonged exercise. While athletes undertaking recreational or light training activities will normally meet their protein needs within population DRIs, for heavily training athletes the guidelines for protein intake have been increased to 1.2–1.6 g/kg BM/day. These guidelines apply to both strength-trained and endurance athletes (for review see Lemon 1991). It is expected that these intakes would be met within the increased energy allowances that accompany training. Indeed, most dietary surveys show that athletes report protein intakes within or above these goals when protein is consumed at levels providing 12–18% of dietary intake. As a result, it is considered unnecessary for athletes who undertake strength or resistance training to eat excessive amounts of protein-rich foods or buy expensive protein supplements, although sports foods such as liquid meal supplements and sports bars may be useful to allow the athlete to achieve high energy needs.

Vitamins and minerals play important roles as cofactors for key reactions in energy metabolism or the synthesis of new tissues. Athletes are interested to know if a heavy program of exercise increases the requirement for micronutrients, and if the intake of additional amounts of vitamins and minerals will enhance performance by 'supercharging' these key reactions. The key factors that underpin the general adequacy of an athlete's diet are a varied eating plan based on nutrient-rich foods and a moderate-to-high energy intake. Dietary surveys of athletes show that when these factors are in place, the reported intakes of vitamins and minerals are well in excess of population DRIs and are likely to meet any increases in micronutrient demand caused by training. Furthermore, research has failed to show clear evidence of an increase in performance following vitamin supplementation, except in the case where a pre-existing deficiency was corrected (for review see Fogelholm 2000). On this basis, routine vitamin supplementation by athletes is not justified.

However, not all athletes achieve variety or adequate energy intake in their eating plans. Situations of suboptimal intake of micronutrients may occur in athletes who are restrained or disordered eaters and those following fad diets. Other risk factors for a restricted food range include poor practical nutrition skills, inadequate finances and an overcommitted lifestyle that limits access to food and causes erratic meal schedules. The best long-term management plan is to educate athletes to improve the quality and quantity of their food intake. However, a vitamin/mineral supplement, providing a broad range of micronutrients in doses similar to DRIs, may be useful when the athlete is unwilling or unable to make dietary changes, or when the athlete is travelling to places with an uncertain food supply and eating schedule.

Iron deficiency anaemia and sport

Minerals are the micronutrients at most risk of inadequate intake in the diets of athletes. Inadequate iron status can reduce exercise performance via suboptimal levels of haemoglobin and, perhaps, iron-related muscle enzymes (see Deakin 2000). Finding the true prevalence of problematic iron deficiency in people who undertake strenuous training is difficult, since it is hard to distinguish true iron deficiency from alterations in iron status measures that are caused by exercise itself (e.g. changes in plasma volume, acute phase responses to training). Reduction of blood haemoglobin concentrations due to plasma volume expansion, often termed 'sports anaemia', does not impair exercise performance (see Deakin 2000). Further issues to consider in making a diagnosis of iron deficiency in athletes are:

- At what stage of iron depletion are impairments to exercise performance observed?
- What is optimal iron status for an athlete, particularly in endurance sports where oxygen delivery to the muscle is important?

At present, we do not have definitive answers to these questions. Although it is easy to detect a haemoglobin level that is below reference ranges, it is difficult to confirm optimal iron status from a single blood test when values fall within the normal limits. Although the effects of gradually reduced haemoglobin on performance have not been systematically studied, it is possible that even a small decline in haemoglobin levels (e.g. 1–2 mg/100 mL) will reduce the competition performance of athletes (Eichner 2000). It is possible that athletes may show a haemoglobin level that is within reference standards but below the level that is 'usual' for them and required for their optimal performance. It is useful to collect a long-term history of iron status results from individual athletes to establish a feel for what is normal for them, and how parameters may vary across the training season or with different interventions. Athletes often believe that the 'more is better' principal applies to haemoglobin levels per se. However, in the absence of haemoconcentration due to dehydration, very high haemoglobin levels are usually explained by genetic individuality or drug use (e.g. erythropoietin [EPO]) and are not possible for most athletes to achieve.

Currently, there is no clear evidence that iron depletion in the absence of anaemia (i.e. reduced serum ferritin concentrations) is a cause of impaired exercise performance (for review see Deakin 2000). However, studies have failed to address the complaint commonly made by athletes with reduced iron stores, namely that they feel fatigued and fail to recover between a series of competition or training sessions. Since low ferritin levels may become progressively lower and eventually lead to iron-deficiency anaemia, there is merit in monitoring the iron status of athletes deemed to be at high risk of iron depletion and implementing an intervention as soon as iron status appears to decline substantially or to symptomatic levels. Evaluation and management of iron status should be undertaken on an individual basis by a sports medicine expert. Prevention and treatment of iron deficiency may include iron supplementation. However, the management plan should be based on long-term interventions to reverse negative iron balance—interventions that reduce or prevent excessive iron losses and dietary counselling to increase the intake of bioavailable iron. Risk factors that commonly lead to iron depletion in athletes are summarised in Table 8.2.

Although iron supplements are available as over-the-counter medications, there are dangers in self-prescription or long-term supplementation in the absence of medical follow-up. Iron supplementation is not a replacement for medical and dietary assessment and therapy since it typically fails to correct underlying problems that have caused iron drain. Chronic supplementation with high doses of iron carries a risk of iron overload, especially in males for whom the genetic traits for haemochromatosis are more prevalent. Iron supplements can also interfere with the absorption of other minerals, such as zinc and copper.

Dietary interventions to improve iron status not only need to increase total iron intake but need to increase the bioavailability of dietary iron. The heme form of iron found in red meat, liver and shellfish is better absorbed

TABLE 8.2 Risk factors for iron deficiency in athletes

PREDICTORS OF INCREASED IRON REQUIREMENTS	PREDICTORS OF INCREASED IRON LOSSES OR IRON MALABSORPTION	PREDICTORS OF INADEQUATE INTAKE OF BIOAVAILABLE IRON
■ Recent growth spurt in adolescents. ■ Pregnancy (current or within the past year).	■ Sudden increase in heavy training load, particularly running on hard surfaces, causing an increase in intravascular haemolysis. ■ Gastrointestinal bleeding due to chronic use of some anti-inflammatory drugs, ulcers or other problems. ■ Gastrointestinal malabsorption problems (e.g. Crohn's disease, ulcerative colitis, parasitic infestation). ■ Heavy menstrual blood losses. ■ Excessive blood losses, such as frequent nose bleeds, recent surgery, substantial contact injuries. ■ Frequent blood donation.	■ Chronic low energy intake (<2000 kcal or 8 MJ per day). ■ Vegetarian eating—especially poorly constructed diets in which alternative food sources of iron are ignored (e.g. legumes, nuts and seeds). ■ Fad diets or erratic eating patterns. ■ Restricted variety of foods in diet, and failure to promote matching of iron-containing foods with dietary factors that promote iron absorption. ■ Over-consumption of micronutrient-poor convenience foods and sports foods (high-CHO powders, unfortified bars and gels). ■ Very high CHO diet with high fibre content and infrequent intake of meats/fish/chicken. ■ Natural food diets: failure to consume iron-fortified cereal foods, such as commercial breakfast cereals and bread.

than organic or non-heme iron found in plant foods, such as fortified and wholegrain cereal foods, legumes and green leafy vegetables. However, iron bioavailability can be manipulated by matching iron-rich foods with dietary factors promoting iron absorption (e.g. vitamin C and other food acids, 'meat factor' found in animal flesh) and reducing the interaction with iron inhibitory factors (e.g. phytates in fibre-rich cereals, tannins in tea). Of course, changes to iron intake must be achieved with eating patterns that are compatible with the athlete's other nutrition goals (e.g. achieving fuel requirements for sport, achieving desired physique). Such education is often a specialised task requiring the expertise of a sports dietitian.

Calcium and bone health in athletes

Some athletes are at risk of problems with calcium status and bone health. Low bone density in athletes seems contradictory since exercise is considered to be one of the best protectors of bone health. However, a serious outcome of the menstrual disturbances frequently reported by female athletes is the high risk of either direct loss of bone density or failure to optimise the gain of peak bone mass that should occur during the 10–15 years after the onset of puberty. The exact cause of menstrual dysfunction in athletes is not clear but a major risk factor appears to be 'energy drain'—chronic periods of restricted energy intake in conjunction with high-energy expenditure (Loucks et al. 1998). Disordered eating and food-related stress are also often associated with menstrual dysfunction. The cluster of eating disorders, menstrual disturbances and suboptimal bone density has become known as 'the female athlete triad' (Yeager et al. 1993) in recognition that female athletes are at increased risk of developing one or more of these problems, and that the causes and outcomes are often closely linked. Individually, or in combination, these problems can directly impair athletic performance. Significantly, they reduce athletes' career span by increasing their risk of illness and injury, including stress fractures. Long-term problems, such as an increased risk of osteoporosis in later life, and chronic inadequate nutritional status might also be expected.

The prevention and management of the female athlete triad, or individual elements within it, require expertise and, ideally, the teamwork of sports doctors, dietitians, psychologists and the coach/fitness adviser. Dietary intervention is important to correct factors that underpin the menstrual dysfunction, as well as those that contribute to suboptimal bone density. Adequate energy intake and the reversal of disordered eating or inadequate nutrient intake are important. Adequate calcium intake is important for bone health, and requirements may be increased to 1200–1500 mg/day in athletes with impaired menstrual function. Where adequate calcium intake cannot be met through dietary means, usually through the use of low-fat dairy foods or calcium-enriched soy alternatives, a calcium supplement may be considered.

Acute nutrition strategies for competition

The nutritional challenges of competition vary according to the length and intensity of the event, the environment and the factors that influence the recovery between events or the opportunity to eat and drink during the event itself. To achieve optimal performance, the coach and athlete should identify factors that are likely to cause fatigue during the event and undertake nutrition strategies before, during and after the event that minimise or delay the onset of this fatigue. Various goals of competition nutrition are summarised in Table 8.1 and generally involve strategies to overcome dehydration and electrolyte imbalances, or carbohydrate depletion. Of course, these physiological challenges also occur during exercise sessions undertaken in the training phase. Therefore, the pre-, during- and post-event nutrition strategies discussed in this section should also be built into the training program. This will allow the athlete to achieve optimal performance and adaptations to training. In addition, they can practise any intended competition strategies to identify and fine-tune a successful plan.

Dehydration is a likely outcome in most sports events, with the effects being directly related to the degree of fluid deficit, the type of exercise and the environmental conditions. Dehydration of as little as 2% of body mass (1.5–2 L for most athletes) is sufficient to cause detectable changes to work output and perception of effort, especially when exercise is carried out in a hot environment; other penalties of fluid deficits include impairment of thermoregulation, reductions in skill and decision-making abilities and an increased risk of gastrointestinal problems (see Chapter 4).

CHO depletion can manifest as central fatigue (hypoglycaemia: blood glucose concentrations < 3 mmol/L) and/or peripheral fatigue (glycogen depletion in the working muscles). When CHO-intake strategies enhance or maintain CHO availability during exercise, they clearly enhance endurance or exercise capacity (for review see Hargreaves 1999). It is much more difficult to undertake studies that measure the effect on exercise *performance*, especially when it involves real-life competition, team sports or sports involving complex decision-making and motor skills. Nevertheless, when such studies are undertaken, many show benefits to various parameters of performance following strategies to enhance CHO availability.

Fuelling up before an event

The normal resting glycogen concentrations of the trained athlete (100–120 mmol/kg wet weight [ww]) appear adequate to meet the fuel needs of events lasting 60–90 minutes in duration. In the absence of severe muscle damage, such stores can be achieved by 24 hours of rest and an adequate CHO intake (7–10 g/kg BM/day) (Costill et al. 1981). In view of the typical rate of glycogen synthesis at 5 mmol/kg ww/h, athletes should allow 24–36 hours following their last training session to normalise fuel stores prior to non-endurance events. For many athletes this might be as simple as scheduling a day of rest or light training before the event while continuing to follow high-CHO eating patterns. However, not all athletes eat sufficient CHO in their usual diets to maximise glycogen storage, particularly females who restrict their total energy intake to control body fat levels. These athletes may need education or encouragement to relax their dietary restraint temporarily and prioritise refuelling as the major dietary goal on the day before competition. Similarly, some athletes may need to reorganise their training programs to allow a lighter training day or rest on the day prior to their event.

CHO loading for endurance events

The term 'CHO loading' is applied to nutrition practices that aim to maximise or supercompensate muscle glycogen stores prior to a competitive event that would otherwise deplete these fuel reserves. CHO loading strategies may elevate muscle glycogen stores to >160 mmol/kg ww. The earliest protocols were an outcome of a series of studies undertaken in the late 1960s by Scandinavian sports scientists, using muscle biopsy techniques to determine muscle glycogen stores following various exercise and dietary manipulations (Ahlborg et al. 1967; Bergstrom & Hultman 1966; Bergstrom et al. 1967; Hermannsen et al. 1967). These studies showed that pre-exercise muscle glycogen stores determined endurance or capacity for prolonged moderate-intensity exercise. In particular, a dietary protocol involving several days of a low CHO diet and exercise followed by several days of high CHO intake was found to supercompensate muscle glycogen stores and increase cycling time to exhaustion. These pioneering studies produced the classic seven-day model of CHO loading, involving a three to four day 'depletion' phase of hard training and low CHO intake, and finishing with a three to four day 'loading' phase of high CHO intake and exercise taper. Early field studies of prolonged running events showed that CHO loading enhanced sports performance, not by allowing the athlete to run faster but by prolonging the time that race pace could be maintained (Karlsson & Saltin 1971).

The extension of studies to include well-trained subjects enabled a 'modified' CHO loading strategy to be developed. Sherman and colleagues (1981) showed that runners were able to elevate their muscle glycogen stores with three days of taper and high CHO intake, regardless of whether this was preceded by a depletion phase or a more typical diet and training preparation. Thus, for well-trained athletes at least, CHO loading may be achieved simply as an extension of 'fuelling up' strategies (rest and high CHO intake) over one to three days prior to an event. The modified CHO loading protocol offers a more practical strategy for competition preparation by avoiding the fatigue and complexity of extreme diet and training requirements associated with the previous depletion phase.

Theoretically, CHO loading could enhance the performance of exercise or sporting events that would otherwise be limited by severe glycogen depletion. An increase in pre-event glycogen stores can prolong the duration for which moderate intensity exercise can be undertaken before fatiguing. It may also enhance the performance of a set amount of work (i.e. a set distance) by preventing the decline in pace or work output that would otherwise occur as glycogen stores decline towards the end of the task. In a recent review of CHO loading studies, Hawley et al. (1997) summarised that supercompensation of glycogen stores is beneficial for the performance of exercise of greater than 90 minutes duration, with the majority of studies investigating exercise protocols involving cycling or running. Typically, CHO loading will postpone fatigue and extend the duration of steady-state exercise by approximately 20%, and improve performance over a set distance or workload by 2–3% (Hawley et al. 1997).

It is more difficult to assess the effects of glycogen supercompensation on prolonged events of intermittent high-intensity exercise, such as team sports, even though they may be associated with significant glycogen depletion in at least some players. While it is intuitive that performance in such sports would be enhanced by supercompensation of muscle glycogen stores, it is extremely difficult to measure the 'performance' of sports that are variable and unpredictable or based on complex skills. On one hand, some studies have shown that pre-event enhancement of fuel stores is of benefit to the performance of the movement patterns in a soccer-simulated trial (Bangsbo et al. 1992), an indoor soccer game (Balsom et al. 1999) and a real-life ice hockey game (Akermark et al. 1996). In contrast, other studies have failed to detect significant improvement in the performance of skill-based tasks in a simulation of a soccer match (Abt et al. 1998). Decisions about the benefits of CHO loading may be specific not only to the sport but to the individual athletes, depending on the requirements of their position or style of play. Of course, the logistics of competition in many of these sports, where games may be played daily to twice a week, would prevent a full CHO loading preparation before each event. Nevertheless, athletes in these sports should fuel up prior to each competition as well as is practical and perhaps experiment with an extended preparation before the most important games, such as the final of the tournament.

The pre-event meal

Foods and drinks consumed in the pre-event meal (i.e. 1–4 h prior to exercise) have a role in fine-tuning competition preparation to meet the goals summarised in Table 8.3.

The pre-event meal menu should include CHO-rich foods and drinks (see Table 8.4 for suggestions), especially in the case where body CHO stores are suboptimal or where the event is of sufficient duration and intensity to challenge these stores. CHO availability is enhanced by increasing muscle and liver glycogen stores (Coyle et al. 1985), as well as by the storage of glucose in the gastrointestinal space for later release. Since liver glycogen stores are labile and may be substantially depleted by an overnight fast, pre-exercise CHO intake on the morning of an event may be important for maintaining blood glucose levels via hepatic glucose output during the latter stages of prolonged exercise. Compared to trials undertaken after an overnight fast, the intake of a substantial amount of CHO (200–300 g) in the 2–4 hours before exercise has been shown to prolong cycling endurance (Wright et al. 1991) and enhance performance of an exercise test undertaken at the end of a standardised cycling task (Neufer et al. 1987; Sherman et al. 1989).

In the field it is not always practical to consume a substantial CHO-rich meal or snack in the 4 hours before a sporting event. For example, it is unlikely that an athlete will want to sacrifice sleep to eat a large meal before an early morning race start. Most would settle for a lighter meal or snack before the event and consume CHO throughout the event to balance missed fuelling opportunities. A smaller pre-event meal may also make sense for athletes predisposed to gastrointestinal discomfort. Foods with a low-fat, low-fibre and low–moderate protein content are the preferred choice for the pre-event menu since they are less prone to cause gastrointestinal upsets (Rehrer et al. 1992). Liquid meal supplements or CHO-containing drinks and bars are useful for athletes who suffer from pre-event nerves or an uncertain pre-event timetable.

TABLE 8.3 Goals of the pre-event meal (adapted from Burke 2000a)

1 Continue to fuel muscle glycogen stores if they have not fully restored or loaded since the last exercise session.

2 Restore liver glycogen content, especially for events undertaken in the morning where liver stores are depleted from an overnight fast.

3 Ensure that the athlete is well-hydrated.

4 Prevent hunger, yet avoid the gastrointestinal discomfort and upset often experienced during exercise.

5 Include foods and practices that are important to the athlete's psychology or superstitions.

TABLE 8.4 Practical CHO-rich food choices to meet special situations in sport

CHO-RICH CHOICES FOR PRE-EVENT MEALS

Breakfast cereal + low-fat milk + fresh/ canned fruit

Muffins or crumpets + jam/honey

Pancakes + syrup

Toast + baked beans (this is a high-fibre choice)

Creamed rice (made with low-fat milk)

Rolls or sandwiches with banana filling

Fruit salad + low-fat fruit yoghurt

Spaghetti with tomato or low-fat sauce

Baked potatoes with low-fat filling

Fruit smoothie (low-fat milk + fruit + yoghurt/ ice-cream)

Liquid meal supplement (e.g. Sustagen Sport)

CHO-RICH FOODS SUITABLE FOR INTAKE DURING EXERCISE (50 G PORTIONS)

600–800 mL Sports drink

2 sports gels

1–1.5 sports bars

2 cereal bars or breakfast bars

Large bread roll filled with jam/honey/cheese

2 bananas or 3 medium pieces of other fruit

100–120 g cake or muffin

100 g fruit bread or bun

60 g jelly/jube confectionery

450 mL cola soft drinks

80 g chocolate bar

POST-EXERCISE RECOVERY SNACKS

(Each serve provides 50 g CHO + valuable source of protein and micronutrients.)

250–350 mL of liquid meal supplement or milkshake/fruit smoothie

Sports bar + 200 mL sports drink

Cup of breakfast cereal + milk + banana or tinned fruit

250 g tin of baked beans or spaghetti on 2 slices of toast or in jaffle

1 round of sandwiches with cheese/meat/chicken filling + 1 piece of fruit

1.5 cups fruit salad with 100 g fruit-flavoured yoghurt or custard

Carton of fruit-flavoured yoghurt + muesli bar or breakfast bar

2 crumpets or English muffins with thick spread of peanut butter

250 g (large) baked potato with cottage cheese or grated cheese filling

200 g thick crust pizza with lean meat/chicken/ seafood and vegetable toppings

330 g creamed rice (1.5 cups)

PORTABLE CHO-RICH FOODS SUITABLE FOR THE TRAVELLING ATHLETE

Breakfast cereal (+ skim milk powder)

Cereal bars, breakfast bars

Dried fruit

Rice crackers, dry biscuits

Spreads—jam, honey, etc.

Sports bars

Liquid meal supplements—powder and ready-to- drink Tetra packs

Sports drink

Athletes should also be conscious of fluid needs and consume adequate fluid to ensure that they are well-hydrated at the start of the event. This is particularly important for events that are conducted in the heat, especially for lengthy periods or at high intensities, or for situations where the athlete is recovering from dehydration caused by previous exercise or 'weight-making attempts'. In these situations, athletes may need to be proactive with rehydration strategies or even undertake hyperhydration strategies in preparation for their event (see Chapter 4).

Since competition often occurs away from home, athletes should have a flexible pre-event meal plan that can be adapted to the available food supply and catering options. Many special or important foods can be taken by athletes to their competition location; portable and easy-to-prepare options include breakfast cereal, sports bars, cereal bars and liquid meal supplements (see Table 8.4). Above all, athletes should choose a strategy that suits their individual situation and their past experiences, which can be fine-tuned with further experimentation.

CHO intake in the hour before exercise

Despite the benefits previously discussed, the issue of CHO intake prior to exercise is not straightforward. CHO eaten in the hours prior to exercise causes a series of metabolic perturbations: the stimulation of insulin following CHO intake suppresses lipolysis and subsequent fat utilisation during exercise, while increasing CHO oxidation compared to exercise in a fasted state. These effects can be seen when CHO is consumed up to 4 hours before exercise (Coyle et al. 1985) but are most pronounced when CHO is consumed in the final hour prior to exercise. Typical outcomes include a transient drop in plasma glucose levels at the start of exercise and an increased rate of muscle glycogen utilisation. In most athletes, these metabolic perturbations are either minor or transient and are not detrimental to performance. In most cases, the decline in blood glucose level observed during the first 20 minutes of exercise is self-corrected with no apparent effects on the athlete. In fact, many studies show that CHO intake in the hour prior to exercise can enhance performance by enhancing body CHO status (for review of the literature see Hawley & Burke 1997).

Nevertheless, there seems to be a small proportion of athletes who respond negatively to CHO intake in the hour before exercise. These athletes experience an exaggerated CHO oxidation and decrease in blood glucose concentrations at the start of exercise, suffering symptoms of hypoglycaemia and a rapid onset of fatigue. Precisely why some athletes experience such an extreme reaction is unclear. Risk factors identified in a recent study include the intake of small amounts of CHO (< 50 g), increased sensitivity to insulin, a lower sympathetic-induced counter-regulation and a low–moderate workload in the subsequent exercise bout (Kuipers et al. 1999). Not all athletes who experience a major decline in blood glucose concentrations experience hypoglycaemic symptoms; there is preliminary evidence that sensitisation to low glucose levels may adapt the athlete to an increased threshold before symptoms are reported (Kuipers et al. 1999).

Nevertheless, these effects are so clear-cut that at-risk athletes will be identified easily. Preventative action for this group includes a number of options, which are summarised in Table 8.5.

It has been proposed that pre-event meals based on CHO sources with a low glycaemic index (GI) will provide a performance benefit for all athletes undertaking prolonged exercise (Thomas et al. 1991) by achieving an attenuation of the post-meal insulin response and better maintenance of CHO throughout the exercise bout. The literature shows that CHO meals based on low GI foods achieve a lower post-prandial blood glucose response and a generally attenuated decline in blood glucose concentrations at the onset of exercise (see Burke 2000a). There is also some, but not complete, evidence that CHO availability and oxidation is better maintained throughout the exercise compared with the consumption of a high GI CHO meal. However, most studies fail to show performance benefits arising from the consumption of a low GI pre-event meal in comparison to a high GI CHO meal, even when metabolism has been altered throughout the exercise (see Burke 2000a). Importantly, one study has shown that when CHO is consumed during exercise according to sports nutrition guidelines, the effects of pre-exercise CHO intake on both metabolism and cycling performance are diminished (Burke et al. 1998).

Individual athletes must judge the benefits and the practical issues associated with pre-exercise CHO intake in their particular sporting situation. In cases where athletes may not be able to consume CHO during a prolonged event or workout, they may find it useful to choose a menu based on low GI CHO foods to promote a more sustained release of CHO throughout exercise. However, there is no evidence of universal benefits from such menu choices, particularly when athletes are able to refuel during their session, or where their favoured and familiar food choices have a high GI. In the overall scheme, pre-event eating needs to balance a number of factors, including the athlete's food likes, availability of choices and gastrointestinal comfort.

TABLE 8.5 Strategies for athletes who experience an extreme reaction to CHO consumed in the hour prior to exercise

1   Experiment to find the critical time before exercise that CHO intake should be avoided.

2   Consume a substantial amount of CHO in the pre-event snack/meal (> 70 g).

3   Choose CHO-rich choices with a low glycaemic index in the pre-event menu, as these have an attenuated and sustained blood glucose and insulin response.

4   Include some high-intensity sprints during the warm-up to the event to stimulate hepatic glucose output.

5   Consume CHO during the event.

Fluid and CHO during the event

In events lasting longer than 30 minutes there is likely to be both a need and an opportunity for replacement of fluid and CHO during the session. The benefits of consuming fluid to reduce the fluid deficit incurred via sweating have already been discussed in Chapter 4. This chapter focuses on changes in guidelines for fluid and CHO intake that have occurred over the past decades. Despite the evidence, at least in some situations of exercise, that the benefits of consuming CHO and fluid are independent and additive (Below et al. 1995), in the past there have been some difficulties in finding ways to integrate these strategies.

Sports drinks became commercially available in the early 1970s, with the aim of replacing the fluid and electrolytes lost in sweat in a sweetened (palatable) form. At that time, the main scientific concern regarding endurance sport was to prevent dehydration by consuming fluids that were readily emptied and absorbed into the body. The available studies showed that compared to the ingestion of water, drinks containing CHO in concentrations greater than 2% (2 g/100 mL) slowed the rate of gastric emptying (Costill & Saltin 1974). Therefore, the official guidelines from expert bodies such as the American College of Sports Medicine (ACSM) during the 1970s and 1980s (ACSM 1975, 1987) promoted water as the best drink to consume during prolonged exercise and recommended that if CHO–electrolyte drinks were used, they should be diluted from 6–8% CHO to 2% CHO concentrations. Based on such official advice, sports drinks were labelled as too concentrated and too salty.

The results of research during the 1980s and 1990s, often funded by sports drink companies, helped to change this official position. Information collected in these studies 'rediscovered' the benefits of CHO intake during exercise on the performance of endurance events and team games, and even high-intensity exercise of 60 minutes duration (for review see Hargreaves 1999). Based on these findings, current sports nutrition guidelines recommend a CHO intake of 30–60 g/h during exercise of more than 60 minutes, with CHO intake starting well in advance of fatigue or depletion of body CHO stores. The major mechanisms to explain the benefits of CHO intake during prolonged exercise are the maintenance of plasma glucose concentration and high rates of CHO oxidation when muscle CHO stores become depleted (Coyle et al. 1986). The recent evidence that CHO intake may benefit shorter duration endurance events lasting about 1 hour (e.g. Jeukendrup et al. 1997) is puzzling, since in these situations muscle CHO stores are not thought to be limiting. Further research is needed to confirm and explain these observations.

There is some evidence that the benefits from combining two strategies that enhance CHO availability—for example, a combination of eating a high CHO meal before the event and consuming CHO during the event—are additive (Chryssanthopoulos & Williams 1997; Wright et al. 1991; Febbraio et al. 2000). Recently Febbraio et al. (2000) investigated the effects of CHO ingestion before and during exercise and in combination on glucose kinetics, metabolism and performance. These workers observed that pre-exercise ingestion of CHO improved performance only when CHO ingestion was maintained throughout exercise, and that even when CHO was ingested in large quantities before and during exercise, the amount of glucose disappearance was relatively minor compared to the overall rates of CHO oxidation (Febbraio et al. 2000). They concluded that the maintenance of high plasma glucose concentrations throughout exercise was important and appeared to increase exercise performance. Clearly, further studies of single CHO strategies or combinations of strategies need to be conducted over a greater range of sports and exercise events so that scientists can give more detailed advice to athletes.

Although the original guidelines warned against adding substantial amounts of CHO to fluids consumed during exercise, these concerns have been overcome by research using better techniques of measuring gastric emptying and intestinal uptake or monitoring whole-body fluid balance. These newer studies showed that drinks of 4–8% CHO were able to promote effective rehydration as well as deliver a useful fuel source. In addition, it was recognised that voluntary intake of fluid, which provides an important determinant of rehydration in real-life activities, is enhanced by adding sodium and a palatable flavour to water. Thus, the most recent guidelines on rehydration during exercise from bodies such as the ACSM now encourage commercially available sports drinks (4–8% CHO solutions, 10–25 mmol/L sodium) as an effective way to provide fluid and CHO during a range of sports and exercise activities (ACSM 1996). In practice, athletes use a variety of drinks and food choices (see Table 8.4) as well as sports drinks to achieve fluid and CHO needs.

Official guidelines for fluid and CHO intake strategies during exercise have also evolved in terms of how athletes are educated to achieve optimal practice. Early guidelines for fluid intake during prolonged events were focused on distance running and the availability of aid stations to provide drinks to participants at regular intervals (ACSM 1975, 1987). It was felt that athletes were assisted by guidelines based on prescriptive examples, such as the amount of fluid that should be drunk at various time intervals or spaces between aid stations (e.g. 150–250 mL every 2–3 km). Although these guidelines might have been proposed as an example or a useful starting point, they were often interpreted as a definite rule. In fact, they have been shown to be impractical if applied literally, leading to severe dehydration in some athletes and discomfort from excessive fluid intake in others (Coyle & Montain 1992). Furthermore, they did not take into account the wide variety of sports and exercise activities in which fluid intake will benefit the safety, enjoyment and performance of the session.

Accordingly, the most recent guidelines for fluid intake during exercise recognise the variable nature of sport and exercise activities and individual differences that occur between people (ACSM 1996). Issues that must be taken into account include individual sweat rates and fluid needs, sports-specific opportunities for fluid intake and practical challenges, such as making fluid available, preventing gastrointestinal discomfort and being aware of fluid needs. Recent guidelines for fluid intake during exercise (ACSM 1996) recognise that since dehydration has a progressive effect on exercise performance (Montain & Coyle 1992), the achievement of an improvement in fluid balance is worthwhile. Therefore, emphasis is no longer on absolute fluid intakes but on individual opportunities to improve on previous fluid intake practices. Newer guidelines emphasise attitudes and behaviours that can be changed to increase fluid intake and enhance fluid balance during sport and exercise. There is also consideration that individuals can experiment with their own fluid intake plans and learn to make this a comfortable habit.

Post-exercise recovery

Recovery after exercise poses an important challenge to the modern athlete who may be required to undertake two training sessions a day or compete in events with heats and finals (e.g. swimming or track and field events) or multi-day competition (e.g. tennis tournaments or cycling stage races). Recovery encompasses a complex range of nutrition-related issues, including restoration of muscle and liver glycogen stores, replacement of fluid and electrolytes lost in sweat, and regeneration, repair and adaptation processes following the catabolic stress and damage caused by the exercise. In many situations, optimal recovery after training or competition will only occur with a specific and organised nutrition plan. After all, thirst and voluntary fluid intake are unlikely to keep pace with large sweat losses. In addition, typical Western eating patterns are unlikely to provide CHO intakes that reach the threshold of daily glycogen storage. These plans must be made in recognition of the practical factors that interfere with an athlete's post-exercise fluid and food intake plans (Table 8.6). This is particularly important for travelling athletes, who may be challenged by an inaccessible and foreign food supply and should consider taking their own food supplies (see Table 8.4).

TABLE 8.6 Practical factors interfering with post-exercise fluid and food intake

- Fatigue—interfering with ability/interest to obtain or eat food.
- Loss of appetite following high-intensity exercise.
- Limited access to (suitable) foods at exercise venues.
- Other post-exercise commitments and priorities (e.g. coach's meetings, drug tests, equipment maintenance, warm-down activities).
- Traditional post-competition activities (e.g. excessive alcohol intake).

Factors promoting rehydration

Despite improved fluid intake practices during exercise, most athletes can expect to be at least mildly dehydrated at the end of their session (e.g. fluid losses equal to 2–5% BM). It may take 6–24 hours for complete rehydration following such losses. Issues of fluid balance are covered in greater detail in Chapter 4. In essence, the success of post-exercise rehydration is dependent on how much the athlete drinks, and then how much of this fluid is retained and re-equilibrated within body fluid compartments. When it is important to encourage voluntary fluid intake, flavoured drinks have been shown to encourage greater intake than plain water (Carter & Gisolfi 1989). Urine losses appear to be minimised by the timely replacement of lost electrolytes, particularly sodium (Shirreffs et al. 1996). The inclusion of sodium in a rehydration drink is an important strategy in the rapid recovery of moderate–high fluid deficits. However, the optimal sodium level is about 50–80 mmol/L, as found in oral rehydration solutions used in the treatment of diarrhoea. This is considerably higher than the concentrations found in commercial sports drinks and may be unpalatable to many athletes.

Creatively planned meals and snacks may be consumed with fluids to fulfil all post-event recovery needs simultaneously; for example: salty CHO-rich foods such as bread and breakfast cereals, or rice and pasta meals with added salt. Since caffeine and alcohol increase diuresis, consumption of alcoholic and caffeine-containing drinks during post-exercise recovery may result in greater fluid losses compared to other fluids (González-Alonso et al. 1992; Shirreffs & Maughan 1997). However, the increased fluid losses may be more than offset by an increased voluntary intake of fluids that are well-liked by the athlete. Of course, intakes of large amounts of alcohol may interfere with recovery, particularly by distracting athletes from undertaking their recommended dietary practices and promoting high-risk behaviour (Burke & Maughan 2000).

Factors promoting muscle glycogen restoration

Maximal rates of post-exercise muscle glycogen storage reported during the first 12 hours of recovery are within the range of 5–10 mmol/kg ww/h (Blom et al. 1987; Ivy et al. 1988b; Reed et al. 1989). Coyle (1991) has noted that with a mean glycogen storage rate of 5–6 mmol/kg ww/h, 20–24 hours of recovery are required for normalisation of muscle glycogen levels following exercise-induced depletion. However, the training and competition schedules of many athletes often provide considerably less time than this. Since performance in subsequent exercise sessions may depend on the success of muscle CHO restoration strategies, many athletes may compromise subsequent performance by beginning with inadequate muscle fuel stores. Several factors that are within the control of the athlete and can enhance or impair the rate of muscle glycogen storage are shown in Table 8.7.

The main dietary factor involved in post-event refuelling is the amount of CHO consumed, with a daily threshold for muscle glycogen storage being 7–10 g/kg BM/day for the typical athlete (Costill et al. 1981), although in some cases of very well-trained athletes, CHO intakes of 12 g/kg BM/day may further increase muscle glycogen stores (Coyle et al. 2001). There is some evidence that moderate and high GI CHO-rich foods and drinks may be more favourable for glycogen storage than some low GI food choices (Burke et al. 1993). Since glycogen storage may occur at a slightly faster rate during the first couple of hours after exercise, athletes are often advised to begin refuelling immediately after exercise. However, the main reason for promoting CHO-rich meals or snacks soon after exercise is that effective refuelling does not start until a substantial amount of CHO (~1 g/kg BM) is consumed (Ivy et al. 1988a). Rapid refuelling strategies are important when there is less than 8 hours between exercise sessions, but when recovery time is longer, immediate intake of CHO after exercise is unnecessary and athletes should choose their preferred meal/snack schedule for achieving total CHO intake goals (Parkin et al. 1997).

The form of the CHO intake—fluids or solids—does not appear to affect glycogen synthesis (Keizer et al. 1986; Reed et al. 1989). Similarly, the frequency of meals—several large meals or regular small snacks—has little impact on rates of glycogen storage over a day as long as CHO intake targets are met (Costill et al. 1981; Burke et al. 1996). Whereas earlier research

TABLE 8.7 Factors affecting restoration of muscle glycogen stores
(from Burke 2000b)

FACTORS THAT ENHANCE THE RATE OF RESTORATION	FACTORS THAT HAVE MINIMAL EFFECT ON RATE OF RESTORATION	FACTORS THAT REDUCE THE RATE OF RESTORATION
■ Depleted stores—the lower the stores the faster the rate of recovery.	■ Gentle exercise during recovery.	■ Damage to the muscle (contact injury or delayed-onset muscle soreness caused by eccentric exercise).
■ Immediate intake of CHO after exercise.	■ Spacing of meals and snacks (provided total amount of CHO is adequate).	■ Delay in intake of CHO after exercise.
■ Adequate amounts of CHO:	■ Other food at meals (e.g. fat- or protein-rich foods) provided that the total amount of CHO is adequate.	■ Inadequate amounts of CHO.
• 1–1.5 g CHO/kg BM immediately after exercise		■ Reliance on CHO-rich foods with a low GI.
• 7–10 g CHO/kg BM/ 24 h.		■ Prolonged and high-intensity exercise during recovery.
■ Focus on CHO-rich foods with a high GI.		

indicated that glycogen synthesis was enhanced by co-ingestion of protein with CHO intake immediately after exercise (Zawadzki et al. 1992), these findings have been refuted in recent studies in which the energy content of test meals was better matched (Tarnopolsky et al. 1997; Jentjens et al. 2001; van Hall et al. 2000). However, there is evidence of benefits to protein balance after exercise when CHO and protein sources are consumed in combination after exercise (Rasmussen et al. 2000; Tipton et al. 2001). Foods providing a substantial source of protein and CHO, as well as other micronutrients, are suggested in Table 8.4. Although the timing and amount of foods consumed after exercise may enhance aspects of post-exercise recovery, it is important that athletes are able to follow eating plans that meet the practical challenges of their busy days and their total nutrition goals.

Summary

Sports nutrition combines science and practice to assist athletes to be healthy, to be able to train effectively and to compete to the best of their ability. Specific requirement needs for individual nutrients must be met within a busy daily timetable and in conjunction with other nutrition goals. Special fluid and food intake strategies before, during and after exercise can improve performance and enhance subsequent recovery and a return to training and/or competition.

References

Abt G, Zhou S, Weatherby R. The effect of a high-carbohydrate diet on the skill performance of midfield soccer players after intermittent treadmill exercise. *J Sci Med Sport* 1998;1:203–12.

Ahlborg B, Bergstrom J, Brohult J. Human muscle glycogen content and capacity for prolonged exercise after difference diets. *Foersvarsmedicin* 1967;85–99.

Akermark C, Jacobs I, Rasmusson M, Karlsson J. Diet and muscle glycogen concentration in relation to physical performance in Swedish elite ice hockey players. *Int J Sport Nutr* 1996;6:272–84.

American College of Sports Medicine. Position statement of the American College of Sports Medicine: prevention of heat injuries during distance running. *Med Sci Sports Exerc* 1975;7:vii–ix.

American College of Sports Medicine. Position stand of the American College of Sports Medicine: the prevention of thermal injuries during distance running. *Med Sci Sports Exerc* 1987;19:529–33.

American College of Sports Medicine. Position stand: exercise and fluid replacement. *Med Sci Sports Exerc* 1996;28:i–vii.

Balsom PB, Wood K, Olsson P, Ekblom B. Carbohydrate intake and multiple sprint sports: with special reference to football (soccer). *Int J Sports Med* 1999;20:48–52.

Bangsbo J, Norregaard L, Thorsoe F. The effect of carbohydrate diet on intermittent exercise performance. *Int J Sports Med* 1992;13:152–7.

Barr SI. Women, nutrition and exercise: a review of athletes' intakes and a discussion of energy balance in active women. *Prog Food Nutr Sci* 1987;11:307–61.

Below PR, Mora-Rodriguez R, González-Alonso J, Coyle EF. Fluid and carbohydrate ingestion independently improve performance during 1 h of intense exercise. *Med Sci Sports Exerc* 1995;27:200–10.

Bergstrom J, Hermansen L, Hultman E, Saltin B. Diet, muscle glycogen and physical performance. *Acta Physiol Scand* 1967;71:140–50.

Bergstrom J, Hultman E. Muscle glycogen synthesis after exercise: an enhancing factor localised to the muscle cells in man. *Nature* 1966;210:309–10.

Blom PSC, Hostmark AT, Vaage O, Kardel KR, Maehlum S. Effect of different post-exercise sugar diets on the rate of muscle glycogen synthesis. *Med Sci Sports Exerc* 1987;19:491–6.

Brownell KD, Steen SN, Wilmore JH. Weight regulation practices in athletes: analysis of metabolic and health effects. *Med Sci Sports Exerc* 1987;19:546–56.

Burke L. Preparation for competition. In: Burke L, Deakin V, eds. *Clinical Sports Nutrition*. 2nd edn. Sydney: McGraw-Hill, 2000a: 341–68.

Burke L. Nutrition for recovery after competition and training. In: Burke L, Deakin V, eds. *Clinical Sports Nutrition*. 2nd edn. Sydney: McGraw-Hill, 2000b:396–427.

Burke LM. Energy needs of athletes. *Can J Appl Physiol* 2001;26 (suppl.):S202–S219.

Burke LM, Claassen A, Hawley JA, Noakes TD. Carbohydrate intake during prolonged cycling minimizes effect of glycemic index of preexercise meal. *J Appl Physiol* 1998;85:2220–6.

Burke LM, Collier GR, Davis PG, Fricker PA, Sanigorski AJ, Hargreaves M. Muscle glycogen storage following prolonged exercise: effect of the frequency of carbohydrate feedings. *Am J Clin Nutr* 1996;64:115–19.

Burke LM, Collier GR, Hargreaves M. Muscle glycogen storage following prolonged exercise: effect of the glycaemic index of carbohydrate feedings. *J Appl Physiol* 1993;75:1019–23.

Burke LM, Cox GR, Cummings NK, Desbrow B. Guidelines for daily CHO intake: do athletes achieve them? *Sports Med* 2001;31:267–99.

Burke LM, Maughan RJ. Alcohol in sport. In: Maughan RJ, ed. *IOC Encyclopaedia on Sports Nutrition*. London: Blackwell, 2000: 405–14.

Carter JE, Gisolfi CV. Fluid replacement during and after exercise in the heat. *Med Sci Sports Exerc* 1989;21:532–9.

Chryssanthopoulos C, Williams C. Pre-exercise carbohydrate meal and endurance running capacity when carbohydrates are ingested during exercise. *Int J Sports Med* 1997;18:543–8.

Costill DL, Saltin B. Factors limiting gastric emptying during rest and exercise. *J Appl Physiol* 1974;37:679–83.

Costill DL, Sherman WM, Fink WJ, Maresh C, Witten M, Miller JM. The role of dietary carbohydrates in muscle glycogen resynthesis after strenuous running. *Am J Clin Nutr* 1981;34:1831–6.

Coyle EF. Timing and method of increased carbohydrate intake to cope with heavy training, competition and recovery. *J Sports Sci* 1991;9(special issue):29–52.

Coyle EF, Coggan AR, Hemmert MK, Ivy JL. Muscle glycogen utilisation during prolonged strenuous exercise when fed carbohydrate. *J Appl Physiol* 1986;61:165–72.

Coyle EF, Coggan AR, Hemmert MK, Lowe RC, Walters TJ. Substrate usage during prolonged exercise following a pre-exercise meal. *J Appl Physiol* 1985;59:429–33.

Coyle EF, Jeukendrup AE, Oseto MC, Hodgkinson BJ, Zderic TW. Low-fat diet alters intramuscular substrates and reduces lipolysis and fat oxidation during exercise. *Am J Physiol Endocrin Metab* 2001;280:E391–E398.

Coyle EF, Montain SJ. Carbohydrate and fluid ingestion during exercise: are there trade-offs? *Med Sci Sports Exerc* 1992;24:671–8.

Deakin V. Iron depletion in athletes. In: Burke L, Deakin V, eds. *Clinical Sports Nutrition*. 2nd edn. Sydney: McGraw-Hill, 2000: 273–311.

Edwards JE, Lindeman AK, Mikesky AE, Stager JM. Energy balance in highly trained female endurance runners. *Med Sci Sports Exerc* 1993;25:1398–404.

Eichner ER. Minerals: iron. In: Maughan R, ed. *Nutrition in Sport*. London: Blackwell Science, 2000: 326–38.

Febbraio MA, Chiu A, Angus DJ, Arkinstall MJ, Hawley JA. Effects of carbohydrate ingestion before and during exercise on glucose kinetics and performance. *J Appl Physiol* 2000;89:2220–6.

Fogelholm M. Vitamins: metabolic functions. In: Maughan RJ, ed. *Nutrition in Sport*. Oxford: Blackwell Science, 2000: 266–80.

Fogelholm GM, Kukkonen-Harjula TK, Taipale SA, Sievanen HT, Oja P, Vuori IM. Resting metabolic rate and energy intake in female gymnasts, figure-skaters and soccer players. *Int J Sports Med* 1995;16:551–6.

González-Alonso J, Heaps CL, Coyle EF. Rehydration after exercise with common beverages and water. *Int J Sports Med* 1992;13:399–406.

Hargreaves M. Metabolic responses to CHO ingestion: effect on exercise performance. In: Lamb DR, Murray R, eds. *Perspectives in Exercise Science and Sports Medicine.* Vol. 12. *The Metabolic Basis of Performance in Exercise and Sport.* Carmel, IN: Cooper Publishing, 1999: 93–124.

Hawley JA, Burke LM. Effect of meal frequency and timing on physical performance. *Br J Nutr* 1997;77(suppl.):S91–S103.

Hawley JA, Schabort EJ, Noakes TD, Dennis SC. Carbohydrate-loading and exercise performance: an update. *Sports Med* 1997;24:73–81.

Hermanssen L, Hultman E, Saltin B. Muscle glycogen during prolonged severe exercise. *Acta Physiol Scand* 1967;129–39.

Ivy JL, Katz AL, Cutler CL, Sherman WM, Coyle EF. Muscle glycogen storage after exercise: effect of time of carbohydrate ingestion. *J Appl Physiol* 1988a;65:1480–5.

Ivy JL, Lee MC, Bronzinick JT, Reed MC. Muscle glycogen storage following different amounts of carbohydrate ingestion. *J Appl Physiol* 1988b:65:2018–23.

Jentjens RL, van Loon LJC, Mann CH, Wagenmakers AJM, Jeukendrup AE. Addition of protein and amino acids to carbohydrates does not enhance postexercise muscle glycogen synthesis. *J Appl Physiol* 2001;91:839–46.

Jeukendrup A, Brouns F, Wagenmakers AJM, Saris WHM. Carbohydrate–electrolyte feedings improve 1 h time trial cycling performance. *Int J Sports Med* 1997;18: 125–9.

Karlsson J, Saltin B. Diet, muscle glycogen, and endurance performance. *J Appl Physiol* 1971;31:203–6.

Keizer HA, Kuipers H, van Kranenburg G, Guerten, P. Influence of liquid and solid meals on muscle glycogen resynthesis, plasma fuel hormone response, and maximal physical work capacity. *Int J Sports Med* 1986;8:99–104.

Kerr D. Kinanthropometry: physique assessment of the athlete. In: Burke L, Deakin V, eds. *Clinical Sports Nutrition.* 2nd edn. Sydney: McGraw-Hill, 2000: 69–89.

Kuipers H, Fransen EJ, Keizer HA. Pre-exercise ingestion of carbohydrate and transient hypoglycemia during exercise. *Int J Sports Med* 1999;20:227–31.

Lemon PWR. Effect of exercise on protein requirements. *J Sports Sci* 1991;9:53–70.

Lemon PWR. Effects of exercise on protein metabolism. In: Maughan RJ, ed. *Nutrition in Sport.* Oxford: Blackwell Science, 2000: 133–52.

Loucks AB, Verdun M, Heath EM. Low energy availability, not stress of exercise, alters LH pulsatility in exercising women. *J Appl Physiol* 1998;84:37–46.

Manore M, Thompson J. Energy requirements of the athlete: assessment and evidence of energy efficiency. In: Burke L, Deakin V, eds. *Clinical Sports Nutrition.* 2nd edn. Sydney: McGraw-Hill, 2000: 124–45.

Montain SJ, Coyle EF. Influence of graded dehydration on hyperthermia and cardiovascular drift during exercise. *J Appl Physiol* 1992;73:1340–50.

Neufer PD, Costill DL, Flynn MG, Kirwan JP, Mitchell JB, Houmard J. Improvements in exercise performance: effects of carbohydrate feedings and diet. *J Appl Physiol* 1987;62:983–8.

O'Connor H, Sullivan T, Caterson I. Weight loss and the athlete. In: Burke L, Deakin V, eds. *Clinical Sports Nutrition.* 2nd edn. Sydney: McGraw-Hill, 2000: 146–84.

Parkin JAM, Carey MF, Martin IK, Stojanovska L, Febbraio MA. Muscle glycogen storage following prolonged exercise: effect of timing of ingestion of high glycemic index food. *Med Sci Sports Exerc* 1997;29:220–4.

Rasmussen BB, Tipton KD, Miller SL, Wolf SE, Wolfe RR. An oral essential amino acid–carbohydrate supplement enhances muscle protein anabolism after resistance exercise. *J Appl Physiol* 2000;88:386–92.

Reed MJ, Brozinick JT, Lee MC, Ivy JL. Muscle glycogen storage postexercise: effect of mode of carbohydrate administration. *J Appl Physiol* 1989;66:720–6.

Rehrer NJ, Van Kemenade M, Meester W, Brouns F, Saris WHM. Gastrointestinal complaints in relation to dietary intake in triathletes. *Int J Sport Nutr* 1992;2: 48–59.

Schulz LO, Alger S, Harper I, Wilmore JH, Ravussin E. Energy expenditure of elite female runners measured by respiratory chamber and doubly labeled water. *J Appl Physiol* 1992;72:23–8.

Sherman WM, Brodowicz G, Wright DA, Allen WK, Simonsen J, Dernbach A. Effects of 4 h pre-exercise carbohydrate feedings on cycling performance. *Med Sci Sports Exerc* 1989;21:598–604.

Sherman WM, Costill DL, Fink WJ, Miller JM. Effect of exercise-diet manipulation on muscle glycogen and its subsequent utilisation during performance. *Int J Sports Med* 1981;2:114–18.

Shirreffs SM, Maughan RJ. Restoration of fluid balance after exercise-induced dehydration: effects of alcohol consumption. *J Appl Physiol* 1997;83:1152–8.

Shirreffs SM, Taylor AJ, Leiper JB, Maughan RJ. Post-exercise rehydration in man: effects of volume consumed and drink sodium content. *Med Sci Sports Exerc* 1996;28:1260–71.

Steen SN, Brownell KD. Patterns of weight loss and regain in wrestlers: has the tradition changed? *Med Sci Sports Exerc* 1990;22:762–8.

Tarnopolsky MA, Bosman M, Macdonald JR, Vandeputte D, Martin JD, Roy BD. Post-exercise protein–carbohydrate and carbohydrate supplements increase glycogen in men and women. *J Appl Physiol* 1997;83:1877–83.

Thomas DE, Brotherhood JE, Brand JC. Carbohydrate feeding before exercise: effect of glycemic index. *Int J Sports Med* 1991;12:180–6.

Thompson JL, Manore MM, Skinner JS, Ravussin E, Spraul M. Daily energy expenditure in male endurance athletes with differing energy intakes. *Med Sci Sports Exerc* 1995;27:347–54.

Tipton KD, Rasmussen BB, Miller SL, et al. Timing of amino acid-carbohydrate ingestion alters anabolic response of muscle to resistance exercise. *Am J Physiol Endocrinol Metab* 2001;281:E197–E206.

van Hall G, Shirreffs SM, Calbert JAL. Muscle glycogen resynthesis during recovery from cycle exercise: no effect of additional protein ingestion. *J Appl Physiol* 2000;88:1631–6.

Walberg-Rankin J. Making weight in sports. In: Burke L, Deakin V, eds. *Clinical Sports Nutrition.* 2nd edn. Sydney: McGraw-Hill, 2000: 185–209.

Walsh RM, Noakes TD, Hawley JA, Dennis SC. Impaired high-intensity cycling performance time at low levels of dehydration. *Int J Sports Med* 1994;15:392–8.

Wright DA, Sherman WM, Dernbach AR. Carbohydrate feedings before, during, or in combination improve cycling endurance performance. *J Appl Physiol* 1991;71: 1082–8.

Yeager KK, Agostini R, Nattiv A, Drinkwater B. The female athlete triad: disordered eating, amenorrhea, osteoporosis. *Med Sci Sports Exerc* 1993;25:775–7.

Zawadzki KM, Yaspelkis BB, Ivy JL. Carbohydrate-protein complex increases the rate of muscle glycogen storage after exercise. *J Appl Physiol* 1992;72:1854–9.

CHAPTER 9

Sports supplements and sports foods

Louise M. BURKE

Introduction

The sports world is filled with products that claim to prolong endurance, enhance recovery, reduce body fat, increase muscle mass, minimise the risk of illness, or achieve other goals that enhance sports performance. According to surveys, athletes are major consumers of supplements and an important target group for the multi-billion dollar supplement industry (for review see Burke et al. 2000). It is easy to understand why promises of improved performance are attractive to athletes and coaches in elite competition, where very small differences separate the winners from the rest of the field (Hopkins et al. 1999). Yet the fame and fortune of Olympic gold medals and world records provides only part of the drive to find a 'magic bullet' because even non-elite and recreational athletes are avid consumers of sports foods and supplements (Burke et al. 2000). Athletes provide each other with testimonials or hearsay about the benefits that are attributed to supplements and sports foods. They fear that their competitors might have a secret weapon, and even in the absence of firm evidence to support a product, they may feel compelled to take it to maintain a 'level playing field'.

Sports scientists are also interested in supplements and sports foods as part of their search for new strategies to enhance training and recovery, and competition performance. Many scientists undertake the applied sports nutrition research that has helped to develop new products and investigate the specific ways in which they can be used to optimise performance (see Burke et al. 2000). Unfortunately, the many challenges to undertaking such research mean that it is impossible to keep pace with the number of new products that appear on the sports market. In reality, the majority of products are either untested or have failed to live up to expectations in the preliminary studies that have been conducted. Scientists believe that well-controlled research should underpin the promotion of any sports nutrition practice and are understandably frustrated that producers of supplements often make impressive claims about their products without adequate or, in some cases, any proof. However, in most countries, legislation regarding supplements or sports foods is either minimal or unenforced, allowing unsupported claims to flourish and products to be manufactured with poor compliance to labelling and composition standards. Athletes are usually unaware of these lapses.

This chapter reviews the range of nutritional products that are currently available to athletes, noting items that have true value as part of an athlete's nutrition program and compounds that have been proven to be ergogenic (work enhancing) by rigorous scientific testing. It also looks at an approach used by the Australian Institute of Sport for educating athletes and coaches about supplements and managing the provision of supplements to athletes and teams.

Sports foods and supplements

The distinction between a sports food and a supplement is often arbitrary. If the definition were based on the *form* of the product, supplements would include pills, potions, capsules or powders, whereas sports foods would take a more traditional form of energy-containing bars, drinks and other edible products. If the definition were based on *function*, sports foods could be seen as products containing nutrients in amounts found in everyday foods to meet known nutritional needs, whereas supplements might target the provision of nutrients or other compounds in supra-physiological amounts. However, the definitions differ between countries according to the way that food and pharmaceutical products are regulated. In this chapter we consider sports foods to be energy-containing products manufactured in a food-like form (e.g. bars, drinks, gels or modified versions of everyday foods).

Sports foods: an overview

Despite the availability of sophisticated guidelines for sports nutrition (see Chapter 8), many dietary surveys have found that athletes fail to make appropriate food choices and eating plans. This is often due to practical challenges associated with the use of everyday foods, creating a need for foods with special properties. A number of special characteristics of a sports food could be of true value to the athlete or person undertaking exercise (Table 9.1). Although food products that are tailor-made for the practical challenges of feeding athletes are useful, often the most tempting characteristic for manufacturers is the inclusion of special ingredients claimed to enhance sports performance. Practical and compositional characteristics of sports foods can often be fine-tuned to a specific need in sport or even a specific type of sport; however, it is often impossible to turn such a niche food into a commercially viable product.

In some countries, there are provisions for sports foods within the national food standards codes. For example, in Australasia, sports foods are included among the foods under the regulation of Food Standards Australia and New Zealand (FSANZ). Standards might make provision for a range of acceptable formulations and permitted additives, as well as a list of permitted or compulsory education messages for presentation on product packaging. Although such standards might exist, the responsibility for adopting them into food laws or checking that these laws are upheld is often dispersed. For example, in Australia, this responsibility is given to individual states rather than the Federal government. In reality, some sports foods do not meet the relevant standards, either by containing ingredients that are in contravention to the code or by carrying illegal claims. This is generally not the case for the larger number of mainstream products, such as commercial sports drinks and bars. However, there are some sports foods, usually produced by smaller manufacturers targeting a niche market of athletes, which fail to comply. When food standards codes rely on a largely self-regulated industry of food manufacture and marketing, there is a greater likelihood that sports foods will contain non-permitted substances and/or incomplete or inaccurate labelling information.

TABLE 9.1 Potentially valuable characteristics of a sports food

■ Communicates an education message related to sports nutrition goals.

■ Packages a precise or compact 'dose' of nutrient(s), especially to meet nutrient recommendations for a specialised situation in sports nutrition (e.g. pre-event, during event, or post-event nutrition).

■ Provides a good source of nutrient(s) 'at risk' in the diets of athletes or subgroups of athletes.

■ Has simple preparation/storage needs, low perishability.

■ Is portable and conveniently packaged.

■ Can be easily consumed with a low risk of gastrointestinal upsets or discomfort.

■ Contains special ergogenic compounds known to enhance sports performance in specific situations.

The dietary supplement industry: an overview

The availability and marketing of dietary supplements fitting the description of pills, powders or other non-food forms varies between countries. In Australia, a country with more comprehensive regulation, these products fall within the jurisdiction of the Therapeutic Goods Administration (TGA) under the *Australian Therapeutic Goods Act 1989*. This Act distinguishes two classes of products: drugs and therapeutic devices, with the latter group being further classified into categories of 'registrable' and 'listable' products. Although dietary supplements may be packaged in a way suggesting medical or scientific rigour, most fall into the 'listable' group, meaning that they receive considerably less regulation and attention than prescription pharmaceutical products. Although they need to comply with relevant statutory standards (e.g. to exclude ingredients banned by Australian Customs laws), they are considered low-risk self-medications and are not subjected to a comprehensive review of quality, safety and efficacy. They are expected to comply with good manufacturing practice and, according to advertising regulations, to make limited therapeutic claims. In practice, these products receive little investigation of quality and advertising claims unless they are the subject of serious complaints regarding health and safety issues.

In other countries, non-food forms of supplements fall under the same regulatory bodies as food products. For example, in the United States, supplements fall under the jurisdiction of the Food and Drug Administration (FDA) and the *Dietary Supplement Health and Education Act* of 1994. This Act reduced the regulation of supplements and broadened the category to include new ingredients, such as herbal and botanical products, and constituents or metabolites of other dietary supplements. Most importantly, the Act shifted responsibility from the manufacturer to the FDA to enforce safety and claim guidelines. Since then, good manufacturing practice has not been enforced and non-compliant products or manufacturers are free to flourish unless there is specific intervention by the FDA.

Athletes need to have a global understanding of the regulation of dietary supplements, since regular travel and modern conveniences such as mail order and the Internet provide them with easy access to products that fall outside the scrutiny of their own country's system. They should also understand that in the absence or minimisation of rigorous government evaluation, the quality control of supplement manufacture is trusted to supplement companies. Large companies that produce conventional supplements, such as vitamins and minerals, particularly to manufacturing standards used in the preparation of pharmaceutical products, are likely to achieve good quality control. This includes precision with ingredient levels and labelling, and avoidance of undeclared ingredients or contaminants. However, this does not appear to be true for all supplement types or manufacturers, with many examples of poor compliance with labelling laws (Gurley et al. 1998; Hahm et al. 1999; Parasrampuria et al. 1998) and the presence of contaminants and undeclared ingredients.

Although manufacturers are not meant to make unsupported claims about health or performance benefits elicited by supplements, product advertisements and testimonials show ample evidence that this aspect of supplement marketing is unregulated and exploited. For example, a survey of five issues of body building magazines found 800 individual performance claims for 624 different products within advertisements (Grunewald & Bailey 1993). It is easy to see how enthusiastic and emotive claims provide a false sense of confidence about the products. Most consumers are unaware that such advertising is not regulated. Therefore, athletes are likely to believe that claims about supplements are medically and scientifically supported, simply because they believe that untrue claims would not be allowed to exist.

Balancing the use of sports foods and supplements

Ultimately, the decision to use a supplement is a personal choice made by athletes, often in consultation with their coach. Before making a decision, athletes and coaches should consider the likely benefits, balanced against the cost of the supplementation program and the risk of negative outcomes such as side-effects or a positive doping outcome. It is important that athletes and coaches are empowered to make a decision by having unbiased information about any scientifically documented benefits of the supplement use, as well as the potential risk of short- and long-term harmful effects. They should also be well-educated about the specific ways in which the supplement or sports food can be used to achieve nutritional goals or enhance performance. The advice of sports scientists or sports nutrition authorities should be sought to provide such information.

Positive outcomes from the use of sports foods and supplements

Some supplements and sports foods offer real advantages to the athlete. Some products work by producing a direct performance-enhancing (ergogenic) effect. Other products can be used by athletes to meet their nutritional goals and, as an indirect outcome, allow athletes to achieve optimal performance. Some ergogenic effects or guidelines of sports nutrition are also so well known and easily demonstrated that beneficial uses of sports foods or supplements are clear-cut. But even when indirect nutritional benefits or true ergogenic outcomes from supplement use are small, they are often worthwhile in the competitive world of sport (Hopkins et al. 1999). Of course, athletes need to be aware that it is the use of the product as much as the product itself that leads to the beneficial outcome. Therefore, education about specific situations and strategies for the use of supplements and sports foods is just as important as the formulation of the product.

Even where a sports food or supplement does not produce a true physiological or ergogenic benefit, an athlete might attain some performance benefit because of a psychological boost or 'placebo' effect. The placebo effect describes a favourable outcome arising simply from an individual's belief that he/she has received a beneficial treatment. In a clinical environment, a placebo is often given in the form of a harmless but inactive substance or treatment that satisfies the patient's symbolic need to receive a 'therapy'. In a sports setting, an athlete who receives enthusiastic marketing material about a new supplement or hears glowing testimonials from other athletes who have used it is more likely to report a positive experience. Despite our belief that the placebo effect is real and potentially worthwhile, only a few studies have tried to investigate the application of the placebo effect in sport (Ariel & Saville 1972; Clark et al. 2000). Additional well-controlled studies are needed to better describe the potential size and duration of this effect and whether it applies equally to all athletes and across all types of performance. In the meantime we can accept that the placebo effect exists and may explain, at least partially, why athletes report performance benefits after trying a new supplement or dietary treatment.

Problems associated with the use of sports foods and supplements

The Supplement Panel of the Australian Institute of Sport, formed in 2000, assessed the supplement use by athletes in its programs and identified a list of problems (Table 9.2). An obvious issue with extensive supplement use is the expense, which in extreme cases can equal or exceed the athlete's weekly food budget. The situation is compounded for teams and sports programs that need to supply the needs of a group of athletes. Supplements and sports foods generally provide nutrients or food constituents at a higher price than everyday foods. This is the result of the costs of special ingredients, research and development, marketing, specialist packaging or processing, higher unit costs for niche products and, sometimes, the profit margin that the sports people seem willing to pay for their dreams of winning performances.

Supplement use, even when it provides a true performance advantage, is an expense that athletes must acknowledge and prioritise appropriately within their total budget. At times, it may be deemed money well spent, particularly when the supplement or sports food provides the most practical and palatable way to achieve a nutrition goal, or when ergogenic benefits have been well documented. On other occasions the athlete may choose to limit the use of expensive products to the most important events or training periods. There are often lower cost alternatives to some supplements and sports foods that the budget-conscious athlete can use on less critical occasions.

A more subtle outcome of reliance on supplements is the displacement of the athlete's real priorities. Successful sports performance is the product of superior genetics, long-term training, optimal nutrition, state-of-the-art equipment and a committed attitude. These factors cannot be replaced by the use of supplements, but often appear less exciting or more demanding than the enthusiastic and emotive claims made for many supplements and sports foods. Athletes can sometimes be side-tracked from the true elements of success in search of short-cuts from bottles and packets.

TABLE 9.2 Problems with current supplement practices by athletes, as evaluated by the Australian Institute of Sport

- Strategies that genuinely enhance performance (e.g. specialised training, sound nutrition practice, good equipment, adequate rest/sleep, mental preparation) are overlooked in favour of supplement use.
- Athletes are drawn to new supplements with marketing hype rather than supplements and sports foods that might have true value in achieving nutrition goals.
- Ad-hoc use of supplements often means that valuable supplements are not used in a manner that achieves optimal outcomes.
- Products with little value are a drain of resources (i.e. money, time, interest are all limited assets).
- Use of unproven supplements by well-known or successful athletes (and institutions) provides 'endorsement' in the eyes of other athletes and continues false expectations.
- Risk of side-effects.
- Risk of inadvertent positive 'doping' outcome.

Since most supplements are considered by regulatory bodies to be relatively safe, in many countries there are no official or mandatory accounting processes to document adverse side-effects arising from the use of these products. Nevertheless, information from medical registers (Kozyrskyj 1997; Perharic et al. 1994; Shaw et al. 1997) shows that while the overall risk to public health from the use of supplements and herbal and traditional remedies is low, cases of toxicity and side-effects include allergic reactions to some products (e.g. royal jelly), overexposure as a result of self-medication and poisoning due to contaminants. During the 1980s, deaths and medical problems resulted from the use of tryptophan supplements (Roufs 1992); products containing ephedrine and caffeine are a more recent source of medical problems, sometimes causing deaths in susceptible individuals. Many reports call for better regulation and surveillance of supplements and herbal products, and increased awareness of potential hazards (Kozyrskyj 1997; Perharic et al. 1994; Shaw et al. 1997).

'Inadvertent doping' through supplement use has emerged as a major concern for athletes who participate in sporting competitions governed by an anti-doping code. Some supplements and sports foods contain ingredients from the Proscribed Lists of the Anti-doping Movement Code (International Olympic Committee [IOC] 2002a) and an athlete may have a positive drug test after unintentionally consuming a banned substance found in such products. Since supplements are regarded as 'harmless' or 'alternatives to drugs', some athletes may not carefully read product labels to check the ingredient list for banned substances. In addition, there is now growing evidence that many supplements or sports foods contain banned substances as undeclared ingredients or contaminants.

A number of studies have reported the undeclared presence of ephedrine and related stimulants, or pro-hormones such as dehydroepiandrosterone (DHEA), or androstenedione in a range of supplement products (Catlin et al. 2001; Cui et al. 1994; Geyer et al. 2000; Kamber et al. 2001; Ros et al. 1999). The most recently reported study of 634 products manufactured by 215 different providers in the United States and Europe found that 94 (15%) contained ingredients that were not listed on any label which would cause a positive doping test (IOC 2002b). These ingredients included prohormone precursors of the anabolic steroid, nandrolone, as well as precursors of testosterone. Another 10% of products returned borderline results for various unlabelled substances. Although supplements have been publicly blamed for a number of cases of positive nandrolone tests in high-profile athletes, the IOC reminds athletes that under the Olympic Movement's rule of strict liability, full responsibility for a positive drug test rests with the athlete, regardless of circumstance (IOC 2002b). As a result, the IOC Medical Commission has issued a recommendation that elite athletes should not take nutritional supplements and notes that the unwitting ingestion of hormone precursors should be a matter of public health concern.

A system for managing the use of supplement and sports foods by athletes

In some cases, sporting organisations or institutions make policies or programs for supplement use on behalf of athletes within their care. This may range from a single sporting team, to an entire sports program such as the National Collegiate Athletics Association (Burke 2001). Since 2000, the Australian Institute of Sport (AIS) has implemented a supplement program for athletes within its funding program with the stated goals of:

- allowing its athletes to focus on the sound use of supplements and special sports foods as part of their special nutrition plans
- ensuring that supplements and sports foods are used correctly and appropriately to deliver maximum benefits to the immune system, recovery and performance
- giving its athletes the confidence that they receive 'cutting edge' advice and achieve 'state of the art' nutrition practices
- ensuring that supplement use does not lead to an inadvertent doping offence.

A key part of the AIS program is a ranking system for supplements and sports foods, based on a risk:benefit analysis of each product by a panel of experts in sports nutrition, medicine and science (AIS 2002). This ranking system has four tiers, each of which has a prescribed level of use by AIS-funded athletes. Although the hierarchy of categories was developed for long-term use, there is a regular assessment of supplements and sports foods to ensure that they are placed in the category that best fits the available scientific evidence. Table 9.3 provides a summary of the AIS supplement program at the time of publication. The remainder of this chapter provides a summary of the current scientific support for a range of products within the various supplement categories.

TABLE 9.3 Australian Institute Sport Supplement Program[a]

SUPPLEMENT CATEGORY AND EXPLANATION OF USE WITHIN THE AIS SUPPLEMENT PROGRAM	PRODUCTS WITHIN THIS CATEGORY
GROUP A *Approved supplements* ■ Provide a useful and timely source of energy and nutrients in the athlete's diet. ■ Or have been shown in scientific trials to provide a performance benefit, when used according to a apecific protocol in a specific situation in sport **AIS Sports Supplement Panel position** We know that athletes and coaches are interested in using supplements to achieve optimal performance. Our 2002 supplement project aims to focus this interest on products and protocols that have documented benefits, by: ■ Making these supplements available and accessible to the AIS athletes who will benefit from their appropriate use. In particular, to provide these supplements at no cost to AIS sports programs, through systems managed by appropriate sports science/medicine departments. Strategies to provide products will range from individual 'prescription' of supplements requiring careful use (e.g. creatine) to creative programs that make valuable sports foods and everyday foods accesible to athletes in situations of nutritional need (e.g. 'recovery bars', providing foods and drinks for sonsumption after exercise). ■ Providing education to athletes and coaches about the beneficial use of these supplements/sports foods and their appropriate use, with the emphasis on state of the art sports nutrition. We also aim to ensure that supplements/sports foods used by AIS athletes carry a minimal risk of doping safety problems.	Sports drinks Liquid meal supplements Sports gels Sports bars Cereal bars Creatine Bicarbonate Anitoxidants: vitamin C, vitamin E Sick pack (zinc and vitamin C) Multivitamin/mineral supplement Iron supplement Calcium supplement Glycerol (for hyperhydration) Glucosamine
GROUP B *Supplements under consideration* Supplements may be classified Category B if they have no substantial proof of health or performance benefits, but: ■ remain of interest to AIS coaches or athletes ■ are too new to have received adequate scientific attention ■ have preliminary data which hint at possible benefits. **AIS Sports Supplement Panel position** ■ These supplements can be used at the AIS under the auspices of a controlled scientific trial or a supervised therapeutic program.	Echinacea Glutamine Hydroxy-methylbutyrate (HMB) Colostrum Probiotics Ribose Melatonin

(continues)

TABLE 9.3 Australian Institute Sport Supplement Program[a] (*continued*)

SUPPLEMENT CATEGORY AND EXPLANATION OF USE WITHIN THE AIS SUPPLEMENT PROGRAM	PRODUCTS WITHIN THIS CATEGORY

GROUP C

Supplements that have no proof or beneficial effects and are therefore not to be provided to official AIS programs

- This category contains the majority of supplements and sports products promoted to athletes.

- These supplements, despite enjoying a cyclical pattern of popularity and widespread use, have not been proven to enhance sports performance or health.

- In some cases these supplements have been shown to impair sports performance or health, with a clear mechanism to explain these results.

AIS Sports Supplement Panel position

In the absence of proof of benefits, these supplements should not be provided to AIS athletes from AIS program budgets.

If an individual athlete or coach wishes to use a supplement from this category, they may do so providing:

- they are responsible for payment for this supplement,

- any sponsorship arrangements are acknowledged to AIS marketing,

- the supplement brand has been assessed for doping safety and determined to be 'low risk'

- the athlete reports their use to the AIS Department of Medicine, and

- the athlete records their use in their supplement and medication diary.

Products within this category:

Amino acids (these can be provided by foods or some Group A products)

Ginseng

Garlic

Cordyceps

Ginkgo biloba

Coenzyme Q10

Cytochrome *c*

Carnitine

Bee pollen

Gamma-oryzanol and ferulic acid

Chromium picolinate

Vitamin B_{12} injections

Oral vitamin B_{12}

Intravenous Iron

All supplements from network marketing companies

GROUP D

Banned supplements

These supplements are directly banned by the IOC doping rules or provide a high risk of producing a positive doping outcome.

AIS Sports Panel position

These supplements should not be used by AIS athletes.

Products within this category:

Androstenedione

DHEA

19-norandrostenedione and 19-norandrostenediol

Tribulus terristris and other herbal testosterone supplements

Ephedra

Strychnine

Caffeine is banned when urinary levels are detected >12 µg/mL

(*a*) Australian Institute of Sport, 2002.

Valuable sports foods and supplements

Sports foods, by providing a practical way to meet goals of sports nutrition, are among the most valuable special products available to athletes. Table 9.4 summarises the major classes of sports foods together with the situations or goals of sports nutrition that they can be used to address. The substantiation for many of these nutrition goals is well accepted (see Chapter 8) and includes situations where a measurable enhancement of performance can be detected as a result of the correct use of the sports food. Although most of these products have specialised uses in sport, some have crossed successfully into the general market (e.g. sports drinks). As long as consumers are prepared to pay an increased price for such a product and sports nutrition messages are left intact, most nutrition experts are not unduly concerned by this outcome. In fact, sports nutritionists have been quick to defend the use of sports drinks by 'weekend warriors' and recreational exercisers, since the benefits of fluid intake and carbohydrate replacement during a workout are determined by the physiology of exercise rather than the calibre of the person who is exercising. It should also be noted that most studies of supplements such as sports drinks have been undertaken on moderately-to-well-trained performers rather than elite athletes; therefore, where evidence of performance benefit does exist, it is directly relevant to these sub-elite populations.

Creatine

In one decade, creatine has gone from being a muscle fuel written about in textbooks to the world's fastest selling and best-investigated ergogenic aid. Its introduction to the sports world included testimonials from gold medal winning sprinters at the 1992 Barcelona Olympic Games and the almost simultaneous publication of data showing that oral intake of large doses of creatine increased muscle creatine stores (Harris et al. 1992). The combination of athletic promise, scientific intrigue and new communication channels offered by the Internet has helped to create a phenomenon in the world of sports nutrition. Today, creatine is the subject of a textbook (Williams et al. 1998) and over 150 peer-reviewed studies, review papers and position statements (American College of Sports Medicine 2000; Greenhaff 2000; Hespel et al. 2001; Juhn & Tarnopolsky 1998a, 1998b; Kraemer & Volek 1999) and has amassed annual sales of more than 5 million kilograms (Hespel et al. 2001).

Creatine (Cr, methylguanidine-acetic acid) is stored primarily in skeletal

TABLE 9.4 Sports foods and their uses by athletes[a]

SUPPLEMENT	FORM	COMPOSITION	SPORTS-RELATED USE
Sports drink	Powder Liquid	5–7% CHO 10–25 mmol/L sodium	Optimum delivery of fluid + CHO during exercise Post-exercise rehydration Post-exercise refuelling
Sports gel	Gel 30–40 g sachets or larger tubes	60–70% carbohydrate (~25 g per sachet) Some contain medium-chain triglycerides or caffeine	Supplement high-CHO training diet CHO loading Post-exercise recovery—provides CHO CHO source during exercise, especially when CHO needs exceed fluid requirements
High CHO supplement	Powder Liquid	10–25% carbohydrate (+ some B vitamins)	Supplement high-CHO training diet CHO loading Post-exercise CHO recovery—provides carbohydrate May be used during exercise when CHO needs exceed fluid requirements
Liquid meal supplement	Powder (mix with water or milk) Liquid	1–1.5 kcal/mL 15–20% protein 50–70% carbohydrate low–moderate fate vitamins/minerals: 0.5–1 L supplies RDIs	Supplement high energy/CHO/nutrient diet (especially during heavy training/competition or weight gain) Low-bulk meal replacement (especially pre-event meal) Post-exercise recovery—provides CHO, protein and micronutrients Portable nutrition for travelling athlete
Sports bar	Bar (50–60 g)	40–50 g carbohydrate 5–10 g protein Usually low in fat Vitamins/minerals: can supply 50–100% of DRIs May contain creatine, amino acids	CHO source during exercise Post-exercise recovery—provides CHO, protein and micronutrients Supplement high energy/CHO/nutrient diet Portable nutrition for the travelling athlete

(a) Adapted from Burke et al. 2000.

muscle at typical concentrations of 100–150 mmol/kg dry weight (dw) of muscle. In its phosphorylated form, creatine phosphate (PCr) provides a rapidly available but small source of phosphate for the resynthesis of ATP during maximal exercise and is therefore an important fuel source in maximal sprints or 'all-out' muscular effort lasting up to 5–10 seconds. Other metabolic functions of PCr include the buffering of hydrogen ions produced during anaerobic glycolysis and an ATP shuttle, by which ATP generated by aerobic metabolism is transported from the muscle cell mitochondria to the cytoplasm where it can be utilised for muscle contraction.

The daily turnover of Cr (1–2 g/day) is replaced either through dietary Cr intake (from animal-derived tissues such as meat) or through endogenous synthesis in the liver from amino acid precursors (arginine, glycine and methionine). Creatine is transported into the muscle against a high concentration gradient via saturable transport processes that are insulin stimulated (Green et al. 1996 a, b). The typical carnivorous diet provides approximately 2 g Cr per day, but vegetarians have reduced body Cr stores, suggesting that endogenous production cannot totally compensate for the lack of dietary intake (Green et al. 1997). High dietary intakes temporarily suppress endogenous Cr production. The reason for the variability of muscle Cr concentrations between individuals is uncertain but may be related to gender, age or fibre type (for review see Hespel et al. 2001).

It has been known for over 50 years that oral Cr doses are largely maintained in the body (Chanutin 1926). However, it is only recent studies using skeletal muscle biopsy procedures and imaging techniques that have documented changes in muscle Cr and PCr content following supplementary Cr intake. In the watershed study of 1992, Harris and colleagues showed that muscle Cr levels were increased following repeated doses of oral Cr large enough to sustain plasma Cr levels above the threshold for maximal transport into the muscle cell (Harris et al. 1992). Their loading protocol— four to six doses of 5 g Cr (monohydrate) for 5 days—increased total muscle Cr concentrations by an average of 20% to reach a muscle 'threshold' of 150–160 mmol/kg dw. About 20% of the increased muscle Cr content was stored as PCr and saturation occurred after 2–3 days. Increases in muscle Cr stores were greatest in those individuals who had the lowest pre-supplementation concentrations and when coupled with intensive daily exercise (Harris et al. 1992). Such a protocol has become known as 'rapid Cr loading'.

Further studies have found that a daily Cr dose of 3 g will achieve a slow loading over 28 days and that elevated muscle Cr stores are maintained by continued daily supplementation of 2–3 g (Hultman et al. 1996). Across studies there is evidence of a continuum of Cr loading response, with about 30% of individuals being 'non-responders'—that is, they fail to increase muscle Cr stores by a sufficiently large amount so that differences in muscle metabolism are detectable (Spriet 1997; Greenhaff 2000). Co-ingestion of substantial amounts of carbohydrate (CHO, 75–100 g) with Cr doses has been shown to enhance Cr accumulation (Green et al. 1996 a, b) and to assist individuals to reach the muscle Cr threshold of 160 mmol/kg dw. Further, prior Cr loading has been shown to augment the response to a CHO loading protocol (Nelson et al. 2001). In the absence of continued supplementation, it takes 4–5 weeks for muscle Cr to return to resting concentrations (Hultman et al. 1996). Many studies have reported an acute gain in body mass (BM) of about 1 kg during rapid Cr loading. This is likely to be primarily a gain in body water and is mirrored by a reduction in urine output during the loading days (Hultman et al. 1996).

Many studies have investigated the effect of Cr supplementation on muscle function and exercise performance. Studies vary according to the characteristics of subjects (gender, age, training status), the mode of exercise, and whether supplementation involved an acute loading intervention, or a chronic effect on training adaptations. Most studies are undertaken using an experimental–placebo design, since the long wash-out period makes a crossover design impractical to conduct. The magnitude of the literature on Cr supplementation is too large to allow a summary of individual studies. However, readers are directed to the following reviews that have tabulated or summarised the literature (Burke et al. 2001; Greenhaff 2000; Juhn & Tarnopolsky 1998 a, b; Kraemer & Volek 1999). Our current understanding of the effect of Cr supplementation on exercise performance is listed below (Burke et al. 2001).

1 The major benefit of Cr supplementation is an increase in the rate of PCr resynthesis during the recovery between bouts of high-intensity exercise, producing higher PCr levels at the start of the subsequent exercise bout. Creatine supplementation can enhance the performance of repeated 6–30 s bouts of maximal exercise, interspersed with short recovery intervals (20 s–5 min), where it can attenuate the normal decrease in force or power production that occurs over the course of the session.

2 Oral Cr supplementation cannot be considered ergogenic for single bout or first-bout sprints because the contribution of PCr to this first exercise effort is not a limiting factor to performance and any likely benefit is too small to be consistently detected.

3 Performance responses to Cr supplementation vary considerably between subjects in a study and between studies.

4   The exercise situations that have been most consistently demonstrated to benefit from Cr supplementation are laboratory protocols of repeated high-intensity intervals involving isolated muscular efforts or weight-supported activities such as cycling.

5   Theoretically, acute Cr supplementation might be beneficial for a single competitive event in sports involving repeated high-intensity intervals with brief recovery periods. This description includes team games and racquet sports. Similarly, chronic Cr supplementation may enhance training performance and long-term adaptation to exercise programs based on repeated high-intensity exercise. These benefits may apply to the across-season performance of athletes in team and racquet sports, as well as the preparation of athletes who undertake interval training and resistance training (e.g. swimmers and sprinters).

6   In many sports, these benefits remain theoretical since few studies have been undertaken with elite athletes or as 'field studies'. Performance enhancements will only occur in weight-bearing (e.g. running) and weight-sensitive sports (e.g. light-weight rowing) if gains in muscular output compensate for increases in body mass. The present literature involving these weight-related sports shows inconsistent results. Performance enhancements may not always occur in complex games and sports; even if changes in strength or speed are achieved by Cr-assisted training, these may not translate into improvements in game outcomes (i.e. goals scored).

7   Evidence that Cr supplementation is of benefit to aerobic endurance exercise is absent.

8   Whether the long-term gains in muscle mass reported in studies of resistance training are caused by direct stimulation of increased myofibrillar protein synthesis by Cr, an enhanced ability to undertake resistance training, or a combination of both factors remains to be determined. Although direct stimulation of muscle protein synthesis was originally discounted, there are some newer data showing that Cr supplementation affects myogenic transcription factors (see review by Hespel et al. 2001).

The enthusiasm with which Cr has been embraced by the sports world raises some concerns over the potential for side-effects or harmful outcomes, particularly associated with long-term use of large Cr doses. There have been anecdotal reports of nausea, gastrointestinal upset, headaches and muscle cramping/strains. Some of these adverse effects are plausible, particularly in the light of increased water retention within skeletal muscle (and perhaps brain) cells. The currently available literature has not found evidence of an increased prevalence or risk of these problems among Cr users. However, it should be noted that studies of long-term use, particularly self-medication with doses far in excess of the recommended Cr usage protocols, have not been conducted. Although it is commonly suggested that Cr supplementation may cause renal impairments, the few case reports of such a problem have occurred in patients with pre-existing renal dysfunction (Pritchard & Kalra 1998). Poortmans and Francaux (1999) found Cr intake had no detrimental effects on renal responses. Until long-term and large population studies can be undertaken, bodies such as the American College of Sports Medicine (2000) have taken a cautious view on the benefits and side-effects of Cr supplementation. However, a recent suggestion from the French food safety agency that Cr supplementation is carcinogenic has been discredited by several other sources charged with public education or safety (see Hespel et al. 2001).

Bicarbonate and citrate

Anaerobic glycolysis provides the primary fuel source for exercise of near maximal intensity lasting longer than approximately 20–30 seconds. The total capacity of this system is limited by the progressive increase in the acidity of the intracellular environment, caused by the accumulation of lactate and hydrogen ions (see Chapter 5). When intracellular buffering capacity is exceeded, lactate and hydrogen ions diffuse into the extracellular space, perhaps aided by a positive pH gradient. Since the 1930s it has been recognised that dietary strategies that decrease blood pH (e.g. intake of acid salts) impair high-intensity exercise, while alkalotic therapies improve such performance (Dennig et al. 1931; Dill et al. 1932). In theory, an increase in extracellular buffering capacity should delay the onset of muscular fatigue during prolonged anaerobic metabolism by increasing the muscle's ability to dispose of excess hydrogen ions.

The two most popular buffering agents are sodium bicarbonate and sodium citrate. Athletes have practised 'soda loading' or 'bicarbonate loading' for over 70 years, with sodium bicarbonate being ingested in the form of the household product 'bicarb soda' or as pharmaceutical urinary alkalinisers such as Ural. The general protocol for bicarbonate loading is to ingest 0.3 g of sodium bicarbonate/kg BM 1–2 hours prior to exercise; this equates to 4–5 teaspoons of bicarb powder. Bicarbonate loading is not considered to pose any major health risk, although some individuals suffer gastrointestinal distress such as cramping or diarrhoea. Consuming sodium bicarbonate with plenty of water (e.g. a litre or more) may help to prevent hyperosmotic diarrhoea. Sodium citrate is also usually ingested in doses of 0.3–0.5 g/kg BM.

Bicarbonate or citrate loading may be a useful strategy to enhance the performance of athletic events that are conducted at near maximum intensity for the duration of 1–7 minutes (e.g. 400–1500 m running, 100–400 m swimming, kayaking, rowing and canoeing events). Sports that are dependent on repeated anaerobic bursts might also benefit from bicarbonate loading. Bicarbonate or citrate intake is not considered a banned practice for human performances, although it is not permitted in dog or horse racing. It is difficult to detect the use of bicarbonate or citrate loading strategies by athletes, since urinary pH varies according to dietary practices such as vegetarianism and high CHO intake (Heigenhauser & Jones 1991).

It is beyond the scope of this chapter to review individually the 50 or more studies of the effects of bicarbonate/citrate loading on athletic or exercise performance in humans (for reviews see Heigenhauser & Jones 1991; Linderman & Fahey 1991; Maughan & Greenhaff 1991; McNaughton 2000). However, a meta-analysis (Matson & Tran 1993) of the data in the bicarbonate supplementation literature provides some interesting insights. This analysis included 29 randomised double-blind crossover investigations of bicarbonate loading and physical performance, examining 35 effect sizes (some studies included multiple investigations within their design) from a total pool of 285 subjects (mainly healthy male college students). There was some variation in the protocols of bicarbonate loading, with different doses and times of ingestion being employed. While cycling was the most frequently used mode of exercise, there were a variety of exercise protocols (single efforts of 30 s to 5–7 min of near maximal intensity, or repeated intervals of 1 min with short rest times between) and a variety of performance outcomes (changes in power over a given time period, total work performed in a specified time or time to exhaustion at a specific exercise intensity).

Overall, this meta-analysis concluded that the ingestion of sodium bicarbonate has a moderate positive effect on exercise performance, with a weighted effect size of 0.44—that is, the mean performance of the bicarbonate trial was, on average, 0.44 standard deviations better than the placebo trial. Overall, there was only a weak relationship reported between the increased blood alkalinity (increase in pH and bicarbonate) attained in the bicarbonate trial and the performance outcome. However, ergogenic effects were related to the level of metabolic acidosis achieved during the exercise, suggesting the importance of attaining a threshold pH gradient across the cell membrane from the combination of the accumulation of intracellular H^+ and the extracellular alkalosis. Significant variability within studies suggests that bicarbonate ingestion has an individual effect on different subjects, and that the effect on performance is more complicated than the simple mechanisms suggested above. Popular theories include the likelihood that anaerobically trained athletes would show less response to bicarbonate/citrate loading due to better intrinsic buffering capacity, and the risk that performance of *prolonged* high-intensity exercise will be impaired if bicarbonate/citrate supplementation leads to increased rates of glycogen utilisation. However, the few studies that have examined bicarbonate or citrate loading using sports specific protocols and well-trained subjects (Table 9.5) fail to support these theories. Some, but not all, studies of well-trained athletes have found performance improvements following bicarbonate/lactate loading prior to brief (1–10 min) or prolonged (30–60 min) events involving high-intensity exercise (see Table 9.5).

Until further research can clarify the range of exercise activities that might benefit from bicarbonate or citrate enhancement, individual athletes are advised to experiment in training and minor competitions to judge their own case. It is important that experimentation is conducted in a competition-simulated environment, including the need to undertake multiple loading strategies for heats and finals of an event; the athlete needs to discover not only the potential for performance improvement but also the likelihood of unwanted side-effects.

Glycerol

Glycerol, a three-carbon alcohol, provides the backbone to the triglyceride molecule. It is released during lipolysis and slowly metabolised via the liver and kidneys. Athletes are interested in glycerol not for its energy potential but, rather, its role as a hyperhydration agent. Oral intake of glycerol, via glycerine or special hyperhydration supplements, achieves a rapid absorption and distribution of glycerol around all body fluid compartments, adding to osmotic pressure. When a substantial volume of fluid is consumed simultaneously with glycerol, there is an expansion of the fluid spaces and retention of this fluid. Effective protocols for glycerol hyperhydration are 1–1.5 g/kg glycerol with an intake of 25–35 mL/kg of fluid. Typically, such a protocol achieves a fluid expansion or retention of about 600 mL above a fluid bolus alone via a reduction in urinary volume (see review by Robergs & Griffin 1998).

Glycerol hyperhydration may be useful in the preparation for events that challenge fluid status and thermoregulation; for example, exercise at high

TABLE 9.5 Studies of bicarbonate or citrate loading on sports specific performance: double-blind crossover designed studies

REFERENCE	SUBJECTS	DOSE	EXERCISE PROTOCOL	ENHANCED PERFORMANCE	SUMMARY
McNaughton et al. 1999	10 well trained male cyclists	300 mg/kg sodium bicarbonate	Cycling 60 min TT[a]	Yes	14% more work completed with bicarbonate.
Potteiger et al. 1996a	8 male cyclists	500 mg/kg sodium citrate	Cycling 30 km TT	Yes	Reduction in TT time (57:36 v 59:22 min). Sodium citrate raised pH values from 10 km onwards and improved power output in the initial 25 min.
Stephens et al. 2002	8 endurance-trained male cyclists	300 mg/kg sodium bicarbonate	Cycling 30 min @ 77% VO_{2max} + TT (~30 min)	No	Increase in blood lactate but no difference in muscle glycogen utilisation or lactate.
Schabort et al. 2000	8 endurance-trained male cyclists	200 mg/kg, 400 mg/kg and 600 mg/kg sodium citrate	Cycling 40 km TT including 500 m, 1 km and 2 km sprints	No	Increasing citrate dose increased blood pH but had no effect on sprint performances or overall 40 km TT performance (58:46, 60: 24, 61:47 and 60:02 min for citrate (200, 400 and 600 mg/kg doses) and placebo.
Tiryaki & Atterbom 1995	11 collegiate female runners + 4 untrained controls	300 mg/kg sodium citrate or sodium bicarbonate	Running 600 m	No	No performance effect despite significant changes to acid–base status.
Goldfinch et al. 1988	6 trained males	400 mg/kg sodium bicarbonate	Running 400 m	Yes	Improved running time (56.94 v 58.63s (placebo) and 58.46 (control)). Elevated post-exercise values for pH and base excess.
Wilkes et al. 1983	6 varsity track male athletes	300 mg/kg sodium bicarbonate	Running 800 m	Yes	Improved running time (2:02.9 v 2:05.1 min (placebo) and 2:05.8 (control)) Elevated post-exercise values for pH, lactate and blood bicarbonate.

(continues)

TABLE 9.5 Studies of bicarbonate or citrate loading on sports specific performance: double-blind crossover designed studies (*continued*)

REFERENCE	SUBJECTS	DOSE	EXERCISE PROTOCOL	ENHANCED PERFORMANCE	SUMMARY
Potteiger et al. 1996b	7 well-trained male runners	300 mg/kg sodium bicarbonate and 500 mg/kg sodium citrate	Running 30 min @ LT[b] + time to exhaustion @ 100% LT	No	Both citrate and bicarbonate supplementation increased blood pH during steady-state run. No differences in run to exhaustion: 287 s, 172.8 s, 222.3 s for bicarbonate, citrate and placebo.
Shave et al. 2001	7 elite male + 2 elite female athletes	500 mg/kg sodium citrate	Running 3000 m	Yes	Performance time significantly faster ($P < 0.05$) for citrate trial (610.9 s) compared with placebo trial (621.6 s). High risk of gastrointestinal distress.
Gao et al. 1988	10 US collegiate swimmers	250 mg/kg sodium bicarbonate	Swimming 5 × 100 yd swim, 2 min rest	Yes	Faster times in 4th and 5th swim.
McNaughton & Cedaro 1991	5 elite male rowers	300 mg/kg sodium bicarbonate	Rowing 6 min max effort on ergometer	Yes	Increased work and distance rowed (1861 v 1813 m). Increased lactate levels.

[a] TT = time trial   [b] LT = lactate threshold.

intensity and/or in hot and humid environments, where sweat losses are high and opportunities to replace fluid are substantially less than the rates of fluid loss. It may also be useful to enhance the recovery of a moderate-to-large fluid deficit; for example, in brief recovery periods between events or important training sessions, or between the weigh-in and competition following 'weight making' strategies in weight division sports. Scientific investigations have focused on its potential for hyperhydrating prior to an endurance event (see Table 9.6).

Some of the apparent inconsistency in the results of these investigations occurs because of differences in study methodologies. For example, some studies have investigated the effect of glycerol in assisting the body to retain larger amounts of a fluid bolus consumed in the hours before exercise, while others have used protocols in which glycerol is consumed with only a modest fluid intake (Inder et al. 1998). At present, the best-supported scenario involves the use of glycerol to maximise the retention of fluid bolus just prior to an event in which a substantial fluid deficit cannot be prevented. In some, but not all, studies of this type, glycerol hyperhydration has been associated with performance benefits, particularly in well-trained athletes (Anderson et al. 2001; Coutts et al. 2002; Hitchins et al. 1999). However, the mechanism for this effect is not clear since the theoretical advantages of increased sweat losses, greater capacity for heat dissipation, and attenuation of cardiac and thermoregulatory challenges are not consistently seen. Further investigation is needed to replicate and explain performance benefits.

Side-effects reported by some subjects following glycerol use include nausea, gastrointestinal distress and headaches resulting from increased intracranial pressure. Fine-tuning of protocols may reduce the risk of these problems, however some individuals may remain at a greater risk than others. At the present time, although glycerol hyperhydration seems to show some promise for the performance of endurance exercise in hot conditions, it should remain an activity that is supervised and monitored by appropriate sports science/medicine professionals and only used in competition situations after adequate experimentation and fine-tuning has occurred.

Colostrum

Colostrum is a protein-rich substance secreted in breast milk in the first few days after a mother has given birth. It is high in nutrients, immunoglobulins and insulin-like growth factors (IGFs). Unlike the adult gut, the gut of a baby has 'leaky' junctions that allow it to absorb whole proteins, including immunoglobulins, thus developing the immunocompetence

TABLE 9.6 Studies of glycerol hyperhydration and performance

STUDY	SUBJECTS	GLYCEROL DOSE	EXERCISE PROTOCOL	ENHANCED PERFORMANCE	COMMENTS
Anderson et al. 2001	6 well-trained male cyclists Crossover design	1 g/kg with 20 mL/kg low joule cordial (compared with low joule cordial overload)	Cycling 90 min @ 98% LT + 15 min TT Hot environment (35∞C)	Yes	Glycerol allowed retention of additional 400 mL of fluid above hyperhydration with cordial alone. 5% improvement in work done in 15 min TT. No change in muscle metabolism. Reduced rectal temperature at 90 min with glycerol trial.
Hitchins et al. 1999	8 well-trained male cyclists Crossover design	1 g/kg with 22 mL/kg dilute sports drink, 2.5 h pre-exercise (compared with sports drink overload)	Cycling 30 min @ fixed power + 30 min TT Hot environment (32∞C)	Yes	Glycerol treatment expanded body water by 600 mL and increased (5%) work achieved in TT. This was achieved largely by preventing the drop in power seen at the start of placebo TT. No difference in power profile at end of TTs. No difference in cardiovascular, thermoregulatory, RPE[a] between trials despite differences in power output.
Inder et al. 1998	8 highly trained male triathletes Crossover design	1 g/kg with 500 mL water, 4 h pre-exercise (compared with 500 mL water)	Cycling 60 min @ 70% VO_{2max} + incremental ride to exhaustion	No	Glycerol was consumed with a modest fluid load. No increase in pre-exercise hydration status, sweat losses or urine production during exercise. No difference in time to exhaustion or workload reached. 3 subjects experienced gastrointestinal problems with glycerol.
Montner et al. 1996	11 active male and female cyclists 7 active male and female cyclists Crossover designs	1.2 g/kg with 26 mL/kg water, 1 h pre-exercise same pre-treatment + sports drink during exercise	Cycling Cycling @ 60% W_{max} until exhaustion	Yes	Reduced heart rate and increased time to exhaustion with pre-exercise glycerol treatment by ~20%.

(continues)

TABLE 9.6 Studies of glycerol hyperhydration and performance (*continued*)

STUDY	SUBJECTS	GLYCEROL DOSE	EXERCISE PROTOCOL	ENHANCED PERFORMANCE	COMMENTS
Latzka et al. 1998	8 heat-acclimatised men Crossover design	1.2 g/kg lean BM + 29 mL/kg water, 1 h pre-exercise (compared with water hyperhydration or control)	Running Treadmill running at 55% VO$_{2max}$ until exhaustion or high rectal temperature Hot environment (35°C) without further fluid intake	Yes (better than control but equal to water hyperhydration)	Both hyperhydration trials increased body fluid by ~1400 mL. Time to exhaustion longer in both trials compared with control. Performance changes not explained by differences in sweat losses, cardiac output or temperature control. Some gastrointestinal and headache symptoms with glycerol.
Coutts et al. 2002	7 male + 3 female well-trained triathletes Crossover design Difference in conditions: Hot day (30°C) Warm day (25°C)	1.2 g/kg BM + 25 mL/kg sports drink, 2 h pre-exercise (compared with sports drink placebo)	Olympic distance triathlon (field conditions) Hot conditions 25–30∞C	Yes	Decrease in triathlon performance (especially run time) between warm and hot conditions was greater in placebo group (11:40 min) than glycerol group (1:47 min). Greatest difference in times between placebo and glycerol group was found on hot day. Hyperhydration increased fluid retention of drink and reduced diuresis.

(a) RPE = rating of perceived exertion.

needed to survive outside the uterus. Recently, companies have developed supplements rich in colostrum derived from cows for use by humans.

In 1997, a peer-reviewed scientific publication reported that 8 days of supplementation with a colostrum product (Bioenervie™) increased serum IGF-1 levels in an athletic population (Mero et al. 1997). These findings raised two controversial interpretations: that adults can absorb an intact protein, and, specifically, that the supplement provides a viable dietary source of IGF-1, an anabolic hormone whose intentional intake is banned by the IOC. It is suggested that issues with the measurement of IGF-1 levels could have contributed to the results of this study. Three further investigations have failed to show either acute (Kuipers et al. 2002) or chronic (Buckley et al. 2002; Coombes et al. 2002; Kuipers et al. 2002) changes in blood levels of IGF-1 following supplementation by athletes with larger doses (60 g/day) of colostrum from a different source (Intact™). However, one study has reported a 17% increase in serum IGF-1 following 2 weeks of supplementation by athletes with 20 g/day of colostrum from yet another colostrum product (Dynamic™) (Mero et al. 2002). In this investigation, a separate absorption study indicated that most of the IGF-1 in the supplement was degraded in the gastrointestinal tract rather than absorbed, suggesting that the source of the increase in plasma IGF-1 following oral intake of colostrum was enhanced stimulus of human IGF-1 synthesis. Colostrum is not on the list of banned substances of the IOC/World Anti-Doping Agency, and one study has reported that 4 weeks of colostrum supplementation (60 g/day) was not seen to cause a positive doping outcome based on urine testing (Kuipers et al. 2002).

The recent nature of the interest in colostrum means that it will take time for a large bank of studies to be conducted and published in the peer-reviewed literature. However, several studies have been published in the last 12 months; the results of studies available as of October 2002 are summarised in Table 9.7. Several studies have involved long-term supplementation (8–9 weeks) in subjects ranging from 'active' (Buckley et al. 2002) to nationally competitive athletes (Brinkworth et al. 2002; Hofman et al. 2002), with good control of training and diet. Such studies are hard to conduct and require a large commitment from both researchers and subjects. The summary of available literature shows that performance benefits are not universal or consistently seen following such long-term colostrum use (see Table 9.7).

There are few data in the present studies to explore a viable mechanism by which colostrum supplementation might achieve performance benefits. Some authors have suggested that colostrum might enhance nutrient

TABLE 9.7 Studies of colostrum supplementation and performance: experimental: placebo design

STUDY	SUBJECTS	COLOSTRUM DOSE AND TRAINING	EXERCISE PROTOCOL	ENHANCED PERFORMANCE	COMMENTS
Buckley et al. 2002	30 active male (colostrum = 17; placebo = 13) Experimental–placebo design	8 weeks @ 60 g/day colostrum or placebo (whey protein) 45 min running @ 3/week	Tests at baseline, 4 weeks and 8 weeks • 2 × treadmill VO_{2max} tests (~30 min) separated by 20 min	4 weeks—no for either run 8 weeks—no for first run, yes for second run	Performance measured as peak effective running speed achieved in running max test. Training improved peak running speed in both groups at week 8. No differences between groups in either run at week 4 although trend to lower peak speed in second run with colostrum group. At week 8, no difference in peak speed in first run, but greater speed in second run in colostrum group ($P < 0.05$), suggesting better recovery between runs.
Coombes et al. 2002	28 trained male cyclists (high dose colostrum = 10; low dose colostrum = 9; placebo = 9) Experimental–placebo design	8 weeks @ 60 g/day colostrum or 20 g/day colostrum or placebo (40 g/day whey protein) 1.5 h/day cycling	Tests at baseline and 8 weeks on separate days: • 2 × VO_{2max} tests (~20 run) separated by 20 min • 2 h @ 65% VO_{2max} + ~ 12 min TT	No for either cycling max test Yes	Performance measured in VO_{2max} test protocol as total work done in the second test. A small but non-significant increase in VO_{2max} seen in all groups at the end of 8 weeks, but no difference between groups. Greater improvement at week 8 in TT following 2 h submaximal ride in both colostrum groups (4%; 19%; 16% $P < 0.05$ for placebo, low dose and high dose)
Brinkworth et al. 2002	13 elite female rowers (colostrum = 6; placebo = 7) Experimental–placebo design	9 weeks @ 60 g/day of colostrum or placebo (whey protein) 18 h/week rowing + 3/week resistance training	Tests at baseline and 9 weeks: • 2 × incremental rowing tests with 15 min recovery interval (each = 3 × 4 min submaximal workloads + 4 min maximal effort.)	No	Rowing performance increased by week 9 in both groups. No difference between groups at week 9 for either maximal rowing performance. Higher value for index of blood buffering capacity at week 9 in colostrum group.

(continues)

TABLE 9.7 Studies of colostrum supplementation and performance: experimental: placebo design (*continued*)

STUDY	SUBJECTS	COLOSTRUM DOSE AND TRAINING	EXERCISE PROTOCOL	ENHANCED PERFORMANCE	COMMENTS
Hofman et al. 2002	17 female + 18 male elite hockey players (colostrum = 9 female + 9 male; placebo = 8 female + 9 male) Experimental–placebo design	8 weeks @ 60 g/day of colostrum or placebo (whey protein) 3/week training + 1/week game	Tests at baseline and 8 weeks: • 5 × 10 m sprint • vertical jump • shuttle run • 'suicide' agility test	Yes No No No	No improvements in shuttle run, jump or agility run over 8 weeks in either group. Significant improvement in sprint performance for both groups with larger improvement in colostrum group (0.64 v 0.33 × P < 0.05). Similar increases in lean BM in both groups.
Antonio et al. 2001	14 male + 8 female resistance-trained subjects Experimental–placebo design	8 weeks @ 20 g/day of colostrum or placebo (whey protein) 3/week aerobic and resistance training	Tests at baseline and 8 weeks: • treadmill run to exhaustion • bench press: 1 repetition maximal • submaximal repetitions to exhaustion	No No No	Colostrum group experienced significant increase in lean BM (1.5 kg) as measured by DEXA, while placebo group showed increase in BM (2 kg) without any change in lean BM.
Mero et al. 1997	9 male sprinters and jumpers Crossover design with 13 day wash-out	8 days @ 25 mL/day colostrum or 125 mL/day or placebo (milk whey) 6 sessions speed & resistance training	Tests at day 6 of each program: • countermovement jump	No	Serum IGF increased over time with colostrum supplementation (although still within physiological ranges) compared with placebo. No change in serum or saliva immunoglobulins between treatments.

DEXA = dual-energy X-ray absorptiometry

absorption from the gut by stimulating intestinal mucosal growth; however, this remains speculative. The effect of colostrum supplementation on blood levels of IGF-1 is inconsistent but is a possible source of enhancement of muscle protein synthesis. One study (Mero et al. 2002) has reported an increase in salivary immunoglobulin A (IgA), a factor that is important in the defence against viruses causing upper respiratory tract infections; however, this is in contradiction to the findings of an earlier study by the same group (Mero et al. 1997). In any case, studies that report a favourable metabolic or physiological response to colostrum supplementation often fail to find any transfer into a performance benefit (Antonio et al. 2001, Brinkworth et al. 2002; Mero et al. 1997). Changes in body mass or composition (e.g. increase in lean body mass or decrease in fat free mass) following colostrum supplementation are not consistent, with one study reporting an increase in lean body mass in colostrum users compared with a placebo group (Antonio et al. 2001), while other studies have not found any differences in changes in body mass or body composition between supplement and placebo groups over the duration of the study (Brinkworth et al. 2002; Buckley et al. 2002; Coombes et al. 2002; Hofman et al. 2002).

Clearly colostrum is a 'hot' supplement in the athletic world and merits further research. However, there is insufficient evidence at present to support definite performance benefits or to define the target group who might benefit from colostrum use. With commercial supplements costing A$25–70 per week to provide a dosage of 20–60 g/day, and the suggestion that it may take at least 4 weeks to show benefits, athletes and coaches are reminded that colostrum supplementation involves a considerable expense.

HMB

β-hydroxy-β-methylbutyrate (HMB), a metabolite of the amino acid leucine, is claimed to increase the gains in strength and lean body mass associated with resistance training and enhance recovery from exercise (see Slater & Jenkins 2000). HMB is claimed to act as an anti-catabolic agent, minimising protein breakdown and the cellular damage that occurs with high-intensity exercise. It has been proposed that the anti-catabolic effects sometimes seen associated with leucine feeding during times of stress are mediated by HMB. Interest in HMB supplementation stemmed from animal studies, with some but not all investigations finding that HMB supplementation increased gains in carcass weight or feed efficiency, defined as weight gain per unit feed, during periods of growth (for review see Slater & Jenkins 2000). HMB supplements were first introduced to the sports market in the

TABLE 9.8 Studies of HMB supplementation on training adaptations and performance

STUDY	SUBJECTS	HMB DOSE AND TRAINING	EXERCISE PROTOCOL	ENHANCED PERFORMANCE	COMMENTS
Slater et al. 2001	27 elite male rowers and male water polo players Experimental–placebo design	0, 3 g/day conventional or time-release HMB for 6 weeks Resistance training 3/weeks + sports related training Nutritional advice + CHO/protein supplement	Tests at baseline, 3 weeks and 6 weeks: • bench press • leg press • chin-ups	No No No	All groups increased strength and lean BM with no differences in response between groups. No differences in urinary 3-MH[a] or plasma CK[b] crude markers of muscle breakdown and damage between groups.
Jowko et al. 2001	40 untrained males Experimental–placebo design	0, 3 g/day HMB, 3 g/day HMB-creatine, or creatine for 3 weeks Resistance training	Tests at baseline and 3 weeks: • strength in various resistance exercises	Yes	Creatine caused greater increase in lean BM and strength than placebo group. Greater strength and trend to greater increase in lean BM with HMB than placebo. Effects were additive. HMB reduced plasma CK levels and urea, suggesting nitrogen sparing.
Vukovich et al. 2001	8 trained male cyclists Crossover study (2 week wash-out)	Placebo, 3 g/day leucine or 3 g/day HMB Cycling training	Tests pre- and post- each 2 week supplementation: – VO_{2peak}	Yes	Significant increase in VO_{2peak} following HMB supplementation but not other supplementation periods.
Panton et al. 2000	39 males and 36 females of varying training status Experimental–placebo design	0 or 3 g/day HMB for 4 weeks Resistance training 3/week	Tests at baseline and 4 weeks: • strength in various resistance exercises	Yes	Data pooled across training status and gender. HMB group showed greater increase in upper body strength, and a trend to greater gains in lean BM, and loss of body fat than placebo, regardless of gender or training status

(continues)

TABLE 9.8 Studies of HMB supplementation on training adaptations and performance (*continued*)

STUDY	SUBJECTS	HMB DOSE AND TRAINING	EXERCISE PROTOCOL	ENHANCED PERFORMANCE	COMMENTS
Gallagher et al. 2000	37 untrained males Experimental–placebo design	0, 3 g/day or 6 g/day HMB for 8 weeks Resistance training 3/week	Tests at baseline and 8 weeks: • 1 repetition maximal in 10 different exercises • peak isometric torque and peak isokinetic torque	No Yes	No differences in 1 repetition maximal strength gains between treatments. Some greater increases in peak isokinetic or isometric torque and greater increase in lean BM with 3 g/day HMB than placebo or 6 g/day. Decrease in plasma CK rise with HMB than placebo.
Kreider et al. 1999	40 resistance trained males (6 mg HMB, 3 mg HMB, placebo) Experimental–placebo design	0, 3 or 6 g/day HMB for 4 weeks Resistance training 7 h/week	Tests at baseline and 4 week: • bench press • leg press	No No	No difference in improvements in strength between groups, or changes in lean BM or body fat levels. No differences between plasma CK level and LDH[c] levels (another marker of catabolism).
Nissen et al. 1996	41 untrained males (placebo, 1.5 mg HMB, 3 mg HMB further subdivided into control or high protein groups) Experimental–placebo design	0, 1.5 g/day or 3 g/day for 3 weeks Resistance training 3/week 117 or 175 g/day protein	Tests at baseline and 3 weeks: • weight lifted in training session	Yes	HMB associated with decrease in urinary 3-MH and plasma CK. Trend to increased gain in lean BM with HMB. Dose-responsive increase in weight lifted during training session with HMB compared with placebo.
Nissen et al. 1996	Resistance trained males Experimental–placebo design	3 g/day for 7 weeks Resistance training 2–3 h/day	Tests at baseline and 7 weeks: • bench press • squat • clean	Yes No No	Control group was stronger at baseline in upper body strength; gains made by HMB group simply caused groups to be equal in upper and lower body strength at end of study. Greater increase in lean BM during early part of study in HMB group was absent by 7 weeks. Effects of HMB diminish over time. Diet not controlled.

(a) 3-MH = 3-methylhistidine. (b) CK = creatine kinase. (c) LDH = lactate dehydrogenase.

mid-1990s and by 1998 were achieving annual sales of US$30–50 million in the United States alone (Slater & Jenkins 2000).

Although a number of scientific investigations of HMB supplementation and exercise performance have been undertaken, only those that have been published in full in peer-reviewed journals are summarised in Table 9.8. In these studies, outcomes from HMB supplementation protocols have been measured in terms of changes in body composition and strength; there is mixed support for a role for HMB in enhancing the response to resistance training. A recent meta-analysis of these studies found that HMB supplementation led to a net increase in lean BM (0.28% per week) and strength gains (1.4% per week) but the effect of these changes was less than 0.2, where such a change is considered small (Nissen & Sharp, 2003). Other studies that have simply monitored indices of muscle damage following eccentric exercise have found that HMB supplementation either reduced (Knitter et al. 2000) or failed to change the normal responses (Paddon-Jones et al. 2001).

It is difficult to find a common thread to the findings of the present HMB research. One theory is that HMB supplementation might be most valuable in the early phases of a new training program, or when previously untrained subjects undertake resistance training, where it is able to reduce the large catabolic response or damage produced by unaccustomed exercise. However, once adaptation to training occurs, reducing the residual catabolism/damage response, HMB supplementation no longer provides a detectable benefit. If this were the case, it would explain why HMB tends to produce favourable results in novice resistance trainers rather than well-trained subjects, and why positive results are reported in shorter studies (i.e. 2–4 weeks) but not at the end of longer studies (i.e. 8 weeks). Further well-controlled studies are required to clarify if, and under what circumstances, HMB is a useful training aid.

Ribose

Ribose is a pentose sugar that provides part of the structure of a variety of important chemicals in the body, including the adenine nucleotides ATP, AMP and ADP. It is found in the diet but purified forms have also recently been released onto the market, finding their way into sports supplements. Oral ribose is quickly absorbed and tolerated even at intakes of 100 g, however at A$700 per kg, ribose powders represent an expensive form of CHO.

In the body, the pentose phosphate pathway is a rate-limiting pathway for the interconversion of ribose-5-phosphate and glucose; ribose-5-phosphate can be converted to phosphoribosyl pyrophosphate (PRPP), which is then involved in the synthesis or salvaging of the adenine nucleotide pool. It has been suggested that suboptimal amounts of PRPP may limit these processes, and ribose infusion has been shown to enhance ATP recovery and exercise function in animal models of myocardial ischaemia (see Op' T Eijnde et al. 2001). High-intensity exercise has been shown to cause a reduction in the muscle ATP content and the total adenine nucleotide pool, possibly because the rate of nucleotide salvaging and synthesis falls behind the massive rates of nucleotide degradation. It has been suggested that oral intake of ribose might increase the rate of nucleotide salvaging/synthesis and achieve quicker recovery of exercise-mediated reductions in muscle total adenine nucleotides. Sports supplements, typically providing 3–5 g doses of ribose, have been produced with claims of 'dramatically reducing recovery from 72 h to 12 h' and, in synergy with creatine, providing 'the most sophisticated energy support systems'. Several studies of ribose supplementation in athletes undertaking repeated bouts of high-intensity exercise have appeared in conference abstract form.

To date, only one such study has been published in full in the peer-reviewed literature (see Op' T Eijnde et al. 2001). This study investigated muscle adenine content and muscle power/force characteristics after two intermittent training sessions 24 hours apart on two occasions; the first occasion was a baseline measure on active subjects, while the second test set followed a 7-day training program involving two bouts of intermittent exercise each day while taking ribose (four doses of 4 g/day) or placebo. The first exercise bout in each testing occasion caused a decrease in muscle total adenine nucleotide with muscle ATP content being reduced by 20% at the time of the second bout. However, ribose supplementation did not alter the loss or recovery of ATP resulting from this exercise protocol, nor did it change muscle force or power characteristics during maximal testing (Op' T Eijnde et al. 2001). The authors acknowledged that plasma ribose concentrations achieved by the supplementation were too low to achieve a significant change in nucleotide synthesis/salvage. However, the doses used in the study were already higher than that recommended by most supplement manufacturers. Further work is needed to explore this area, but the ultimate outcome might be challenged by the practicality and expense of consuming larger doses of oral ribose.

L-carnitine

The first reports on carnitine in the early 1900s described it as a vitamin (essential component of the diet). Following the discovery that carnitine can be manufactured in the liver and kidney from amino acid precursors (lysine and methionine), it is now considered to be a non-essential nutrient. Most animal foods provide a dietary source of carnitine, but due to losses in cooking and preparation of foods there are few data on the total content of the diet. Carnitine ingested or synthesised by humans is in the L-isoform and is carried via the blood for storage, predominantly in the heart and skeletal muscle. Within these tissues, carnitine plays a number of roles related to fat and carbohydrate metabolism.

Carnitine is a component of the enzymes carnitine palmityltransferase I (CPT-1), carnitine-palmityltransferase II (CPT-II) and carnitine-acylcarnitine translocase (CAT). These enzymes are involved in the transportation of long chain fatty acids (LCFAs) across the mitochondrial membrane to the site of their oxidation. Because of this function, it has been suggested that carnitine supplementation might enhance fatty acid transport and oxidation. As a result, carnitine is a popular component of supplements claimed to enhance the loss of body fat, and has been embraced by body builders wanting to 'cut up' and other populations interested in weight loss. An increase in fatty acid oxidation during exercise could be of advantage to endurance athletes if it resulted in a sparing of glycogen during events in which CHO stores are otherwise limiting.

During exercise, carnitine also plays the role of a 'sink' for acetyl-CoA production. By converting this to acetyl-carnitine and CoA, carnitine helps to maintain CoA availability and to decrease the ratio of acetyl-CoA:CoA. If carnitine supplementation could increase this function it might enhance flux through the citric acid cycle. Furthermore, it could enhance the activity of the enzyme pyruvate dehydrogenase, which is otherwise inhibited by high levels of acetyl-CoA, thus increasing oxidative metabolism of glucose. If this results in lower lactate production, it might enhance exercise performance in situations that might otherwise be limited by excess lactate and hydrogen ion accumulation. Extensive reviews of carnitine function are available (Cerretelli & Marconi 1990; Clarkson 1992; Heinonen 1996; Wagenmakers 1991).

When muscle carnitine activity is inadequate, as in the case of inborn errors of metabolism, individuals demonstrate lipid abnormalities and reduced exercise capacity. Carnitine supplementation is an established medical therapy for these conditions and helps to attenuate such symptoms.

TABLE 9.9 Studies of carnitine supplementation and metabolism on performance

STUDY	SUBJECTS	CARNITINE DOSE	EXERCISE PROTOCOL	ENHANCEMENT	COMMENTS
Metabolism only					
Barnett et al. 1994	8 untrained males Crossover design—order effect	4 g/day for 14 days	Cycling 4 min ride at 90% VO_{2max} + 5 × 1 min rides at 115% VO_{2max}	No	Supplementation failed to increase muscle carnitine content. No change in lactate accumulation during submaximal and supramaximal performance.
Vukovich et al. 1994	8 untrained males Crossover design	6 g/day for 7 and 14 days	Cycling 60 min at 70% VO_{2max} High-fat pre-trial diet to promote lipid availability	No	No change in muscle carnitine content after supplementation. No effect on substrate utilisation even after dietary strategy to promote fat availability.
Gorostiaga et al.1989	10 endurance trained males and females Crossover design	2 g/day for 28 days	Cycling 45 min at 66% VO_{2max} + 60 min seated recovery	Yes	Reduced RER[a] during exercise (P < 0.05). Non-significant trend for higher O_2 uptake, heart rate, blood glycerol and resting plasma FFA.
Soop et al. 1988	7 moderately trained males Crossover design, with order effect	5 g/day for 5 days	Cycling 120 min at 50% VO_{2max}	No	No effect on muscle substrate utilisation during exercise or at rest.
Oyono-Enguelle et al. 1988	10 untrained males Crossover design with 2 control trials and 1 experimental trial. Order effect.	2 g/day for 4 weeks	Cycling 60 min at 50% VO_{2max} + 120 min recovery	No	No change in physiological parameters and blood metabolites. The increased demand for FFA oxidation during exercise is adequately supported by endogenous carnitine.
Decombaz et al. 1993	9 untrained males Crossover design	3 g/day for 7 days	Cycling CHO depletion regimen + 20 min at 60% VO_{2max}	No	Substrate metabolism not affected during submaximal exercise even after glycogen depletion and situation of high lipid flux

(continues)

TABLE 9.9 Studies of carnitine supplementation and metabolism on performance (*continued*)

STUDY	SUBJECTS	CARNITINE DOSE	EXERCISE PROTOCOL	ENHANCEMENT	COMMENTS
Siliprandi et al. 1990	10 moderately trained males Crossover design	Acute administration 2 g @ 1 h before exercise	Cycling Cycle to exhaustion	Yes	Increased time to exhaustion. Carnitine reduced the increase in plasma lactate and pyruvate after maximal progressive work. However, dose and time frame for uptake into muscle seems unrealistic.
Vecchiet et al. 1990	10 moderately trained males Crossover design	Acute administration 2 g @ 1 h before exercise	Cycling Incremental cycling to exhaustion	Yes	Increase in time (and work) until exhaustion. Decrease in lactate production and oxygen consumption at same workload. However, dose and time frame for uptake into muscle seems unrealistic.
Greig et al. 1987	9 untrained males and females 10 untrained males and females Crossover design	2 g for 4 weeks 2 g/day for 2 weeks	Cycling Progressive test to exhaustion	No	No significant physiological changes. Changes in performance were small and inconsistent.
Trappe et al. 1994	20 highly trained male collegiate swimmers Experimental–placebo design	4 g/day for 7 days	Swimming 5 × 91.4 m swims	No	No difference in performance times between trials or between groups.
Colombani et al. 1996	7 endurance-trained male athletes Crossover design	2 g @ 2 h before run and at 20 km mark	Running Marathon run + submaximal performance test day after marathon	No	No change in exercise metabolism or marathon running time. No change in recovery and submaximal test performance on following day.
Marconi et al. 1985	6 national class walkers Crossover design	4 g/day for 2 weeks	Running Supramaximal work (jumps) + treadmill VO_{2max} + submaximal run	Yes?	Increase in VO_{2max} by 6%. However, no effects on oxygen utilisation and RER at submaximal loads, or change in lactate accumulation with jumps. Results appear inconsistent.

(a) RER = respiratory exchange ratio.

However, whether additional carnitine intake in healthy individuals enhances metabolism and exercise performance is a different issue. A positive outcome would require one or more of the following scenarios: heavy training causing suboptimal levels of muscle carnitine; carnitine supplementation increasing muscle carnitine content; carnitine being a limiting factor in fatty acid transport; carnitine being a limiting factor in pyruvate dehydrogenase activity or citric acid cycle flux. However, thorough reviews cast doubt on the potential for enhanced metabolic function via enhanced carnitine status (Wagenmakers 1991; Heinonen 1996). These reviews summarise that normal muscle carnitine levels appear to be adequate for maximal function of CPT-I and CPT-II, and that there is no proof that fatty acid transport is the rate-limiting step in fat oxidation. Furthermore, pyruvate dehydrogenase is believed to be fully active within seconds of high-intensity exercise, and additional carnitine is unlikely to stimulate this activity further.

Optimal muscle carnitine content in athletes is probably the most important issue to address. Exercise is known to increase carnitine excretion and it is possible that muscle carnitine content may decrease during intense training. However, a series of reviews conclude that although most human studies find an increase in *plasma* carnitine levels following carnitine supplementation of 1–6 g/day, there is no compelling evidence that *muscle* carnitine levels are enhanced as a result of supplementation (Cerretelli & Marconi 1990; Wagenmakers 1991; Heinonen 1996). Studies that have investigated the effects of carnitine supplementation on exercise metabolism and/or performance are summarised in Table 9.9. On balance, there is little evidence of increased performance during submaximal or high-intensity exercise resulting from carnitine supplementation. The effect of carnitine supplementation on body-fat levels, although widely publicised in supplement advertising, has not been studied in athletes.

Coenzyme Q10

Coenzyme Q10, or ubiquinone, is a non-essential, lipid-soluble nutrient found predominantly in animal foods and in low levels in plant foods. In the body it is located primarily in skeletal and cardiac muscle, inside the mitochondria. Coenzyme Q10 provides a link in the electron transport chain producing ATP, and is part of the mitochondrial antioxidant defence system, preventing damage to DNA and cell membranes. Some cardiac and neuromuscular dysfunction is believed to result from coenzyme Q10 deficiency. Indeed, patients with ischaemic heart disease are often seen

TABLE 9.10 Studies of coenzyme Q10 supplementation and oxidative damage or performance

STUDY	SUBJECTS	COENZYME Q10 DOSE	EXERCISE PROTOCOL	ENHANCEMENT	COMMENTS
Oxidative damage only					
Svensson et al. 1999	17 well-trained males Experimental–placebo design	110 mg/day for 20 days	Cycling 30 s max cycle + 10 × 10 s max cycles	No	Supplementation increased plasma but not muscle coenzyme Q10. Coenzyme Q10 did not affect purine catabolism or plasma malondialdehyde (indication of lipid peroxidation).
Kaikkonen et al. 1998	37 moderately trained male runners Experimental–placebo design	90 mg/day for 3 weeks (+ vitamin E)	Running Marathon (field test)	No	No change in indices of oxidative or muscle damage following marathon run.
Performance					
Nielsen et al. 1999	7 well-trained male triathletes	100 mg/day for 6 weeks (+ vitamin E + vitamin C)	Cycling Incremental VO_{2max} test to exhaustion	No	No effect on maximal oxygen uptake or muscle energy metabolism (determined by nuclear magnetic resonance spectroscopy).
Malm et al. 1997	18 male Experimental–placebo design	120 mg/day for 22 days	Cycling Anaerobic training sessions + anaerobic + submaximal cycling tests undertaken throughout 2 days of supplementation	No[a]	Coenzyme Q10 produced negative effect on anaerobic cycling performance—failure to achieve a training effect. Increased CK levels with coenzyme Q10. No effect on submaximal performance.
Weston et al. 1997	18 trained male cyclists and triathletes Experimental–placebo design	1 mg/kg/day for 28 days	Cycling Normal training undertaken during 28-day supplementation. Incremental test to exhaustion undertaken pre- and post	No	Coenzyme Q10 did not enhance any performance parameters.

(continues)

TABLE 9.10 Studies of coenzyme Q10 supplementation and oxidative damage or performance (continued)

STUDY	SUBJECTS	COENZYME Q10 DOSE	EXERCISE PROTOCOL	ENHANCEMENT	COMMENTS
Malm et al. 1996	15 healthy males Experimental–placebo design	120 mg/day for 22 days	Cycling Anaerobic training sessions + anaerobic + submaximal cycling tests undertaken throughout 22 days of supplementation	No[a]	Coenzyme Q10 produced negative effect on anaerobic cycling performance—failure to respond to training. No effect on submaximal performance.
Laaksonen et al. 1995	11 young and 8 older trained males Crossover design	120 mg/day for 6 weeks	Cycling Prolonged endurance test to exhaustion	No[a]	No change in muscle coenzyme Q10 concentrations or plasma malondialdehyde as a result of coenzyme Q10 supplementation. Negative effect on time to exhaustion (placebo had greater endurance).
Snider et al. 1992	11 highly trained triathletes Crossover design	100 mg/day for 4 weeks (+ vitamin E, inosine, cytochrome c)	Cycling and running 90 min on treadmill @ 70% VO2max + cycling @ 70% VO2max to exhaustion	No	No difference in time to exhaustion between trials. No differences in blood metabolites or RPE.
Braun et al. 1991	10 male cyclists Experimental–placebo design	100 mg/day for 8 weeks	Cycling Incremental test to exhaustion performance pre- and post- supplementation period. Training continued during period	No	Performance increased equally in both groups after training period. Coenzyme Q10 had no effect on cycling performance or any measured parameters. Malondialdehyde concentrations reduced in both groups after training.
Ylikoski et al. 1997	25 national-level cross-country skiers Experimental–placebo design	90 mg/day for 6 weeks	Cross-country skiing Treadmill pole-walking to exhaustion	Yes	Improved VO2max with coenzyme Q10 supplementation. Increase in aerobic and anaerobic thresholds. No control of exercise during supplementation periods.

(a) Decrease in performance.

to have lower plasma coenzyme Q10 concentrations and improve their exercise capacity following coenzyme Q10 supplementation. The marketing campaigns for coenzyme Q10 supplements promote increased vigour and youthfulness as a benefit of their use. For athletes they are claimed to enhance energy production and reduce the oxidative damage of exercise.

Peer-reviewed studies of coenzyme Q10 supplementation on exercise metabolism, oxidative damage caused by exercise and performance are summarised in Table 9.10. There are few data that support an ergogenic benefit of coenzyme Q10 on exercise performance. By contrast, studies undertaken at the Karolinska Institute in Sweden have consistently shown that coenzyme Q10 has an *ergolytic*, or negative, effect on high-intensity performance and training adaptations (Malm et al. 1997; Malm et al. 1996; Svennson et al. 1999). These studies found that coenzyme Q10 supplementation *increased* the oxidative damage produced by high-intensity exercise in previously untrained subjects. Twenty-two days of supplementation, undertaken in conjunction with high-intensity training, was shown to increase oxidative damage, as indicated by higher plasma creatine kinase levels and increased malondialdehyde levels in response to exercise (Malm et al. 1997; Malm et al. 1996). In these circumstances, coenzyme Q10 was believed to act as a pro-oxidant rather than an antioxidant. Training adaptations were impaired in healthy subjects who undertook high-intensity training while taking co-enzyme Q10 supplements, with the placebo group out-performing the coenzyme Q10 group at the end of the supplementation phase (Malm et al. 1997).

Further work is required to investigate the effects of coenzyme Q10 supplementation on exercise performance and training. However, at present there is little to recommend coenzyme Q10 supplementation to athletes undertaking high-intensity training, and we are reminded that the issue of antioxidant supplementation is complex and as yet unsolved.

Ginseng

Ginseng has a long history as a health supplement. There are several species of ginseng: American, Siberian, Korean and Japanese (Bahrke & Morgan 1994). While most of these ginsengs are related, belonging to the *Panax* species, Russian or Siberian ginseng is extracted from a different plant (*Eleutherococcus senticosus*). The root of the plants is considered the most valuable part and a number of chemically similar steroid glycosides or saponin chemicals, known as ginsenosides, have been identified as active ingredients in ginsengs. The chemical composition of commercial supplement products is highly variable due to differences in

TABLE 9.11 Studies of ginseng supplementation and metabolism on performance

STUDY	SUBJECTS	GINSENG DOSE	EXERCISE PROTOCOL	ENHANCEMENT	COMMENTS
Metabolism only					
Engels & Wirth 1997	37 healthy males Experimental–placebo design	200 mg/day or 400 mg/day for 8 weeks	Cycling Submaximal and maximal cycling test	No	No change in RPE, heart rate or RER at submaximal or maximal workloads.
Performance					
Ziemba et al. 1999	15 male soccer players Experimental–placebo design	350 mg/day for 6 weeks	Cycling Incremental test to exhaustion Reaction time measured at each stage	No Yes	No change in lactate threshold or VO_{2max}. However, enhanced reaction time at submaximal workloads.
Allen et al. 1998	28 healthy subjects (male and female) Experimental–placebo design	200 mg/day for 3 weeks	Cycling Incremental test to exhaustion	No	No enhancement of total workload, RPE and lactate at submaximal loads or VO_{2max}.
Morris et al. 1996	8 active subjects (male and female) Crossover design	8 mg/kg/day or 16 mg/kg/day for 1 week standard ginseng preparation	Cycling Time to exhaustion @ 75% VO_{2max}	No	No change in time to exhaustion or metabolic parameters. No change in RPE.
Dowling et al. 1996	20 highly trained runners (male and female) Experimental–placebo design	60 drops/day (maximum recommended dose) of Russian ginseng for 6 weeks	Running 10 min treadmill test at 10-km race pace, maximal treadmill test	No	No change in metabolic characteristics at race pace, treadmill max, RPE. Low statistical power may prevent small changes from being detected.
Pieralisi et al. 1991	Active male subjects Crossover design	2 capsules/day for 6 weeks Ginsana 115 (ginseng, vitamins, bitartrate + minerals)	Running Incremental treadmill test to exhaustion	Yes (was this due to ginseng or other ingredients?)	Increased VO_{2max} and reduced O_2 consumption at submaximal workloads.
McNaughton et al. 1989	30 active subjects (male and female) Crossover design	1 g/day × 6 weeks of Chinese ginseng or Russian ginseng	Physical testing VO_{2max}, grip, pectoral and quadriceps strength	Yes	Significantly greater increase in VO_{2max} and pectoral and grip strength with Chinese ginseng. Trends for enhancement with Russian ginseng.

the genetic nature of the plant source, variation in active ingredients with cultivation and season, differences in the methods of drying and curing, and differences in the process of supplement preparation. Some ginseng preparations also provide additional agents such as vitamins, minerals or other herbal compounds.

Ginseng has been used widely in herbal medicines of oriental cultures to cure fatigue, relieve pain and headaches, and improve mental function and vigour. It has also been described by Eastern-bloc scientists as an 'adaptogen': a substance purported to normalise physiology after exposure to a variety of stresses. An adaptogen is considered to exhibit a lack of specificity in its actions and can either reduce or increase a response that has been altered by a stressor. This theory represents a different philosophy of physiology or medicine to traditional Western understanding.

In athletes, ginseng is claimed to reduce fatigue and improve aerobic conditioning, strength, mental alertness and recovery. Table 9.11 summarises the few fully published studies that have investigated the effect of ginseng and related products on exercise or sports performance. Although other studies are mentioned in reviews or discussions of ginseng supplementation (Bahrke & Morgan 1994; Dowling et al. 1996) these have not been included in the present discussion due to flaws in research design (failure to include a control or placebo group) and an absence of details due to publication in a foreign language journal.

Given the small number of studies and the lack of investigations involving well-trained subjects, it is fair to say that the effect of ginseng supplementation on athletic performance is largely unresearched. However, the variability of the content of commerciawl ginseng supplements creates a major impediment to research. One study of 50 commercial ginseng preparations found that 44 products ranged in ginsenoside concentration from 1.9% to 9.0%, while six preparations failed to produce a detectable level of ginsenosides (Chong & Oberholzer 1988). Therefore, even if scientific evidence showed that ginseng could enhance exercise performance, athletes could not be certain of receiving the appropriate dose and type of active ingredients from all preparations in the commercially available range. Athletes should also be aware that herbal preparations are considered at higher risk of containing contaminants than other supplements. Indeed, two separate studies have found commercial ginseng supplements to contain ephedrine, a stimulant in contravention to doping codes (Chong & Oberholzer 1988; Cui et al. 1994). At the current time there is no substantial evidence to support testimonial claims that ginseng is of benefit to performance or recovery.

Inosine

Inosine is a non-essential nutrient with good dietary sources, including yeast and organ meats. Several theories have suggested mechanisms by which inosine supplementation could benefit exercise performance. Inosine is a precursor of the nucleotide inosine monophosphate (IMP) and could lead to an increase in ATP content. In-vitro tests suggest that inosine may enhance the levels of 2,3-diphosphoglycerate in red blood cells, which theoretically could produce an increased release of oxygen into the muscle via a shift in the oxyhaemoglobin curve. Inosine is believed to have vasodilatory effects and antioxidant properties (for further information on inosine see Williams et al. 1990 and Starling et al. 1996). However, these are only hypothetical situations that have not been supported by research.

The major support for inosine supplementation is testimonial, with reports from athletes, especially from Russian and ex-Eastern-Bloc countries, and muscle building magazines. One popular magazine, *Muscle and Fitness*, published an article describing a 6-week study of inosine supplementation on four trained athletes (Colgan 1988). The report claimed the study was undertaken using a double-blind crossover design and found strength gains as a result of the supplementation. This study has not appeared in a peer-reviewed publication or in adequate detail to judge the validity of these claims. The athletes reported irritability and fatigue while taking the inosine supplements.

Table 9.12 summarises the results of the only three well-controlled studies of inosine supplementation that have been published in the peer-reviewed literature. Inosine was also an ingredient in a multi-compound ergogenic aid (CAPS) that failed to enhance performance of triathletes in a study by Snider and colleagues (1992); this study has been reviewed in the section on coenzyme Q10 above. The three studies of isolated inosine supplementation all failed to find either favourable metabolic changes or performance benefits following inosine supplementation in well-trained subjects (McNaughton et al. 1999; Starling et al. 1996; Williams et al. 1990). There were no data to support any of the theoretical actions of inosine supplementation. Although muscle substrates were not directly measured in these studies, purported changes to ATP concentrations are unlikely to enhance exercise performance since ATP is not depleted by exercise, even at the point of fatigue.

Of note, two studies reported that subjects showed better performance of high-intensity tasks while on the placebo treatment than on the inosine trial, suggesting that inosine supplementation might actually *impair* the

TABLE 9.12 Studies of inosine supplementation and performance

STUDY	SUBJECTS	INOSINE DOSE	EXERCISE PROTOCOL	ENHANCED PERFORMANCE	COMMENTS
McNaughton et al. 1999	7 well-trained males Crossover design	10 000 mg for 5 and 10 days	Cycling 5 × 6 s, 30 s and 20 min TT	No	No improvements in sprint times or TT performance. Increase in plasma uric acid concentrations.
Starling et al. 1996	10 competitive male cyclists Crossover design	5000 mg/day for 5 days	Cycling Wingate bike test, 30-min self-paced cycle, supramaximal sprint to fatigue	No[a]	No difference in Wingate performance or 30-min cycle. Negative effect on time to fatigue. Increase in plasma uric acid concentration.
Williams et al. 1990	9 highly trained male and female endurance runners Crossover design	6000 mg/day for 2 days (maximum recommended dose)	Running Submaximal warm-up run, competitive 3-mile treadmill run, maximal treadmill run.	No[a]	No effect on 3 mile run time, VO$_{2peak}$ or other variables. Negative effect on maximal run.

(a) Decrease in performance.

performance of high-intensity exercise (Starling et al. 1996; Williams et al. 1990). Potential mechanisms for exercise impairment include an increased formation of IMP in the muscle, either at rest or during exercise. High IMP concentrations have been found at the point of fatigue in many exercise studies; furthermore IMP has been shown to inhibit ATPase activity (Sahlin 1992). It is possible that increased resting concentrations of muscle IMP reduced the duration of high-intensity exercise before critically high levels were reached, causing premature fatigue. Such a theory can only be investigated by direct measurements of muscle nucleotides. Another possible mechanism of performance impairment is an increase in levels of uric acid, a product of inosine degradation. In the present studies, two days of inosine supplementation did not change uric acid levels, however 5 days and 10 days of intake doubled blood concentrations to levels above the normal range (McNaughton et al. 1999; Starling et al. 1996; Williams et al. 1990). Thus, chronic inosine supplementation may pose a health risk since high uric acid levels are implicated as a cause of gout. In summary, since there is a lack of evidence of performance benefits, and the possibility of performance decrements and side-effects, there is little to recommend the use of inosine supplements by athletes.

Branched-chain amino acids

During the 1980s, preparations of individual amino acids were the most successfully marketed 'designer' supplement despite a lack of evidence that 'free-form' preparations of amino acids were superior in digestion/absorption than amino acids found in intact proteins (i.e. in everyday foods). Many of these specialised amino acid products are expensive and provide amino acid intakes that can easily be consumed from everyday foods at more reasonable cost. However, popular theories have attributed a special role for particular amino acids in athletic performance and recovery from exercise.

General interest in branched-chain amino acids (BCAA supplements: leucine, isoleucine and valine) is based on their important role in protein metabolism. BCAAs in the muscle are able to transaminate pyruvate to form alanine, which is recycled to glucose in the liver via the Cori cycle. Significant oxidation of these amino acids occurs during exercise, and tracer studies that follow leucine kinetics are often used as an estimation of protein turnover. Supplements containing BCAAs are claimed to enhance recovery after exercise, although there is no proof that BCAA supplements are unique in promoting an enhanced reversal of protein catabolism. Instead, intake of CHO and protein, as provided by everyday foods and supplements such as liquid meal preparations, is the recommended dietary strategy for post-exercise recovery (see Chapter 8).

Supplementation with BCAAs *during* exercise has also been claimed to reduce or delay the onset of 'central fatigue'—fatigue arising from neurotransmitters and the central nervous system rather than the muscle. Since it is difficult to undertake a direct examination of brain function during exercise in humans, studies of central fatigue are reliant on monitoring indirect markers, such as plasma levels of neurotransmitter precursors, or monitoring the effects of drugs that are known agonists or antagonists of neurotransmitter function. One popular theory proposes that central fatigue results from increased brain levels of serotonin, which occurs when greater amounts of free (unbound) tryptophan are able to cross the blood–brain barrier (for review see Davis 1995). A key factor in this increased uptake is an increase in the plasma ratio of free tryptophan to BCAAs, which compete for the same transporters into the brain. The ratio changes during exercise as BCAAs are oxidised by the muscle. However, it also changes because the rise in free fatty acids (FFAs) that occurs during exercise displaces tryptophan from its binding site on the albumin molecule and increases the plasma concentration of free tryptophan. It has been theorised that supplementation of BCAAs during exercise might prevent the drop in plasma BCAA levels, attenuate the rise in free tryptophan:BCAA, and reduce the likelihood of fatigue arising from increased brain serotonin concentrations.

Studies that have investigated the effect of BCAA supplementation immediately before or during endurance exercise are summarised in Table 9.13. Although there appears to be evidence in support of BCAA supplementation, several of the studies can be criticised on methodological grounds (for review see Davis 1995). For example, the field studies failed to control for fluid and CHO intake during the event (Blomstrand et al. 1991a), and found enhancements there were either of questionable applicability to sport (i.e. a general test of cognitive function) or were achieved by undertaking the artificial statistical procedure of subdividing 'randomly selected' subjects according to an arbitrary finishing time (Blomstrand et al. 1991a). Other better-controlled studies have failed to provide clear evidence of an enhancement in the performance of prolonged exercise following BCAA supplementation.

In order to prove convincingly the benefits of BCAA supplementation during prolonged exercise, studies need to be undertaken comparing supplementation with BCAAs, or BCAAs and CHO, against CHO alone. After all, the ingestion of CHO during exercise minimises the unfavourable change in plasma free tryptophan:BCAA by suppressing the rise in FFA

TABLE 9.13 Studies of BCAA supplementation and performance

STUDY	SUBJECTS	BCAA DOSE	EXERCISE PROTOCOL	ENHANCED PERFORMANCE	COMMENTS
Mittleman et al. 1998	13 moderately trained males and females Crossover design	9.4 g (females) or 15.8 g (males)	Cycling in the heat (34∘C) Time to exhaustion at 40% VO_{2max}	Yes	Increased time to exhaustion (153 vs 137 min) with BCAA trial. Increase in plasma BCAA and decrease in plasma tryptophan:BCAA. Trend to higher plasma ammonia. No gender differences.
Blomstrand et al. 1997	7 trained male cyclists Crossover design	90 mg/kg (~6.5 g)	Cycling • 60 min @ 70% VO_{2max} + 20 min TT • Stroop colour word test (CWT) after ride	No Yes	No differences in work done in TT. However, RPE lower in BCAA trial during steady-state phase. Index of cognitive function (Stroop CWT) improved after exercise on BCAA trial.
Madsen et al. 1996	9 well-trained male cyclists Crossover design	3.5 L @ 5% glucose or 5% glucose + 18 g BCAA	Cycling • 100 km TT	No	No performance differences between trials. Plasma BCAA and ammonia levels higher with BCAA trial.
Davis et al. 1999	8 active males and females Crossover design	CHO + 7 g BCAA or CHO or placebo consumed before/ during/after	Running • intermittent shuttle run to exhaustion	No	CHO or CHO + BCAA increased time to fatigue compared with placebo. No further enhancement with addition of BCAA.
Blomstrand et al. 1991a	25 male cross country runners, 193 male marathon runners Experimental–placebo design	16 g (marathon) or 7.5 g (cross-country)	Running Marathon or 30 km cross country race • run time • Stroop CWT given after cross-country run	?Yes Yes	CWT performance improved in BCAA trial after cross-country run. 'Slower runners' ran faster in BCAA group. Note that the methodology of dividing group into slower and faster runners according to arbitrary time point has been criticised on statistical grounds.
Blomstrand et al. 1991b	6 female national soccer players Crossover design	6% CHO + 7.5 g BCAA or CHO alone	Soccer match • Stroop CWT given after match	Yes	Improvement in CWT test after game with CHO + BCAA.

concentrations (Davis et al. 1992). To date, investigations of this type are scarce and the findings are inconsistent, although some commercial sports drinks are already being produced with a combination of CHO and amino acids. According to the website promoting one such product (www.enduroxr4.com), an unpublished study found that the use of a CHO–amino acid drink by well-trained cyclists improved endurance during a 3-hour exercise protocol compared with CHO alone, and water. The mechanism of this performance benefit was claimed to be 'sparing of muscle glycogen' via an amino-acid mediated increase in insulin response and increased plasma glucose utilisation. However, from the brief description of the study methodology, it appears that neither direct nor indirect measurements of glycogen utilisation were collected to address this theory. Although these new products are claimed to represent an 'important advance in sports drink research' and are of great interest to endurance athletes and their coaches, we await the fully published results of well-conducted investigations before a decision can be made.

Medium-chain triglycerides

Medium-chain triglycerides (MCTs) are fats composed of medium-chain fatty acids (MCFA) with a chain length of six to 10 carbon molecules. They are digested and metabolised differently from the long-chain fatty acids that make up most of our dietary fat intake. Specifically, MCTs can be digested within the intestinal lumen with less need for bile and pancreatic juices than long-chain triglycerides, with MCFAs being absorbed via the portal circulation. MCFAs can be taken up into the mitochondria without the need for carnitine-assisted transport. In clinical nutrition, MCT supplements derived from palm kernel and coconut oil are used as an energy supplement for patients who have various digestive or lipid metabolism disorders. In the sports world, MCTs have been positioned as an easily absorbed and oxidised fuel source, and have been marketed to body builders as a fat source that is less likely to deposit as body fat. However, the role of MCTs in the general diet of athletes has not been studied.

Another role for MCTs in sport is to provide a fuel source during endurance and ultra-endurance events that could potentially spare glycogen, and prolong the availability of important CHO stores. Jeukendrup and colleagues (1995) reported that the co-ingestion of MCT with CHO during prolonged exercise increased the rate of MCT oxidation, possibly by increasing its rate of absorption; the maximum rate of MCT oxidation was achieved at around 120–180 minutes of exercise, with values of 0.12 g/min.

TABLE 9.14 Studies of medium-chain triglycerides + CHO supplementation and ultra-endurance performance: crossover design

STUDY	SUBJECTS	MCT DOSE	EXERCISE PROTOCOL	ENHANCED PERFORMANCE	COMMENTS
Angus et al. 2000	8 endurance-trained male cyclists/ triathletes	1 L per h of 6% CHO + 4% MCT (vs 6% CHO or placebo) Total intake of MCT = 42 g per hour or ~120 g	Cycling 100 km TT (~3 h)	No	CHO enhanced performance over placebo, but addition of MCT did not provide further benefits. 4 subjects experienced gastrointestinal problems with MCT. No differences in fat oxidation, plasma FFA between MCT and CHO + MCT. Suppression of fat oxidation may be due to high exercise intensity or pre-trial CHO meal causing high insulin concentrations.
Goedecke et al. 1999	9 endurance-trained male cyclists	1.6 L of 10% CHO or 10% CHO + 1.7% MCT or 10% CHO + 3.4% MCT Total intake of MCT = 26 or 52 g	Cycling 2 h @ 63% VO_{2max} + 40 km TT (~70 min)	No	No differences in TT performance. 2 subjects experienced gastrointestinal distress with higher MCT intake. Higher FFA with MCT but no change in CHO oxidation.
Jeukendrup et al. 1998	9 endurance-trained male cyclists/ triathletes	20 mL/kg of 10% CHO or 10% CHO + 5% MCT or 5% MCT or placebo Total intake of MCT = 86 g	Cycling 2 h @ 60% VO_{2max} + TT (~15 min)	No	No difference between CHO, CHO + MCT or placebo (~14 min) but MCT alone impaired performance (17.3 min). MCT + CHO showed slightly higher fat oxidation than CHO alone. No glycogen sparing.
van Zyl et al. 1996	6 endurance-trained cyclists	2 L of 4.3% MCT or 10% CHO or 10% CHO + 4.3% MCT Total intake of MCT = 86 g	Cycling 2 h @ 60% VO_{2max} + 40 km TT (~70 min)	Yes	MCT + CHO enhanced TT performance times (65.1 min) compared with CHO (66.8 min) and MCT (72.1 min). Increase in FFA and glycogen sparing with MCT + CHO.

Table 9.14 summarises the findings of studies that have examined the effect of the co-ingestion of MCT and CHO on ultra-endurance performance; the results are inconsistent and appear to depend on the amount of MCT that can be ingested and the prevailing hormonal conditions. Studies in which the intake of large amounts of MCT raised plasma FFA concentrations and allowed glycogen sparing reported a performance benefit at the end of prolonged exercise (van Zyl et al. 1996). However, these metabolic (and performance) benefits may be compromised when exercise is commenced with higher insulin levels, as is the case following a CHO-rich pre-exercise meal (Goedecke et al. 1999; Angus et al. 2000). Critical to the whole issue is the ability of subjects to tolerate the substantial amount of MCT oils required to have a metabolic impact. Jeukendrup et al. (1995) found that the gastrointestinal tolerance of MCT is limited to a total intake of about 30 g, which would limit its fuel contribution to 3–7% of the total energy expenditure during typical ultra-endurance events. At greater intakes, subjects report gastrointestinal reactions that range in severity from insignificant (van Zyl et al. 1996) to performance limiting (Jeukendrup et al. 1998). Differences in gastrointestinal tolerance between studies or within studies may reflect differences in the mean chain length of MCTs found in the supplements, or increased tolerance in some athletes due to constant exposure to MCTs. The intensity and mode of exercise may also affect gastrointestinal symptoms.

In summary, although some CHO gels are marketed with the addition of MCTs, there is little evidence to support an ergogenic effect from these special products. Furthermore, the theoretical use is limited to the small population of athletes who undertake ultra-endurance events and have developed gastrointestinal tolerance. Further research may clarify whether MCTs can be a useful supplement for ultra-endurance sports but significant investigation of gastrointestinal concerns is needed before any recommendations can be made.

Chromium picolinate

Chromium is an essential element, required in trace amounts. Dietary sources of chromium include yeast, nuts and legumes, some fruit and vegetables, chocolate, wine and beer. Many countries such as Australia have not set a dietary reference intake (DRI) for chromium, however, the US Food and Nutrition Board have established an Estimated Safe and Adequate Daily Dietary Allowance (ESADDA) within the range of 50–200 µg/day (National Research Council 1989). Dietary surveys often report the estimated chromium intake of many populations to be below this recommended range, however this may be an artefact of the lack of reliable food composition data for chromium. It has also been suggested that the ESADDA ranges for chromium have been set artificially high (for review see Clarkson 1997). There is some evidence that daily training may increase urinary chromium losses, increasing chromium requirements and the risk of suboptimal chromium intakes. However, adaptations may also occur to improve absorption or retention of chromium in compensation (see Clarkson 1997). As is the case for many micronutrients, athletes with restricted energy intakes are most at risk of low chromium intakes.

One of the best-known roles of chromium in the body is to potentiate insulin action and the muscle uptake of glucose and amino acids (for review see Stoecker 1996). Subjects with chromium deficiencies often show improvements in growth or glucose tolerance in response to chromium supplementation (Stoecker 1996). In the case of the athletic population, individuals with inadequate dietary intake of chromium may respond positively to supplemental chromium intake. However, the major market is focused on claims that chromium supplements will enhance handling of glucose, amino acids and fatty acids, allowing dramatic gains in muscle mass and strength, while reducing body fat.

Chromium supplements are available in the form of chromium nicotinate, chloride and picolinate. Chromium picolinate is claimed to be the most biologically active form, and the claims for the efficacy of chromium picolinate have caused an interesting public debate between the patent holders and other trace element/mineral experts (see Evans 1993; Levafi et al. 1992; Levafi 1993). A concern with chromium supplementation is that chromium potentially competes with trivalent iron for binding to transferrin, thus predisposing those with chronically high intakes of chromium to iron deficiency (Lukaski et al. 1996). Some (Lukaski et al. 1996), but not all (Campbell et al. 1997), studies have reported a reduction in iron status as a result of chromium picolinate supplementation.

Table 9.15 summarises the studies of chromium picolinate supplementation and the effect on body composition and exercise performance. This table does not include the studies responsible for motivating the original interest in chromium picolinate, in which supplementation was claimed to cause significant increases in lean body mass in subjects undertaking aerobic exercise classes (Evans 1993) and weight training (Evans 1989). These studies have been criticised for methodological flaws, such as lack of a control group, inadequate control of diet or training status, and the reliance on unreliable and insensitive methods of assessing body composition (Levafi

TABLE 9.15 Studies of chromium picolinate and changes in body composition and performance

STUDY	SUBJECTS	CHROMIUM PICOLINATE DOSE AND TRAINING	OUTCOME MEASURES	BENEFITS	COMMENTS
Walker et al. 1998	20 male collegiate wrestlers Experimental–placebo design	200 mg/day for 14 weeks 14-week resistance and conditioning training program and endurance testing	Testing at baseline and 14 weeks • strength • peak power • body composition • Wingate test • VO_{2max} on run treadmill	 No No No No No	Did not enhance body composition or performance variables beyond improvements seen with training alone.
Lukaski et al. 1996	36 untrained males Experimental–placebo design	3.4 mmol/day (~200 mg/day) chromium picolonate or chloride for 8 weeks 8-week resistance training program	Testing at baseline and 8 weeks • strength • body composition • iron status	 No No No	No beneficial effects on lean BM, body fat or strength above training effect. No difference between chromium preparations. Trend for ↓ iron status (↓ transferrin status) with chromium picolinate.
Hallmark et al. 1996	16 untrained males Experimental–placebo design	200 mg/day for 12 weeks 12-week resistance training program	Testing at baseline and 12 weeks • strength • body composition	 No No	No differences in body composition with training or supplement. Strength increases independent of supplement.
Trent & Thieding-Cancel 1995	95 active-duty Navy personnel (male and female) Experimental–placebo design	400 mg/day for 16 weeks 16-week physical conditioning program	Testing at baseline and 16 weeks • body composition	No	No differences in BM and fat changes between groups. (Note body composition measured by anthropometry.)

(continues)

TABLE 9.15 Studies of chromium picolinate and changes in body composition and performance (*continued*)

STUDY	SUBJECTS	CHROMIUM PICOLINATE DOSE AND TRAINING	OUTCOME MEASURES	BENEFITS	COMMENTS
Clancy et al. 1994	36 male collegiate football (gridiron) players Experimental–placebo design	200 mg/day for 9 weeks 9-week pre-season resistance and conditioning training	Testing at baseline, mid and 9 weeks • strength • body composition	No No	No enhancement of BM, body composition or strength above placebo group.
Hasten et al. 1992	59 male and female college students Experimental–placebo design	200 mg/day for 12 weeks 12-week resistance training program	Testing at baseline and 12 weeks • strength • body composition	No No (but ↑ BM in females)	No differences in strength changes due to chromium picolinate. Greater ↑ in BM in females with chromium but no difference with males. No difference with loss of body fat.

et al. 1992; Levafi 1993). The remaining literature does not provide evidence of gains in strength and lean body mass or loss of body fat other than what can be achieved through training alone. There is certainly no support for the dramatic claims made in some advertisements that position chromium picolinate as a 'legal anabolic' agent. The only situation in which chromium supplementation is likely to be useful is in treating individuals whose dietary intakes are inadequate.

Pro-hormones

Anabolic steroids are controlled pharmaceutical agents and are listed as proscribed (banned) substances by the IOC. However, since the liberalisation of supplement laws following the 1994 passage of the Dietary Supplement Health and Education Act in the United States, the supplement market has been flooded with a new group of products—pro-hormones that can be converted in the body to testosterone or the anabolic steroid nandrolone (Blue & Lombardo 1999). These products include androstenedione, DHEA, 19-norandrostenedione and other metabolites found in the steroid pathways. Theoretically, each has some androgen activity as well as being part of the pathway to testosterone production; it is hypothesised that a dietary intake of these pro-hormones will increase testosterone production. Some herbal compounds such as *Saw palmetto* and *Tribulus terrestris* are also claimed to have anabolic activity, specifically by blocking the aromatisation pathways in which these steroid metabolites are converted to oestradiols in peripheral tissues rather than progressing to testosterone. The evidence behind these theories is limited and historical—for example, the patent for androstenedione is based on the case histories on two female patients from the 1960s (Mahesh & Greenblatt 1962). As a result of the suggested attainment of increased androgenic-anabolic activity, pro-hormone supplements have been promoted for a wide variety of anti-ageing and vigour-achieving activities. In the sports world, they have become a common ingredient or single focus of 'body building' supplements that claim to promote fat loss, enhance gains in muscle mass and strength, increase libido, and enhance immunity.

Products containing pro-hormones are marketed as over-the-counter dietary supplements in countries such as the United States, and even in countries where they don't enjoy this liberalised status they may be available to athletes through Internet or mail-order sales. As stated previously, such products are often badly labelled or produced with a variable content and other supplements are often contaminated with undeclared amounts of pro-hormones. This has important consequences in terms of side-effects arising from supplement use as well as inadvertent doping. Pro-hormones are banned by the IOC, either directly by name or under the umbrella of being a 'related substance' to anabolic-androgenic steroids. However, individual sporting organisations may not include these products within their own list of banned agents. For example, androstenedione shot to public attention when Mark McGwire admitted to taking it during his 1998 record-breaking baseball season; this is not considered illegal under the codes governing professional baseball.

Athletes who are observed, or admit to, using pro-hormone substances may be in breach of an anti-doping code and could face penalties on this evidence. However, there is some confusion about whether the use of these agents will always result in a positive outcome from (urinary) drug screening. To date, excretion studies have produced conflicting results, with some but not all subjects who ingested supplements containing pro-hormones experiencing differential changes in urinary testosterone and epitestosterone concentrations that increased the ratio above the legal cut-off of 6:1 (Bosy et al. 1998; Uralets & Gillette 1999). However, high concentrations of metabolites of nandrolone have been found in urine for 7–10 days following the ingestion of a single dose of 19-norandrostenedione (Uralets & Gillette 1999), and a recent report found that 15% of all dietary supplements sampled in a laboratory analysis study contained sufficient amounts of pro-hormone contaminants to cause an athlete to produce a 'positive' drug test (IOC 2002b).

Table 9.16 summarises the recent studies in which chronic protocols of supplementation with pro-hormones and related products have been investigated in athletes and people undertaking exercise. Since there appears to be considerable variability in the actual content of commercial pro-hormone supplements, it is important that investigators verify the pro-hormone content of treatments used in their investigations. The present literature shows little evidence that the chronic intake of various pro-hormones causes a favourable change in blood testosterone values—at least in healthy male subjects who consume moderate (recommended) doses of these products. Although such ingestion protocols cause a rise in the blood levels of these compounds, the effect appears to be short-lived or unable to convert into an increase in circulating testosterone levels. There may be a more pronounced effect in some subjects at higher doses (Leder et al. 2000). Studies investigating the acute response to moderate intakes of pro-hormone supplements have also failed to produce evidence of testosterone increases following the raised plasma concentration of various testosterone precursors (Brown et al. 1999b; King et al. 1999), except perhaps when larger doses are in use (Earnest et al. 2000). It appears that the major fate of these exogenous metabolites is aromatisation to oestradiols; even the co-ingestion of herbal extracts claimed to reduce this pathway (e.g. *Tribulus terristris*, *Saw palmetto*, chrysin and indole-3-carbinol) has also been shown to fail to increase circulating testosterone levels (Brown et al. 1999a).

Not surprisingly, in the absence of increases in blood testosterone concentrations, most studies have failed to find differences in the response of pro-hormone treatment and placebo groups to a resistance-training program. Another investigative approach, using tracer techniques to study muscle protein kinetics before and after the intake of 100 mg/day androstenedione, found a lack of effect on protein anabolism (Rasmussen et al. 2000). There was a trend towards increased muscle protein turnover (increased synthesis matched by increased breakdown) in the treatment group compared with control subjects. However, differences were small and did not lead to a net protein increase. Of some concern are the consistent reports that supplementation with some pro-hormones can raise blood oestrogen levels and reduce levels of high-density-lipoprotein cholesterol (Ballantyne et al. 2000; Brown et al. 1999a; King et al. 1999; Leder et al. 2000; Rasmussen et al. 2000). These findings, which would be of concern to long-term health, appear to occur with androstenedione supplementation (Ballantyne et al. 2000; Brown et al. 1999a; King et al. 1999; Leder et al. 2000; Rasmussen et al. 2000) but not DHEA supplementation (Brown et al. 1999b). To date, there are few published reports of the effects of 19-norandrostenedione or related compounds on serum hormone concentrations, changes in body composition or exercise performance.

In general, there is no clear evidence that pro-hormone supplements offer an advantage to athletic performance or exercise response. However, it has been pointed out that although the treatment doses used in studies are in excess of the protocols recommended by the manufacturers, they are conservative in comparison to the doses recommended and used by some athletes (Yesalsis 1999). It has also been noted that different effects might be expected in studies of well-trained athletes compared with untrained or novice athlete trainers. For example, the strength gains made by previously untrained men might be sufficiently large and variable so as to mask any effects from pro-hormones, or perhaps only well-trained athletes, who have reached a plateau in the results of their resistance training, could be expected to benefit from pro-hormone supplementation. The effects of pro-hormone supplementation on older subjects, with lower testosterone levels through ageing, or female subjects also deserve investigation. Although the present literature is not supportive of ergogenic benefits, researchers have

TABLE 9.16 Studies of chronic supplementation with pro-hormones and related compounds on sex hormones, body composition and performance

STUDY	SUBJECTS	PRO-HORMONE DOSE	EXERCISE PROTOCOL	ENHANCED PERFORMANCE	COMMENTS
Van Gammeren et al. 2001	16 resistance-trained males Experimental–placebo design	100 mg/day 19-norandrostenedione + 56 mg/day 19-norandrostenediol or placebo (multi-vitamin/mineral) for 8 weeks Resistance training 4 days/week	Tests at baseline, 4 weeks • bench press	No	No difference in strength, body composition or body circumferences between groups or over time with continued training program. No change in vigour or fatigue.
Wallace et al. 1999	40 resistance-trained males Experimental–placebo design	100 mg/day DHEA or 100 mg/day androstenedione or placebo for 12 weweks Resistance training	Tests at baseline, 6, 12 weeks • series of upper and lower body strength measurements	No	Neither DHEA or androstenedione group reported greater improvements in body composition and performance than placebo group. No increase in blood testosterone concentrations following pro-hormones. No changes in lipid profiles.
Brown et al. 1999a	Untrained males Experimental–placebo design	150 mg/day DHEA, 300 mg/day androstenedione and herbals (Tribulus terristris, Saw palmetto, chrysin and indole-3-carbinol) or placebo for 8 weeks Resistance training	Tests at baseline, 4, 8 weeks • series of upper and lower body strength measurements	No	The supplement failed to increase blood testosterone levels. Increases in strength and lean body mass achieved by the resistance training program were not enhanced compared to placebo group. Supplement associated with rise in blood oestrogens and decrease in HDL cholesterol.

(continues)

TABLE 9.16 Studies of chronic supplementation with pro-hormones and related compounds on sex hormones, body composition and performance (*continued*)

STUDY	SUBJECTS	PRO-HORMONE DOSE	EXERCISE PROTOCOL	ENHANCED PERFORMANCE	COMMENTS
Brown et al. 1999b	20 healthy males Experimental–placebo design	150 mg/day DHEA or placebo (rice flour capsule) for 8 weeks Resistance training	Tests at baseline, 4, 8 weeks • series of upper and lower body strength measurements	No	No differences in training-mediated increases in muscle strength and lean BM, or decreases in body fat between groups. No increase in blood testosterone concentrations following DHEA supplementation.
King et al. 1999	20 healthy males Experimental–placebo design	300 mg/day androstenedione or placebo (rice flour capsule) for 8 weeks Resistance training 3 days/week	Tests at baseline, 4, 8 weeks • series of upper and lower body strength measurements	No	No differences in training-mediated increases in muscle strength and lean BM, or decreases in body fat between groups. No increase in blood testosterone following androstenedione supplement; instead increase in oestrogens and decrease in HDL cholesterol.

been reminded that the first scientific position papers regarding anabolic steroids also concluded that they were ineffective in enhancing strength or performance in sport; this was a result of the failure of scientists to investigate the real practices undertaken by athletes (Yesalsis 1999). Nevertheless, given the potential for negative outcomes to lipid and oestradiol profiles, and the evidence of poor manufacturing practices regarding pro-hormones in supplements, many experts are calling for a cessation or overhaul of the sale of these products.

Caffeine

Caffeine is a drug that enjoys social acceptance and widespread use around the world. Caffeine is the best known member of the methyl xanthines, a family of naturally occurring stimulants found in the leaves, nuts and seeds of a number of plants. Major dietary sources of caffeine, such as tea, coffee, chocolate and cola drinks, typically provide 30–100 mg of caffeine per serve, while some non-prescriptive medications contain 100–200 mg of caffeine per tablet. The recent introduction of caffeine (or guarana) to 'energy drinks', confectionery and sports foods/supplements has increased the opportunities for athletes to consume caffeine, either as part of their everyday diet or for specific use as an ergogenic aid.

Several reviews have discussed the various actions of caffeine on the central nervous system, cardiac muscle, diuresis, and epinephrine release and activity (Graham 2001a, b; Spriet 1997; Tarnopolsky 1994). Briefly, caffeine has several effects on skeletal muscle, involving calcium handling, sodium–potassium pump activity, elevation of cyclic AMP and direct action on enzymes such as glycogen phosphorylase. Increased catecholamine action and the direct effect of caffeine on cyclic AMP may both act to increase lipolysis in adipose and muscle tissue, causing an increase in plasma FFA concentrations and an increased availability of intramuscular triglyceride. It has been proposed that an increased potential for fat oxidation during moderate-intensity exercise promotes glycogen sparing. Caffeine may also influence athletic performance via central nervous system effects, such as a reduced perception of effort or an enhanced recruitment of motor units. Breakdown products of caffeine, such as paraxanthine and theophylline, may also have actions within the body. Caffeine supplementation is a complex issue to investigate due to the difficulty in isolating the individual effects of caffeine, and the potential for variability between subjects.

Athletes have used caffeine to enhance performance for at least a century but it is in only the last 40 years that controlled studies have been conducted.

Early research in the 1970s focused on the effects of caffeine on metabolism and performance during endurance events. A resurgence of interest in caffeine supplementation during the 1990s expanded the focus of studies to include exercise performances such as sprints (< 90 s), and short (5 min) and long (20 min) events involving high-intensity effort. It is beyond the scope of this chapter to summarise the large amount of literature on caffeine; instead, readers are directed to recent review papers (Graham 2001a, b; Spriet 1997; Tarnopolsky 1994) and the following emerging points:

1 There is sound evidence that caffeine enhances endurance and provides a small but worthwhile enhancement of performance over a range of exercise protocols. There is still no consensus on the mechanism to explain this performance improvement but it is unlikely to result from the so-called 'metabolic theory' (increase in fat oxidation and 'sparing' of glycogen utilisation during exercise). Instead, altered perception of fatigue and effort, or direct effects on the muscle may underpin performance changes. Most studies of caffeine and performance have been undertaken in laboratories; studies that investigate performance effects in elite athletes under field conditions or during real-life sports events are scarce. Caffeine may enhance competition performance, but is also likely to be a useful training aid, allowing the athlete to undertake better and more consistent training.

2 There is evidence, particularly from recent studies (Cox et al. 2002; Kovacs et al. 1998), that beneficial effects from caffeine intake occur at very modest levels of intake (1–3 mg/kg BM or 70–150 mg caffeine), when caffeine is taken before and/or during exercise. Furthermore, there is no evidence of a dose–response relationship to caffeine; that is, performance benefits do **not** increase with increases in the caffeine dose (Cox et al. 2002; Pasman et al. 1995). This is an advance on previous research that used caffeine intakes of 6–9 mg/kg BM (e.g. 400–600 mg) consumed 1 hour prior to the exercise. Further research is needed to define the range of caffeine intake protocols that provide performance enhancements.

3 The effects of caffeine supplementation differ between individuals. Some people are non-responders and some people experience negative side-effects, such as tremors, increased heart rate and headaches. Such side-effects are more common at higher doses (e.g. exceeding 6–9 mg/kg BM).

In 1984, caffeine was added back to the IOC list of banned substances based on urinary caffeine concentrations from a single urine sample taken after the event. The urinary caffeine concentration initially set as the cut-off for caffeine 'doping' was 15 µg/mL; this was reduced in 1988 to 12 µg/mL. This cut-off value was chosen to exclude 'normal' or 'social' coffee drinking and dietary practices (Delbeke & Debackere 1984). Indeed, studies document that at caffeine doses of 5–6 mg/kg, 'positive' urinary caffeine levels are unlikely and a substantial risk of urinary caffeine values greater than 12 µg/mL does not occur until intakes greater than 9 mg/kg are achieved (Pasman et al. 1995). It is uncertain whether this ban was primarily related to safety concerns over intakes of very large doses of caffeine or the ethics of achieving performance advantages through caffeine use. However, as a result of recent developments in both sports science knowledge and athletic practice, the present situation regarding caffeine use by elite athletes has become confusing and inconsistent. First, the current wording of the Anti-Doping Code's list of Prohibited Substances and Methods regarding caffeine is ambiguous and can be taken to mean, presumably in relation to competition, either that 'caffeine is prohibited at *all* times' or 'caffeine is permitted at doses that produce urinary caffeine concentrations below 12 mg/mL' (IOC 2002a). These interpretations have widely different and far-reaching outcomes; at one extreme it could mean that athletes are unable to consume any caffeine on the day of competition and that the provision of caffeine-containing beverages such as colas and coffee or tea at a sporting venue would be considered 'trafficking' in a banned substance. On the other extreme it could mean that athletes are able to consume large amounts of caffeine as long as their urinary caffeine concentrations are below 12 µg/mL in the official sample provided at drug testing.

Urinary concentration reflects the small amount (~1%) of plasma caffeine that escapes metabolism and is excreted unchanged. Metabolic clearance of caffeine varies widely between athletes and between different occasions of use by the same athlete (Birkett & Miners 1991). Urinary caffeine levels are determined by a variety of factors including the size of caffeine dose, metabolic clearance of caffeine and the timing of the urine sample in relation to the caffeine dose. Since there is huge variation in urinary caffeine content for the same caffeine dose, and neither standardisation of the time between caffeine intake and urine collection nor prevention of opportunities to urinate during/after an event, urinary caffeine levels are not a consistent marker of a particular use of caffeine. The emerging evidence is that performance benefits can be found with very modest caffeine intakes; intakes that are well within, or even below, normal social intakes of caffeine, and likely to produce very low urinary caffeine levels.

In summary, there is clear evidence that caffeine is an ergogenic aid for a variety of types of sport and exercise activities. Caffeine is widely consumed from a variety of sources as part of a normal diet, as well as being available in specialised products for use by athletes. While further studies are needed to define the range of caffeine protocols or sports activities that show evidence of performance enhancement, there is a need for clarification of caffeine use within the present anti-doping codes. Despite being accepted and consumed by a large majority of the population, caffeine provokes a range of attitudes in relation to its use by athletes.

Summary

Sports scientists frequently observe a chaotic pattern of use of supplements and sports foods by athletes and coaches, and an almost never-ending range of products that claim to achieve benefits needed to enhance sports performance. The poor regulation of supplements and sports foods in many countries allows athletes and coaches to be the target of marketing campaigns based on exaggerated claims and hype rather than documented benefits. However, scientific study has identified a number of products that offer true benefits to performance or the achievement of nutritional goals. A systematic approach to educating athletes and coaches about supplements and sports foods, and managing their provision to athletes and teams, can allow sports people to include the successful use of these products with the activities that underpin optimal performance.

References

Allen JD, McLung J, Nelson AG, Welsch M. Ginseng supplementation does not enhance healthy young adults' peak aerobic exercise performance. *J Am Coll Nutr* 1998;17:462–6.

American College of Sports Medicine. Position Statement: The physiological and health consequences of oral Cr supplementation. *Med Sci Sports Exerc* 2000;32:706–17.

Anderson MJ, Cotter JD, Garnham AP, Casley DJ, Febbraio MA. Effect of glycerol-induced hyperhydration on thermoregulation and metabolism in the heat. *Int J Sport Nutr Exerc Metab* 2001;11:315–33.

Angus DJ, Hargreaves M, Dancey J, Febbraio MA. Effect of carbohydrate or carbohydrate plus medium chain triglyceride ingestion on cycling time trial performance. *J Appl Physiol* 2000;88:113–19.

Antonio J, Sanders MS, Van Gammeren D. The effects of bovine colostrum supplementation on body composition and exercise performance in active men and women. *Nutrition* 2001;17:243–7.

Ariel G, Saville W. Anabolic steroids: the physiological effects of placebo. *Med Sci Sports* 1972;4:124–6.

Australian Institute of Sport. AIS Sports Supplement programme, 2002, <http://www.ais.org.au/nutrition/SuppPolicy.htm>.

Bahrke MS, Morgan WP. Evaluation of the ergogenic properties of ginseng. *Sports Med* 1994;18:229–48.

Ballantyne CS, Phillips SM, MacDonald JR, Tarnopolsky MA, MacDougall JD. The acute effects of androstenedione supplementation in healthy young males. *Can J Appl Physiol* 2000;25:68–78.

Barnett C, Costill DL, Vukovich MD, Cole KJ, Goodpaster BH, Trappe SW, Fink WJ. Effect of L-carnitine supplementation on muscle and blood carnitine content and lactate accumulation during high-intensity sprint cycling. *Int J Sport Nutr* 1994;4: 280–8.

Birkett DJ, Miners JO. Caffeine renal clearance and urine caffeine concentrations during steady-state dosing. Implications for monitoring caffeine intake during sports events. *Br J Clin Pharmacol* 1991;31:405–8.

Blue JG, Lombardo JA. Steroids and steroid-like compounds. *Clin Sports Med* 1999;18: 667–89.

Blomstrand E, Hassmen P, Ek S, Ekblom B, Newsholme EA. Influence of ingesting a solution of branched-chain amino acids on perceived exertion during exercise. *Acta Physiol Scand* 1997;159:41–9.

Blomstrand E, Hassmen P, Ekblom B, Newsholme EA. Administration of branched-chain amino acids during sustained exercise—effects on performance and on plasma concentration of some amino acids. *Eur J Appl Physiol* 1991a;63:83–8.

Blomstrand E, Hassmen P, Newsholme EA. Effect of branched-chain amino acid supplementation on mental performance. *Acta Physiol Scand* 1991b;143:225–6.

Bosy TZ, Moore KA, Polkis A. The effect of oral dehydroepiandrosterone (DHEA) on the urine testosterone/epitestosterone (T/E) ratio in human male volunteers. *J Anal Toxicol* 1998;22:455–9.

Braun B, Clarkson PM, Freedson PS, Kohl RL. Effects of coenzyme Q10 supplementation on exercise performance, VO_{2max}, and lipid peroxidation in trained cyclists. *Int J Sport Nutr* 1991;1:353–65.

Brinkworth GD, Buckley JD, Bourdon PC, Gulbin JP, David AZ. Oral bovine colostrum supplementation enhances buffer capacity but not rowing performance in elite female rowers. *Int J Sport Nutr Exerc Metab* 2002; 12:349–63.

Brown GA, Vukovich MD, Reifenrath TA, et al. Effects of anabolic precursors on serum testosterone adaptations to resistance training in young men. *Int J Sports Nutr* 1999a:10;1–30.

Brown GA, Vukovich MD, Sharp RL, Reifenrath TA, Parsons KA, King DS. Effect of oral DHEA on serum testosterone and adaptations to resistance training in young men. *J Appl Physiol* 1999b;87:2274–83.

Buckley JD, Abbott MJ, Brinkworth GD, Whyte PBD. Bovine colostrum supplementation during endurance running training improves recovery, but not performance. *J Sci Med Sport* 2002; 5:65–79.

Burke LM. An interview with Dr Gary Green about supplements and doping problems from an NCAA perspective. *Int J Sport Nutr Exerc Metab* 2001;11:397–400.

Burke L, Desbrow B, Minehan M. Dietary supplements and nutritional ergogenic aids in sport. In: Burke L, Deakin V, eds. *Clinical Sports Nutrition*. 2nd edn. Sydney: McGraw-Hill, 2000: 455–553.

Campbell WW, Beard JL, Joseph LJ, Davey SL, Evans WJ. Chromium picolinate supplementation and resistive training by older men: effects on iron-status and hematologic indexes. *Am J Clin Nutr* 1997;66:644–9.

Catlin DH, Leder BZ, Ahrens B, Starcevic B, Hatton CK, Green GA, Finkelstein JS. Trace contamination of over-the-counter androstenedione and positive urine test results for a nandrolone metabolite. *J Am Med Assoc* 2001;284:2618–21.

Cerretelli P, Marconi C. L-carnitine supplementation in humans. The effects on physical performance. *Int J Sports Med* 1990;11:1–14.

Chanutin A. The fate of creatine when administered to man. *J Biol Chem* 1926;67:29–37.

Chong SKF, Oberholzer VG. Ginseng—is there a clinical use in medicine? *Postgrad Med J* 1988;65:841–6.

Clancy S, Clarkson PM, De Cheke M, Nosaka K, Freedson PS, Cunningham JJ, Valentine B. Effects of chromium picolinate supplementation on body composition, strength, and urinary chromium loss in football players. *Int J Sport Nutr* 1994;4:142–53.

Clark VR, Hopkins WG, Hawley JA, Burke LM. Placebo effect of carbohydrate feedings during a 40-km cycling time trial. *Med Sci Sports Exerc* 2000;32:1642–7.

Clarkson PM. Nutritional ergogenic aids: carnitine. *Int J Sport Nutr* 1992;92:185–90.

Clarkson PM. Effects of exercise on chromium levels. Is supplementation necessary? *Sports Med* 1997;23:341–9.

Colgan M. Inosine—the latest Weider-sponsored research. *Muscle & Fitness* 1988;49(1): 94–6.

Colombani P, Wenk C, Kunz I, Krahenbuhl S, Kuhnt M, Arnold M, Frey-Rindova P, Frey W, Langhans W. Effects of L-carnitine supplementation on physical performance and energy metabolism of endurance-trained athletes: a double-blind crossover field study. *Eur J Appl Physiol* 1996;73:434–9.

Coombes JS, Conacher M, Austen SK, Marshall PA. Dose effects of oral bovine colostrum on physical work capacity in cyclists. *Med Sci Sports Exerc* 2002; 34:1184–8.

Coutts A, Reaburn P, Mummery K, Holmes M. The effect of glycerol hyperhydration on Olympic distance triathlon performance in high ambient temperatures. *Int J Sport Nutr Exerc Metab* 2002;12:105–19.

Cox GR, Desbrow B, Montgomery P, Anderson ME, Bruce CR, Macrides TA, Martin DT, Moquin A, Roberts A, Hawley JA, Burke LM. Difference protocols of caffeine intake enhance performance of prolonged cycling. *J Appl Physiol* 2002; 93:990–9.

Cui J, Garle M, Eneroth P, Bjorkhem I. What do commercial ginseng preparations contain? *Lancet* 1994;344:134.

Davis JM. Carbohydrates, branched-chain amino acids and endurance: the central fatigue hypothesis. *Int J Sport Nutr* 1995;5(suppl.):S29–S38.

Davis JM, Bailey SP, Woods JA, Galiano FJ, Hamilton M, Bartoli WP. Effects of carbohydrate feedings on plasma free tryptophan and branched-chain amino acids during prolonged cycling. *Eur J Appl Physiol* 1992;65:513–19.

Davis JM, Welsh RS, De Volve KL, Alderson NA. Effects of branched-chain amino acids and carbohydrate on fatigue during intermittent, high-intensity running. *Int J Sports Med* 1999;20:309–14.

Decombaz J, Deriaz O, Acheson K, Gmuender B, Jequier E. Effect of L-carnitine on submaximal exercise metabolism after depletion of muscle glycogen. *Med Sci Sports Exerc* 1993;25:733–40.

Delbeke FT, Debackere M. Caffeine: use and abuse in sports. *Int J Sports Med* 1984;5: 179–82.

Dennig H, Talbot JH, Edwards HT, Dill B. Effects of acidosis and alkalosis upon the capacity for work. *J Clin Invest* 1931;9:601–13.

Dill DB, Edwards HT, Talbot JH. Alkalosis and the capacity for work. *J Biol Chem* 1932;97:58–9.

Dowling EA, Redondo DR, Branch JD, Jones S, McNabb G, Williams MH. Effect of *Eleutherococcus senticosus* on submaximal and maximal exercise performance. *Med Sci Sports Exerc* 1996;28:482–9.

Earnest CP, Olson MA, Broeder CE, Brueul KK, Beckham SG. In vivo 4-androstene-3,17-dione and 4-androstene-3β,17β-diol supplementation in young men. *Eur J Appl Physiol* 2000;81:229–32.

Engels HJ, Wirth JC. No ergogenic effects of ginseng (*Panax ginseng* C.A. Meyer) during graded maximal aerobic exercise. *J Am Diet Assoc* 1997;97:1110–15.

Evans GW. The effect of chromium picolinate on insulin controlled parameters in humans. *Int J Biosocial Med Res* 1989;11:163–80.

Evans GW. Chromium picolinate is an effective, efficacious and safe supplement. *Int J Sport Nutr* 1993;3:117–19.

Gallagher PM, Carrithers JA, Godard MP, Schulze KE, Trappe SW. Beta-hydroxy-beta-methylbutyrate ingestion. Part I: effects on strength and fat free mass. *Med Sci Sports Exerc* 2000;32:2109–15.

Gao J, Costill DL, Horswill CA, Park SH. Sodium bicarbonate ingestion improves performance in interval swimming. *Eur J Appl Physiol* 1988;58:171–4.

Geyer H, Henze MK, Mareck-Engelke U, Sigmund G, Schanzer W. Positive doping cases with norandrosterone after application of contaminated nutritional supplements. *Deutsche Zeit für Sportmed* 2000;51:378–82.

Goedecke JH, Elmer-English R, Dennis SC, Schloss I, Noakes TD, Lambert EV. Effects of medium-chain triacylglycerol ingested with carbohydrate on metabolism and exercise performance. *Int J Sport Nutr* 1999;9:35–47.

Goldfinch J, McNaughton L, Davies P. Induced metabolic alkalosis and its effects on 400 m racing time. *Eur J Appl Physiol* 1988;57:45–8.

Gorostiaga EM, Maurer CA, Eclache JP. Decrease in respiratory quotient during exercise following L-carnitine supplementation. *Int J Sports Med* 1989;10:169–74.

Graham TE. Caffeine and exercise: metabolism, endurance and performance. *Sports Med* 2001a;31:765–807.

Graham TE. Caffeine, coffee and ephedrine: impact on exercise performance and metabolism. *Can J Appl Physiol* 2001b;26:S103–S109.

Green AL, Hultman E, Macdonald IA, Sewell DA, Greenhaff PL. Carbohydrate ingestion augments skeletal muscle creatine accumulation during supplementation in man. *Am J Physiol* 1996a;271:E812–E826.

Green AL, Macdonald IA, Greenhaff PL. The effects of creatine and carbohydrate on whole body creatine retention in vegetarians. *Proc Nutr Soc* 1997;56:81A.

Green AL, Simpson EJ, Littlewood JJ, Macdonald IA, Greenhaff PL. Carbohydrate ingestion augments creatine retention during creatine feeding in man. *Acta Physiol Scand* 1996b;158:195–202.

Greenhaff PL. Creatine. In: Maughan RJ, ed. *Nutrition in Sport*. Oxford: Blackwell Science, 2000: 367–78.

Greig C, Finch KM, Jones DA, Cooper M, Sargeant AJ, Forte CA. The effect of oral supplementation with L-carnitine on maximum and submaximum exercise capacity. *Eur J Appl Physiol* 1987;56:457–60.

Grunewald KK, Bailey RS. Commercially marketed supplements for body building athletes. *Sports Med* 1993;15:90–103.

Gurley BJ, Wang P, Gardner SF. Ephedrine-type alkaloid content of nutritional supplements containing *Ephedra sinica* (Ma Huang) as determined by high performance liquid chromatography. *J Pharm Sci* 1998;87:1547–53.

Hallmark MA, Reynolds TH, DeSouza CA, Dotson CO, Anderson RA, Rogers MA. Effects of chromium and resistive training on muscle strength and body composition. *Med Sci Sports Exerc* 1996;28:139–44.

Hahm H, Kujawa J, Ausberger L. Comparison of melatonin products against USP's nutritional supplements standards and other criteria. *J Am Pharm Assoc* 1999;39: 27–31.

Harris RC, Soderlund K, Hultman E. Elevation of creatine in resting and exercise muscle of normal subjects by creatine supplementation. *Clin Sci* 1992;83:367–74.

Hasten DL, Rome EP, Franks BD, Hegsted M. Effects of chromium picolinate on beginning weight training students. *Int J Sport Nutr* 1992;2:343–50.

Heigenhauser GFJ, Jones NJ. Bicarbonate loading. In: Lamb DR, Williams MH, eds. *Perspectives in Exercise Science and Sports Medicine*. Vol 4. *Ergogenics*. Carmel, IN: Cooper Publishing Group, 1991: 183–212.

Heinonen OJ. Carnitine and physical exercise. *Sports Med* 1996;22:109–32.

Hespel P, Op' T Eijnde B, Derave W, Richter EA. Creatine supplementation: exploring the role of the creatine kinase/phosphocreatine system in the human muscle. *Can J Appl Physiol* 2001;26(suppl.):S79–S102.

Hitchins S, Martin DT, Burke LM, Yates K, Fallon K, Hahn A, Dobson GP. Glycerol hyperhydration improves cycle time trial performance in hot humid conditions. *Eur J Appl Physiol* 1999;80:494–501.

Hofman Z, Smeets R, Verlaan G, van der Lugt R, Verstappen PA. The effect of bovine colostrum supplementation on exercise performance in elite field hockey players. *Int J Sport Nutr Exerc Metab* 2002 (in press).

Hopkins WG, Hawley A, Burke LM. Design and analysis of research on sport performance enhancement. *Med Sci Sports Exerc* 1999;31:472–85.

Hultman E, Soderlund K, Timmons JA, Cederblad G, Greenhaff PL. Muscle creatine loading in men. *J Appl Physiol* 1996;81:232–7.

Inder WJ, Swanney MP, Donald RA, Prickett TCR, Hellemans J. The effect of glycerol and desmopressin on exercise performance and hydration in triathletes. *Med Sci Sports Exerc* 1998;30:1263–9.

International Olympic Committee. Olympic Movement Anti-Doping Code. Appendix A. 2002a, <http://www.olympic.org/uk/index_uk.asp>.

International Olympic Committee. Official press release. IOC Nutritional supplements study points to need for greater quality control, 2002b, <http://www.olympic.org/uk/index_uk.asp>.

Jeukendrup AE, Saris WHM, Schrauwen P, Brouns F, Wagenmakers AJM. Metabolic availability of medium-chain triglycerides coingested with carbohydrates during prolonged exercise. *J Appl Physiol* 1995;79:756–62.

Jeukendrup AE, Thielen JJHC, Wagenmakers AJM, Brouns F, Saris WHM. Effects of MCT and carbohydrate ingestion during exercise on substrate utilisation and subsequent performance. *Am J Clin Nutr* 1998;67:397–404.

Jowko E, Ostaszewski P, Jank M, Sacharuk J, Zieniewicz A, Wilczak J, Nissen S. Creatine and beta-hydroxy-beta-methylbutyrate (HMB) additively increase lean body mass and muscle strength during a weight-training programme. *Nutrition* 2001;17:558–66.

Juhn MS, Tarnopolsky M. Oral creatine supplementation and athletic performance: a critical review. *Clin J Sport Med* 1998a;8:286–97.

Juhn MS, Tarnopolsky M. Potential side-effects of oral creatine supplementation: a critical review. *Clin J Sport Med* 1998b;8:298–304.

Kaikkonen J, Kosonen L, Nyyssonen K, Porkkala-Sarataho E, Salonen R, Korpela H, Salonen JT. Effect of combined coenzyme Q10 and d-a-tocopheryl acetate supplementation on exercise-induced lipid peroxidation and muscular damage: a placebo-controlled double-blind study in marathon runners. *Free Radical Res* 1998;29:85–92.

Kamber M, Baume N, Saugy M, Rivier L. Nutritional supplements as a source for positive doping cases? *Int J Sport Nutr Exerc Metab* 2001;11:258–63.

King DS, Sharp RL, Vukovich MD. Effect of oral androstenedione on serum testosterone and adaptations to resistance training in young men. *JAMA* 1999;281:2020–8.

Knitter AE, Panton L, Rathmacher JA, Petersen A, Sharp R. Effects of beta-hydroxy-beta-methylbutyrate on muscle damage after a prolonged run. *J Appl Physiol* 2000;89:1340–4.

Kovacs EM, Stegen JHCH, Brouns F. Effect of caffeinated drinks on substrate metabolism, caffeine excretion, and performance. *J Appl Physiol* 1998;85:709–15.

Kozyrskyj A. Herbal products in Canada. How safe are they? *Can Fam Phys* 1997;43:697–702.

Kraemer W, Volek JS. Creatine supplementation: its role in human performance. *Clin Sports Med* 1999;18:651–66.

Kreider RB, Ferreira M, Wilson M, Almada AL. Effects of calcium β-hydroxy-β-methylbutyrate (MMB) supplementation during resistance-training on markers of catabolism, body composition and strength. *Int J Sports Med* 1999;20:509–9.

Kuipers H, Van Breda E, Verlaan G, Smeets R. Effects of oral bovine colostrum supplementation on serum insulin-like growth factor 1 levels. *Nutrition* 2002; 18:566–7.

Laaksonen R, Fogelholm M, Himberg JJ, Laaksoc J, Salorinne Y. Ubiquinone supplementation and exercise capacity in trained young and older men. *Eur J Appl Physiol* 1995;72:95–100.

Latzka WA, Sawka MN, Montain SJ, Skrinar GS, Fielding RA, Matott RP, Pandolf KB. Hyperhydration: tolerance and cardiovascular effects during uncompensable exercise-heat stress. *J Appl Physiol* 1998;84:1858–64.

Leder BZ, Longcope C, Catlin DH, Ahren B, Schoenfeld DA, Finkelstein JS. Oral androstenedione administration and serum testosterone concentrations in young men. *J Am Med Assoc* 2000; 283:779–782.

Lefavi RG. Response to Evans—chromium picolinate. *Int J Sport Nutr* 1993;3:120–2.

Lefavi RG, Richard AA, Keith RE, Wilson GD, McMillan JL, Stone MH. Efficacy of chromium supplementation in athletes: emphasis on anabolism. *Int J Sport Nutr* 1992;2:111–22.

Linderman J, Fahey TD. Sodium bicarbonate ingestion and exercise performance. *Sports Med* 1991;11:71–7.

Lukaski HC, Bolonchik WW, Siders WA, Milne DB. Chromium supplementation and resistance training: effects on body composition, strength, and trace element status of men. *Am J Clin Nutr* 1996;63:954–65.

Madsen K, MacLean DA, Kiens B, Christensen D. Effects of glucose, glucose plus branched-chain amino acids, or placebo on bike performance over 100 km. *J Appl Physiol* 1996;81:2644–50.

Mahesh VB, Greenblatt RB. The in vivo conversion of dehydroepiandrosterone and androstenedione to testosterone in the human. *Acta Endocrinol* 1962;41:400–6.

Malm C, Svensson M, Ekblom B, Sjodin B. Effects of ubiquinone-10 supplementation and high intensity training on physical performance in humans. *Acta Physiol Scand* 1997;161:379–84.

Malm C, Svensson M, Sjoberg B, Ekblom B, Sjodin S. Supplementation with ubiquinone-10 causes cellular damage during intense exercise. *Acta Physiol Scand* 1996;157:511–12.

Marconi C, Sassi G, Carpinelli A, Cerretelli P. Effects of L-carnitine loading on the aerobic and anaerobic performance of endurance athletes. *Eur J Appl Physiol* 1985: 54:131–5.

Matson LG, Tran ZT. Effects of sodium bicarbonate ingestion on anaerobic performance: a meta-analytic review. *Int J Sports Nutr* 1993;3:2–28.

Maughan R, Greenhaff P. High intensity exercise performance and acid–base balance: the effect of diet and induced alkalosis. In: Brouns F, ed. Advance in Nutrition and Top Sport. *Med Sports Sci* 1991;32:147–65.

McNaughton LR, Cedaro R. The effect of sodium bicarbonate on rowing ergometer performance in elite rowers. *Aust J Sci Med Sport* 1991;23:66–9.

McNaughton L, Dalton B, Palmer G. Sodium bicarbonate can be used as an ergogenic aid in high-intensity, competitive cycle ergometry of 1 h duration. *Eur J Appl Physiol* 1999;80:64–9.

McNaughton L, Egan G, Caelli G. A comparison of Chinese and Russian ginseng as ergogenic aids to improve various facets of physical fitness. *Int Clin Nutr Rev* 1989;9:32–5.

McNaughton LR, Dalton B, Tarr J. Inosine has no effect on aerobic or anaerobic cycling performance. *Int J Sport Nutr* 1999;9:333–44.

McNaughton LR. Bicarbonate and citrate. In: Maughan RJ, ed. *Nutrition in Sport*. Oxford: Blackwell Science Ltd, 2000: 379–92.

Mero A, Kahkonen J, Nykanen T, Parviainen T, Jokinen I, Takala T, Nikula T, Rasi S, Leppaluoto J. IGF-1, IGA and IgG responses to bovine colostrum supplementation during training. *J Appl Physiol* 2002; 93:732–9.

Mero A, Mikkulainen H, Riski J, Pakkanen R, Aalto J, Takala T. Effects of bovine colostrum supplement on serum IGF-1, IgG, hormone and saliva IgA during training. *J Appl Physiol* 1997;83:1144–51.

Mittleman KD, Ricci MR, Bailey SP. Branched-chain amino acids prolong exercise during heat stress in men and women. *Med Sci Sports Exerc* 1998;30:83–91.

Montner P, Stark DM, Riedesel ML, Murata G, Robergs R, Timms M, Chick TW. Pre-exercise glycerol hydration improves cycling endurance time. *Int J Sports Med* 1996;17:27–33.

Morris AC, Jacobs I, McLellan TM, Klugerman A, Wang LCH, Zamecnik J. No ergogenic effects of ginseng ingestion. *Int J Sport Nutr* 1996;6:263–71.

National Research Council. *Recommended Dietary Allowances*. Washington DC: National Academy Press, 1989.

Nelson AG, Arnall DA, Kokkonen J, Day R, Evans J. Muscle glycogen supercompensation is enhanced by prior creatine supplementation. *Med Sci Sports Exerc* 2001;33: 1096–100.

Nielsen AN, Mizuno M, Ratkevicius A, Mohr T, Rohde M, Mortensen SA, Quistorff B. No effect of antioxidant supplementation in triathletes on maximal oxygen uptake, 31P-NMRS detected muscle energy metabolism and muscle fatigue. *Int J Sports Med* 1999;20:154–8.

Nissen SL, Sharp RL. Effect of dietary supplements on lean mass and strength gains with resistance exercise: a meta-analysis. *J Appl Physiol* 2003 (in press).

Nissen S, Sharp R, Ray M, Rathmacher JA, Rice D, Fuller JC, Connelly ASA. Effect of leucine metabolite β-hydroxy-β-methylbutyrate on muscle metabolism during resistance-exercise training. *J Appl Physiol* 1996;81:2095–104.

Op' T Eijnde B, Van Leemputte B, Brouns F, et al. No effects of oral ribose supplementation on repeated maximal exercise and de novo ATP resynthesis. *J Appl Physiol* 2001;91:2275–81.

Oyono-Enguelle S, Freund H, Ott C, Gartner M, Heitz A, Marbach J, Maccari F, Frey A, Bigot H, Bach AC. Prolonged submaximal exercise and L-carnitine in humans. *Eur J Appl Physiol* 1988;58:53–61.

Paddon-Jones D, Keech A, Jenkins D. Short-term β-hydroxy-β-methylbutyrate supplementation does not reduce symptoms of eccentric muscle damage. *Int J Sport Nutr Exerc Metab* 2001;11:442–50.

Panton LN, Rathmacher JA, Baier S, Nissen S. Nutritional supplementation of the leucine metabolite beta-hydroxy beta-methylbutyrate (HMB) during resistance training. *Nutrition* 2000;16:734–9.

Parasrampuria J, Schwartz K, Petesch R. Quality control of dehydroepiandrosterone dietary supplement products. *JAMA* 1998;280:1565.

Pasman WJ, van Baak MA, Jeukendrup AE, de Haan A. The effect of different dosages of caffeine on endurance performance time. *Int J Sports Med* 1995;16:225–30.

Perharic L, Shaw D, Collbridge M, House I, Leon C, Murray V. Toxicological problems resulting from exposure to traditional remedies and food supplements. *Drug Safety* 1994;11:284–94.

Pieralisi G, Ripari P, Vecchiet L. Effects of standardised ginseng extract combined with dimethylaminoethanol bitartrate, vitamins, minerals and trace elements on physical performance during exercise. *Clin Therapeut* 1991;12:373–82.

Poortmans JR, Francaux M. Long-term oral creatine supplementation does not impair renal function in healthy athletes. *Med Sci Sports Exerc* 1999;31:1108–10.

Potteiger JA, Nickel GL, Webster MJ, Haub MD, Palmer RJ. Sodium citrate ingestion enhances 30 km cycling performance. *Int J Sports Med* 1996a;17:7–11.

Potteiger JA, Webster MJ, Nickel GK, Haub MD, Palmer RJ. The effects of buffer ingestion on metabolic factors related to distance running performance. *Eur J Appl Physiol* 1996b;72:365–71.

Pritchard NR, Kalra PA. Renal dysfunction accompanying oral creatine supplements. *Lancet* 1998;351:1252–3.

Rasmussen BB, Volpi E, Gore DC, Wolfe RR. Androstenedione does not stimulate muscle protein anabolism in young healthy men. *J Clin Endocrinol Metab* 2000;85:55–9.

Robergs RA, Griffin SE. Glycerol: biochemistry, pharmacokinetics and clinical and practical applications. *Sports Med* 1998;26:145–67.

Ros JJ, Pelders MG, de Smet PA. A case of positive doping associated with a botanical food supplement. *Pharm World Sci* 1999;21:44–6.

Roufs JB. Review of L-tryptophan and eosinophilia-myalgia syndrome. *J Am Diet Assoc* 1992;92:844–50.

Sahlin K. Metabolic aspects of fatigue in human skeletal muscle. In: Marconnet P, Komi PV, Saltin B, Sejersted OM, eds. *Muscle Fatigue Mechanisms in Exercise and Training*. Vol 34. Basel: Karger, 1992: 54–68.

Schabort EJ, Wilson G, Noakes TD. Dose-related elevations in venous pH with citrate ingestion do not alter 40-km cycling time-trial performance. *Eur J Appl Physiol* 2000;83:320–7.

Shave R, Whyte G, Siemann A, Doggart L. The effects of sodium citrate ingestion on 3,000-meter time-trial performance. *J Strength Cond Res* 2001;15:230–4.

Shaw D, Leon C, Kolev S, Murray V. Traditional remedies and food supplements. A 5-year toxicological study (1991–1995). *Drug Safety* 1997;17:342–56.

Siliprandi N, Di Lisa F, Pieralisi G. Metabolic changes induced by maximal exercise in human subjects following L-carnitine administration. *Biochimica et Biophysica Acta* 1990;1034:17–21.

Slater GJ, Jenkins D. β-hydroxy β-methylbutyrate (HMB) supplementation and the promotion of muscle growth and strength. *Sports Med* 2000;30:105–16.

Slater G, Jenkins D, Logan P, Lee H, Vukovich M, Rathmacher JA, Hahn AG. β-hydroxy-β-methylbutyrate (HMB) supplementation does not affect changes in strength or body composition during resistance training in trained men. *Int J Sport Nutr Exerc Metab* 2001;11:384–96.

Slater GJ, Logan PA, Boston T, Gore CJ, Stenhouse A, Hahn AG. β-hydroxy β-methylbutyrate (HMB) supplementation does not influence the urinary testosterone:epitestosterone ratio in healthy males. *J Sci Med Sport* 2000;3:79–83.

Snider I, Bazzarre TL, Murdoch SD, Goldfarb A. Effects of coenzyme athletic performance system as an ergogenic aid on endurance performance to exhaustion. *Int J Sport Nutr* 1992;2:272–86.

Soop M, Bjorkman O, Cederblad G, Hagenfeldt L, Wahren J. Influence of carnitine supplementation on muscle substrate and carnitine metabolism during exercise. *J Appl Physiol* 1998;64:2394–9.

Spriet LL. Ergogenic aids: recent advances and retreats. In: Lamb DR, Murray R, eds. *Perspectives in Exercise Science and Sports Medicine*: Vol 10. *Optimizing Sports Performance*. Carmel, IN: Cooper Publishing Company, 1997: 185–238.

Starling RD, Trappe TA, Short KR, Sheffield-Moore M, Joszi AC, Fink WJ, Costill DL. Effect of inosine supplementation on aerobic and anaerobic cycling performance. *Med Sci Sports Exerc* 1996;28:1193–8.

Stephens TJ, McKenna MJ, Canny BJ, Snow RJ, McConell GK. Effect of sodium bicarbonate on muscle metabolism during intense endurance cycling. *Med Sci Sports Exerc* 2002;34:614–21.

Stoecker BJ. Chromium. In: Ziegler EE, Filer LJ, eds. *Present Knowledge in Nutrition*. 7th edn. Washington: ILSI Press, 1996: 344–52.

Svennson M, Malm C, Tonkonogi M, Ekblom B, Sjodin B, Sahlin K. Effect of Q10 supplementation on tissue Q10 levels and adenine nucleotide catabolism during high-intensity exercise. *Int J Sport Nutr* 1999;9:166–80.

Tarnopolsky MA. Caffeine and endurance performance. *Sports Med* 1994;18:109–25.

Tiryaki GR, Atterbom HA. The effects of sodium bicarbonate and sodium citrate on 600 m running time of trained females. *J Sports Med Phys Fitness* 1995;35:194–8.

Trappe SW, Costill DL, Goodpaster MD, Fink WJ, The effects of L-carnitine supplementation on performance during interval swimming. *Int J Sports Med* 1994;15:181–5.

Trent LK, Thieding-Cancel D. Effects of chromium picolinate on body composition. *J Sports Med Phys Fitness* 1995;35:273–80.

Uralets VP, Gillette PA. Over-the-counter anabolic steroids 4-androsten-3,17-dione; 4-androsten-3beta,17beta-diol; and 19-nor-4-androsten-3,17-dione: excretion studies in men. *J Anal Toxicol* 1999;23:357–66.

Van Gammeren D, Falk D, Antonio J. The effects of supplementation with 19-nor-4-androstene-3,17-dione and 19-nor-4-androstene-3,17-diol on body composition and athletic performance in previously weight-trained male athletes. *Eur J Appl Physiol* 2001;84:426–31.

van Zyl CG, Lambert EV, Hawley JA, Noakes TD, Dennis SC. Effects of medium-chain triglyceride ingestion on fuel metabolism and cycling performance. *J Appl Physiol* 1996;80:2217–25.

Vecchiet L, Di Lisa F, Pieralisi G. Influence of L-carnitine administration on maximal physical exercise. *Eur J Appl Physiol* 1990;61:486–90.

Vukovich MD, Costill DL, Fink WJ. Carnitine supplementation: effect on muscle carnitine and glycogen content during exercise. *Med Sci Sports Exerc* 1994;26:1122–9.

Vukovich MD, Dreifort GD. Effect of beta-hydroxy beta-methylbutyrate on the onset of lactate accumulation and VO_{2peak} in endurance trained cyclists. *J Strength Cond Res* 2001;15:491–7.

Wagenmakers AJM. L-carnitine supplementation and performance in man. In: Brouns F, ed. *Advances in Nutrition and Top Sport: Medicine and Sport Science*. Basel: Karger, 1991: 110–27.

Walker LS, Bemben MG, Bemben DA, Knehans AW. Chromium picolinate effects on body composition and muscular performance in wrestlers. *Med Sci Sports Exerc* 1998;30:1730–7.

Wallace MB, Lim J, Cutler A, Bucci L. Effects of dehydroepiandrosterone vs androstenedione supplementation in men. *Med Sci Sports Exerc* 1999;31:1788–92.

Weston SB, Zhou S, Weatherby RP, Robson J. Does exogenous coenzyme Q10 affect aerobic capacity in endurance athletes? *Int J Sport Nutr* 1997;7:197–206.

Wilkes D, Gledhill N, Smyth R. Effect of acute induced metabolic acidosis on 800m racing time. *Med Sci Sports Exerc* 1983;15:277–80.

Williams MH, Kreider R, Hunter DW, Somma CT, Shall LM, Woodhouse ML, Rokitski L. Effect of inosine supplementation on 3-mile treadmill run performance and VO_{2peak}. *Med Sci Sport Exerc* 1990;22:517–22.

Williams M, Kreider R, Branch JD. Creatine. Champaign, IL: Human Kinetics, 1998.

Yesalsis CE. Medical, legal, and societal implications of androstenedione. *JAMA* 1999;281:2043–4.

Ylikoski T, Piirainen J, Hanninen O, Penttinen J. The effect of coenzyme Q10 on the exercise performance of cross-country skiers. *Molec Aspects Med* 1997;18: S283–S290.

Ziemba AW, Chmura J, Kaciuba-Uscilko H, Nazar K, Wisnik P, Gawronski W. Ginseng treatment improves psychomotor performance at rest and during graded exercise. *Int J Sport Nutr* 1999;9:371–7.

CHAPTER 10

Exercise in the heat

Mark A. FEBBRAIO

Introduction

It is well established that exercise in the heat results in a reduced endurance capacity. This reduction in endurance capacity is primarily due to the attenuated thermal gradient between the skin and the environment, which results in a reduced rate of body heat dissipation, ultimately leading to greater heat storage. In an effort to delay the onset of acute hyperthermia, a number of thermoregulatory, cardiovascular and metabolic responses are invoked. This chapter summarises recent advances in the physiology of exercise and heat stress.

Cardiovascular alterations during exercise and heat stress: new perspectives

The magnitude of the effects of heat stress on cardiovascular function during exercise depends on many variables, such as the level of hyperthermia (determined by the environmental temperature, the prevailing exercise intensity and the duration of exercise), the state of hydration, training status, degree of acclimatisation and body position. The cardiovascular responses to exercise and heat stress have been the subject of many comprehensive reviews (see Buskirk 1977; Gisolfi & Wenger 1984; Hardy 1961; Nadel 1985; Rowell 1974). However, as will be discussed, some of the major theories regarding the cardiovascular response to exercise and heat stress have been recently challenged (Coyle & González-Alonso 2001a).

It is well established that during exercise in the heat cardiovascular responses begin a time-dependent change as exercise progresses. Termed the 'cardiovascular drift', a progressive decline in stroke volume and a parallel increase in heart rate are observed such that cardiac output is maintained (Ekelund 1967). The traditional viewpoint is that cardiovascular drift is due to a progressive increase in cutaneous blood flow, leading to an increase in cutaneous venous volume and hence decreased venous return, thereby reducing ventricular filling pressure, end diastolic volume and, ultimately, stroke volume (Rowell 1986). However, recent work from Dr Ed Coyle's laboratory at The University of Texas has challenged this concept. Fritzsche et al. (1999) had subjects perform 60 minutes of exercise with and without the ingestion of a β_1-adrenoreceptor blocker. In the control trial, the increase in heart rate was related to an increase in stroke volume but not to an increase in forearm blood flow. In addition, during β_1-receptor blockade, while the heart rate was lower and the stroke volume higher compared with the control trial, forearm blood flow was unaffected. Taken together, these findings suggest that cutaneous flow may not be the mediator of cardiovascular function during exercise and heat stress. Indeed, González-Alonso et al. (1995) have demonstrated that the combination of heat stress and dehydration actually *decreases* cutaneous flow. This has led to an alternative hypothesis being proposed (Coyle & González-Alonso 2001), which is summarised in Figure 10.1.

In this model, the primary mediator of cardiovascular drift during exercise in the heat is progressive dehydration, which occurs as a result of an increased sweat rate.

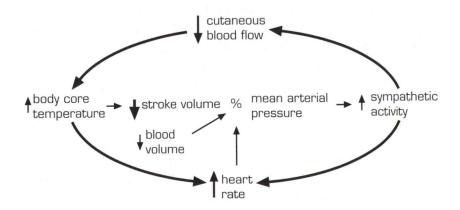

FIG. 10.1 New perspective regarding mechanisms for cardiovascular drift during prolonged exercise and heat stress. From Coyle and González-Alonso (2001) with permission

Metabolic alterations during exercise and heat stress

Substrate metabolism

Compared with exercise in a cooler environment, heat stress results in an augmented utilisation of intramuscular carbohydrate (CHO) stores (Febbraio et al. 1994a; Febbraio et al. 1994b; Fink et al. 1975; González-Alonso et al. 1999; Jentjens et al. 2002). In addition, when the rise in body temperature is attenuated by heat acclimatisation (Febbraio et al. 1994a; King et al. 1985; Kirwan et al. 1987; Young et al. 1985) reducing the ambient temperature (Febbraio et al. 1996b; Parkin et al. 1999), or providing external cooling (Kozlowski et al. 1985), the rate of muscle glycogenolysis and/or whole-body CHO oxidation is/are reduced by preventing dehydration (González-Alonso et al. 1999; Hargreaves et al. 1996b).

Not all studies, however, have observed that heat stress increases CHO use. Factors such as the magnitude of difference in ambient temperature, the acclimatisation status of the subject population and the presence or absence of circulating air will all affect body core temperature responses. It is not surprising, therefore, that in a study by Yaspelkis et al. (1993) glycogenolysis was not altered during exercise in the hot trial because the ambient temperature difference when comparing the two experimental conditions was approximately 10°C and the subject population was heat acclimatised. Consequently, the largest difference in body core temperature at any point when comparing the two experimental trials was 0.4°C, a difference unlikely to have major physiological ramifications.

It is also important to note that the rate of glycogenolysis during submaximal exercise is largely influenced by the pre-exercise glycogen concentration (Chesley et al. 1995; Hargreaves et al. 1995; Hespel & Richter 1992; Steensberg et al. 2002). This occurs because glycogen can bind to phosphorylase, the enzyme responsible for its breakdown, to increase its activity (Johnson 1982). Therefore, it is not surprising that in studies where pre-exercise glycogen levels were higher prior to exercising in cooler, relative to warmer, experimental conditions no differences were observed in intramuscular glycogenolysis (Nielsen et al. 1990; Young et al. 1995). Recently, Maxwell et al. (1999) demonstrated no difference in the glycogenolytic rate when comparing maximal exercise in the heat with that in a cooler environment. As suggested by these authors, the supramaximal nature of the exercise may have increased the energy turnover to a level where heat stress was rendered unimportant. Indeed, muscle lactate accumulation in both trials was > 100 mmol/kg dry mass (Maxwell et al. 1999).

It appears that if exercise in the heat is submaximal in nature and a marked (> 0.5°C) increase in body core temperature is observed, intramuscular CHO utilisation is indeed augmented. If, however, body temperature is not markedly influenced by exercise and heat stress, it is unlikely that metabolic differences will be observed during exercise and heat stress.

The consistent observation of an increased respiratory exchange ratio when comparing exercise in the heat with that in a cooler environment (Dolny & Lemon 1988; Febbraio et al. 1994a; Febbraio et al. 1994b; Hargreaves et al. 1996a; Young et al. 1985) suggests that CHO, in particular glycogen, is also oxidised to a greater extent during exercise and heat stress, possibly at the expense of lipid oxidation. Evidence from both our research group (Hargreaves et al. 1996a) and others (González-Alonso et al. 1999; Jentjens et al. 2002) supports this hypothesis. Using an isotopic tracer method, we have demonstrated that the rate of glucose disappearance (R_d) was not different when comparing exercise at 40°C with that at 20°C. In contrast, estimated rates of CHO oxidation were higher in the heat. If we assume that the R_d-glucose was fully oxidised within contracting skeletal muscle, then the calculated level of intramuscular glycogen oxidation was higher in the 40°C trial (Fig. 10.2).

Recently, Jentjens et al. (2002) have directly measured exogenous glucose oxidation using a carbon-labelled tracer. Despite a lower rate of ingested glucose oxidation, total carbohydrate oxidation tended to be higher in the heat as a result of an increased (25%) muscle glycogenolysis. Likewise, González-Alonso et al. (1999) have demonstrated that the contracting limb respiratory quotient was higher in exercising subjects with dehydration-induced hyperthermia compared with those in a euhydrated state. These authors also observed little difference in glucose uptake to contracting muscle as measured by arteriovenous difference for the two experimental conditions (González-Alonso et al. 1999), which also suggests that glycogen oxidation was augmented (see Fig. 10.2). Taken collectively, these results suggest that flux through the pyruvate dehydrogenase (PDH) pathway is up-regulated during exercise and heat stress because some of the pyruvate formed during exercise is being oxidised.

Recently we tested the hypothesis that PDH is, indeed, up-regulated during exercise and heat stress. Subjects exercised in the heat or cool for 5 minutes at 70% VO_{2max} (Saunders et al. 2001). In this study, we chose to

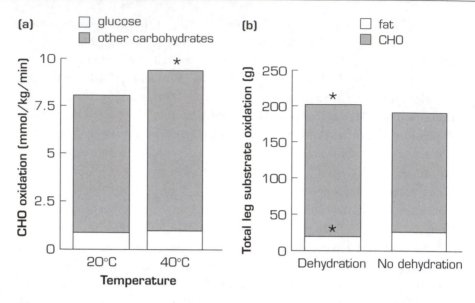

FIG. 10.2 (a) Carbohydrate oxidation during exercise in the heat (40°C) and cool (20°C) and (b) substrate oxidation during exercise in the heat in the presence or absence of dehydration. * denotes difference ($P < 0.05$) when comparing (a) oxidation of other carbohydrate between trials and when comparing (b) fat and carbohydrate oxidation between trials. Values are means—(a) $n = 6$, (b) $n = 7$. Data from (a) Hargreaves et al. (1996a); (b) González-Alonso et al. (1999)

examine the PDH pathway in the transition from rest to exercise because of the previous observation that PDH is activated to its full extent by 1 minute after the onset of exercise when the intensity is 65% VO_{2max} (Howlett et al. 1998b). In our recent study we did not observe an increase in PDH activity when comparing subjects exercising in the heat with those in a cooler environment. However, whether PDH activity is elevated later during exercise requires further clarification.

A few studies have examined lipid metabolism during exercise and heat stress. Plasma free fatty acid (FFA) concentration has been consistently observed to be unaltered by exercise and thermal stress (Fink et al. 1975; Nielsen et al. 1990; Yaspelkis et al. 1993). However, plasma FFAs only reflect a balance between rates of whole body lipolysis and FFA uptake by other tissues and organs during exercise. Of note was the finding of Fink et al. (1975), who observed similar plasma FFA concentrations when comparing subjects exercising in the heat with those in a cooler environment, despite a reduction in intramuscular triacylglycerol utilisation during exercise at 41°C. No subsequent attempts have been made to measure intramuscular triacylglycerol utilisation in human skeletal muscle during exercise and heat stress.

Only two studies have examined the effect of exercise and heat stress on FFA uptake. Nielsen et al. (1990) observed no change in FFA uptake during exercise in the heat when compared with exercise of a similar intensity/duration in a cooler environment. In contrast, González-Alonso et al. (1999) observed a lower FFA uptake during the latter stages of exercise in subjects with dehydration-induced hyperthermia compared with a trial in which subjects were euhydrated and exercising in the heat. Hence, based on the respiratory quotient and FFA flux across the contracting limb, total leg lipid oxidation was lower in subjects with dehydration-induced hyperthermia (González-Alonso et al. 1999), a result consistent with the earlier observations of Fink et al. (1975).

It appears, therefore, that exercise and acute heat stress result in an increase in intramuscular glycogen use via both oxidative and non-oxidative energy pathways. The increase in lactate accumulation in both contracting muscle and plasma results from net intramuscular glycogenolysis and not from increased uptake and oxidation of circulating glucose.

The effect of exercise and heat stress on protein metabolism has not been directly measured due, in part, to the minimal contribution of protein to the total energy turnover and/or the difficulty in measuring protein turnover during exercise. There is indirect evidence that suggests that protein catabolism may be increased during such exercise in the heat. Work from our laboratory has observed increased intramuscular ammonia (NH_3) accumulation in both endurance-trained (Febbraio et al. 1994b) and untrained (Snow et al. 1993) humans. Although a major pathway for NH3 production during exercise is via the deamination of adenosine monophosphate (AMP) to form NH_3 and inosine monophosphate (IMP), NH3 can also be formed in skeletal muscle from the oxidation of branched chain amino acids (Graham et al. 1995). During one study (Febbraio et al. 1994b), the augmented NH_3 accumulation was observed in the absence of any difference in IMP accumulation. In addition, the exercise-induced increase in NH_3 during the hotter experimental condition was fivefold higher than the accumulation of IMP (see Fig. 10.3). These data suggest that protein degradation may be increased during exercise in the heat, although it must be noted that even if this were to be the case, the contribution of protein to total energy turnover would still be minimal.

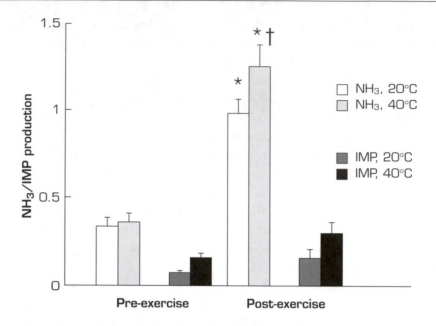

FIG. 10.3 Ammonia (NH_3) and IMP concentrations before and after 40 minutes of exercise at 70% VO_{2peak} in the heat (40°C) and cool (20°C). * indicates difference ($P < 0.05$) for post-exercise compared with pre-exercise; † indicates difference ($P < 0.05$) at 40°C compared with at 20°C. Values are means ± SE ($n = 12$). Data from Febbraio et al. (1994b)

Glucose availability and requirement during exercise and heat stress

Many studies have observed relative hyperglycaemia in athletes during exercise in the heat (Febbraio et al. 1994a; Fink et al. 1975; Hargreaves et al. 1996a; Yaspelkis et al. 1993), which likely reflects an imbalance between glucose production and utilisation. Indeed, using a dye infusion technique, Rowell et al. (1968) have previously demonstrated that hepatic glucose production was augmented in heat-stressed humans. These data have recently been confirmed using both isotopic tracer dilution (Fig. 10.4; Hargreaves et al. 1996a) and arteriovenous balance (González-Alonso et al. 1999) techniques.

The regulation of hepatic glucose production during exercise involves a complex interplay of neural and hormonal factors and both 'feed-back' and 'feed-forward' mechanisms (for review see Kjær 1995). Hence, during submaximal exercise in comfortable ambient conditions, euglycaemia is

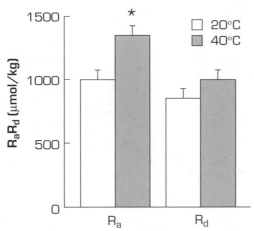

FIG. 10.4 Total hepatic glucose production (R_a) and glucose uptake (R_d) during 40 minutes of exercise at 70% VO_{2peak} in the heat (40°C) and cool (20°C). Values are means ± SE ($n = 6$). * denotes difference ($P < 0.05$) from 20°C. Data from Hargreaves et al. (1996a)

usually maintained as hepatic glucose production is regulated to match the metabolic need for glucose. Consequently, an increasing circulating glucose concentration as a result of exogenous feeding (Jeukendrup et al. 1999; McConell et al. 1994) or glucose infusion (Howlett et al. 1998a) blunts the increase in hepatic glucose production during exercise. However, we have recently conducted an experiment where subjects ingested either a placebo solution or a labelled isotopic glucose solution, while being infused with an alternatively labelled glucose isotope. Our data demonstrate that despite an increase in glucose appearance from the gastrointestinal tract and a concomitant increase in plasma glucose concentration, hepatic glucose production was unaffected by glucose ingestion (Fig. 10.5; Angus et al. 2001). The absence of effective 'feed-back' regulation of hepatic glucose production with CHO ingestion highlights the powerful 'feed-forward' control of glucose homeostasis with thermal stress.

Muscle energy metabolism

Few studies have examined the effect of whole body heat stress on muscle energy metabolism during exercise. A reduction in intramuscular contents of adenosine triphosphate (ATP) and phosphocreatine (PCr) and increases in adenosine diphosphate (ADP) and AMP accumulation have been observed during fatiguing submaximal exercise with heat stress in dogs (Kozlowski et al. 1985). While PCr degradation is augmented during exercise and heat stress

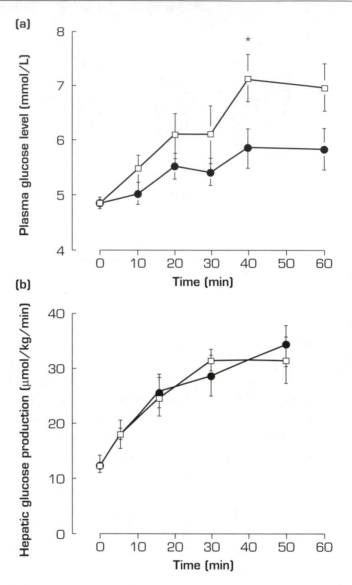

FIG. 10.5 (a) Plasma glucose concentration and (b) hepatic glucose production during 60 minutes of exercise at 70% VO_{2peak} in 35°C with (squares) or without (circles) the ingestion of carbohydrate. * denotes difference ($P < 0.05$) when comparing trials. Values are means ± SE ($n = 6$). Data from Angus et al. (2001)

in humans, total adenine nucleotide metabolism, IMP accumulation and the energy charge potential of the contracting muscle is unaltered in subjects when comparing 40 minutes of exercise in 40°C with similar exercise in 20°C (Febbraio et al. 1994b). While the conflict when comparing these two studies may be related to species differences, they may also be related to the important fact that one protocol required the participants to exercise to exhaustion, while the other was non-fatiguing and of fixed duration.

Limits to exercise performance in the heat

Laboratory studies versus competition performance

Numerous laboratory studies have demonstrated that thermal stress reduces exercise capacity (Booth et al. 1997; Brück & Olschewski 1987; Febbraio et al. 1996a; Galloway & Maughan 1997; González-Alonso et al. 1997; Hessemer et al. 1984; Kozlowski et al. 1985; Kruk et al. 1985; Lee & Haymes 1995; MacDougall et al. 1974; Nielsen et al. 1993; Saltin et al. 1972; Schmidt & Brück 1981; Walsh et al. 1994). In contrast, while reduced athletic performances during competition in the heat have been documented (Terrados & Maughan 1995), it must be noted that in some circumstances athletes can perform well in the heat (Maughan et al. 1994; Noakes et al. 1991; Robinson 1963). This apparent anomaly can be best reconciled by examining the interaction between the exercise intensity or, more importantly, the degree of endogenous heat production and the exogenous heat load. In general, during many endurance athletic events the exercise intensity is moderate and the exogenous heat load is high, but not extreme. Therefore, thermoregulation is adequate and athletes can minimise cardiovascular strain. In these circumstances the heat stress is aptly referred to as 'compensable heat stress' (Montain et al. 1994; Sawka et al. 1992) and can usually be overcome.

In contrast, during laboratory experiments, especially those that adopt a protocol that does not include the utilisation of circulating air, the exercise intensity coupled with the magnitude of the exogenous heat load usually results in 'uncompensable heat stress', a situation where the body's cardiovascular and thermoregulatory capacities are insufficient as a means to cope with the heat load. In these circumstances, body core temperature continues to rise and performance must deteriorate.

Is fatigue during exercise in the heat substrate-dependent?

During prolonged exercise in comfortable ambient temperatures fatigue often coincides with glycogen concentrations < 150 mmol/kg dry weight (Baldwin et al. 1999; Coggan & Coyle 1987; Constantin-Teodosiu et al. 1992; Coyle et al. 1986; Febbraio & Dancey 1999; Sahlin et al. 1990). Given that glycogen utilisation is augmented during exercise in the heat, it is reasonable to suggest that the reduced endurance performance often observed during exercise and heat stress may be related to substrate availability. It is somewhat paradoxical, therefore, that fatigue during exercise with uncompensable heat stress is not related to CHO availability but appears to be related to hyperthermia. In contrast with studies conducted in comfortable ambient temperatures, the glycogen concentration at fatigue during prolonged exercise in the heat is ≥ 300 mmol/kg dry weight in unacclimatised, endurance trained (Parkin et al. 1999) and non-specifically trained (Nielsen et al. 1993) individuals. Furthermore, CHO ingestion during prolonged exercise in the heat, where the heat stress in uncompensable, has no effect on endurance performance (Davis et al. 1988a; Febbraio et al. 1996a; Levine et al. 1991; Millard-Stafford et al. 1990). The results of these studies are in contrast with the well-described ergogenic benefits of CHO supplementation during prolonged exercise in comfortable ambient temperatures (for review see Coyle & Montain 1992). It must be noted, however, that when the heat stress is compensable, CHO ingestion does improve performance (Below et al. 1995; Davis et al. 1988b; Millard-Stafford et al. 1992; Murray et al. 1987). It appears, therefore, that in severe, but not mild, heat stress the limit to exercise performance is not related to substrate availability.

The role of the central nervous system

It has been hypothesised that fatigue during exercise and heat stress is related to negative effects on the motor control centres in the brain (Brück & Olschewski 1987; Nielsen et al. 1990). This hypothesis has not been tested directly, although the concept of a critical body core temperature limiting exercise performance is supported by data from several studies. In 1993, Nielsen et al. conducted a study whereby trained men were heat acclimatised by exercising at 60% VO_{2peak} to fatigue in a hot environment for 9–12 consecutive days. Although exercise capacity increased from 48 ± 2 min to 80 ± 3 min, fatigue occurred at the same body core temperature each day. Of note during this study were the observations of no reduction in muscle or skin blood flow, no lack of available substrate, and no accumulation of lactate or potassium at the point of fatigue when subjects were either unacclimatised or acclimatised. In addition, there was no significant decline in force (measured by a maximal voluntary contraction) at the point of fatigue in either trial.

Two studies conducted in our laboratory also suggest that fatigue may be associated with the attainment of a critical body core temperature leading to a diminished drive to exercise. When subjects ingested CHO beverages of various concentrations during exercise to exhaustion at 33°C, endurance performance was neither increased nor impaired if the change in plasma volume or the rise in body core temperature was not different compared with the ingestion of a placebo. In contrast, when a concentrated (14%) CHO beverage was ingested, the plasma volume was less well maintained and the rise in body core temperature was augmented. In these circumstances performance tended to be diminished. Of note, however, was the observation that in all circumstance, fatigue coincided with a similar body core temperature (Febbraio et al. 1996a).

In a separate study, we have recently examined the effect of heat stress on a 30-minute laboratory time-trial performance in elite road cyclists. Subjects performed two time trials at either 32°C or 23°C. Although mean power output (W) was significantly lower in the trial conducted at 32°C (6.5%), rectal temperature was remarkably similar during both exercise bouts (Tatterson et al. 2000). These data suggest that during self-paced exercise in the heat, athletes may select a power output that coincides with an arbitrary (individual) upper limit in body core temperature. However, the mechanisms underlying such a hypothesis are not clear.

Preparation for exercise in the heat

Heat acclimatisation

As previously discussed, exercise performance in the heat which results in uncompensable heat stress appears to be largely dependent on the attainment of a critical body core temperature (Nielsen et al. 1993). Since heat acclimatisation postpones the onset of this time (Nielsen et al. 1993), athletes should be advised to adopt suitable heat acclimatisation programs prior to competition in the heat. Heat acclimatisation, a process that involves repeated exercise bouts in a hot environment, involves a complex array of adaptations which decrease body core temperature, heart rate, and renal and sweat electrolyte concentrations, and increase total sweat rate and plasma volume (for review see Armstrong & Maresh 1991). Gisolfi (1987) defined the parameters of heat acclimatisation as being mild to moderate activity (20–50% VO_{2max}) for a duration of 90 minutes for a period of 7–14 days. Since the major physiological adaptations plateau after approximately 14 days of heat acclimatisation (Armstrong & Maresh 1991), there is no evidence to suggest that extending the program beyond this time will result in any additional benefit to an acute acclimatisation response. It must be noted, however, that the better performing athletes during athletic competition in the heat often reside in hot environments for prolonged periods, suggesting that some (other) chronic adaptations may take place.

In addition to the beneficial cardiovascular and thermoregulatory adaptations associated with heat acclimatisation, this process also results in reductions in muscle glycogen utilisation and lactate accumulation (King et al. 1985; Kirwan et al. 1987; Febbraio et al. 1994a). In fact, in some studies the glycogen use during exercise after acclimatisation was attenuated by as much as 40% (King et al. 1985; Kirwan et al. 1987). This adaptation, although often overlooked in assessing the benefits of heat acclimatisation, is nonetheless very important from a performance perspective. In circumstances when the heat stress is compensable, performance is likely to be limited by substrate availability and therefore an attenuation of glycogen use can improve exercise capacity. The metabolic adaptations associated with heat acclimatisation are likely to be mediated by the lower muscle temperature and the sympathoadrenal response resulting from heat acclimatisation (Febbraio et al. 1994a).

Despite the fact that heat acclimatisation results in enhanced athletic performance (compared to no acclimatisation), one must exercise caution with respect to dietary intake when undertaking such a program. Athletes who undertake a heat acclimatisation program prior to competition should ensure that their diet contains sufficient CHO. This is important because even though heat acclimatisation reduces net muscle glycogen utilisation during exercise and heat stress, post-acclimatisation glycogenolysis remains somewhat higher than that observed during exercise in cooler conditions (Febbraio et al. 1994a). Although a high CHO diet will reduce thermoregulatory capacity in rats (Francesconi & Hubbard 1986), there is no evidence that this occurs in humans (Schwellnus et al. 1990). Therefore, athletes should not be fearful that such a diet might negate the effects of a heat acclimatisation regimen.

Fluid availability

In addition to dietary modification, one needs to monitor fluid intake carefully when preparing for exercise in the heat. During heat acclimatisation, there is an increased requirement for fluid intake because of the enhanced sweating response (Greenleaf et al. 1983). Exercise-induced dehydration is associated with an increase in body core temperature (Hamilton et al. 1991; Montain & Coyle 1992), reduced cardiovascular function (Hamilton et al. 1991; Montain & Coyle 1992) and impaired exercise performance (Walsh et al. 1994). These deleterious physiological effects are attenuated, if not completely prevented, by fluid ingestion (Candas et al. 1986; Costill et al. 1970; Hamilton et al. 1991; Montain & Coyle 1992), which also improves exercise performance (Maughan et al. 1989; McConell et al. 1997; Walsh et al. 1994). Apart from the adverse physiological effect of dehydration during exercise, such a circumstance also results in increased muscle temperature, sympathoadrenal response and glycogen utilisation (González-Alonso et al. 1997; Hargreaves et al. 1996b). Therefore, if athletes become dehydrated, they also increase their likelihood of depleting their intramuscular CHO stores.

What is the best nutritional preparation for exercise in a hot environment?

As discussed, it is clear that both CHO and fluid are very important when making dietary recommendations for those exercising in the heat. Apart from maintaining a CHO-rich diet and remaining in a euhydrated state in the days leading up to exercise/competition, there are strategies that should be employed during exercise, particularly exercise lasting longer than 60 minutes.

It would be advisable to ingest a CHO/fluid/electrolyte beverage frequently during exercise. Since the relative importance of fluid delivery is increased during exercise in the heat, one may be tempted to ingest water in these circumstances. Such a practice should, however, be avoided since the ingestion of a CHO/electrolyte/fluid beverage empties from the gut at a similar rate to water (Francis 1979; Owen et al. 1986; Ryan et al. 1989) and can spare muscle glycogen during exercise in the heat (Yaspelkis & Ivy 1991). In addition, the relative importance of electrolyte intake is increased during exercise in the heat. It has been suggested that sodium be included in rehydration beverages to replace sweat sodium losses, prevent hyponatraemia, promote the maintenance of plasma volume and enhance intestinal absorption of glucose and fluid (for review see Chapter 4; Maughan 1994). Although the addition of sodium to a fluid beverage has little effect on glucose or fluid bioavailability during exercise (Hargreaves et al. 1994), such an addition will maintain the drive for drinking, help to minimise urinary fluid loss in recovery from exercise, and maintain the extracellular fluid volume space (Maughan & Leiper 1995; Nose et al. 1988; Takamata et al. 1995).

The amount of CHO within a fluid beverage ingested during exercise in the heat appears to have little effect on fluid availability or exercise performance provided the CHO is not too concentrated. As previously discussed, the change in plasma volume and exercise performance in the heat is not different when ingesting beverages containing 4.2% or 7% CHO. However, when a more concentrated (14%) CHO solution is ingested during exercise in the heat, the maintenance of plasma volume is reduced while the rise in rectal temperature tends to be augmented. Accordingly, exercise performance tends to fall (Febbraio et al. 1996a). It is important, therefore, during exercise in the heat to keep the concentration of CHO within a fluid beverage to approximately < 10%, even though CHO utilisation is augmented in these circumstances. In terms of volume and frequency, a practical recommendation would be to ingest approximately 400 mL every 15 minutes since the rate of fluid loss during exercise in the heat is typically close to 1.6 L per hour. The CHO beverage should also be ingested after training/competition (i.e. during recovery) to ensure rapid replenishment of intramuscular glycogen stores, and to promote rehydration, especially during repeated exercise bouts in a hot environment (Terrados & Maughan 1995).

As discussed above, there is some evidence to suggest that protein catabolism is increased during exercise in the heat (Febbraio et al. 1994b; Mittleman et al. 1995; Snow et al. 1993). One may be tempted, therefore, to recommend that protein intake be increased prior to and during such exercise. However, there is a relative paucity of studies that have systematically examined protein requirements during exercise in the heat and more research is required before definitive recommendations can be made. Likewise, there is some evidence to suggest that oxyradical generation may be increased via the combination of exercise and heat stress (Mills et al. 1996) and it may be of some benefit to supplement those undertaking repeated exercise in a hot environment with antioxidants such as alpha-tocopherol (vitamin E) and ascorbic acid (vitamin C). This recommendation is speculative, however, since the hypothesis that such supplementation is advantageous during exercise in the heat is yet to be investigated experimentally.

Glycerol hyperhydration

Since the deleterious effects of dehydration during exercise, especially that conducted in a hot environment, have been well documented, hyperhydration would be desirable prior to exercise in a hot environment. Accordingly, glycerol added to a bolus of water and ingested has been demonstrated by some (Freund et al. 1995; Lyons et al. 1990, Montner et al. 1996) but not all (Latzka et al. 1997; Murray et al. 1991) to increase fluid retention, reduce sweat rate and consequently result in an enhanced thermoregulatory capacity, especially during exercise in a hot environment (Lyons et al. 1990). Although not clearly understood, it appears that the effectiveness of glycerol may be related to an attenuated rate of free water clearance, and/or an increase in the kidney's medullary concentration gradient, resulting in increased glomerular reabsorption (Freund et al. 1995). Only one study, however, has demonstrated lower body core temperature with glycerol hyperhydration (Lyons et al. 1990).

We recently conducted a comprehensive study where we examined the effect of glycerol hyperhydration on thermoregulation and metabolism during exercise in the heat. Subjects ingested either 1 g glycerol in 20 mL H_2O/kg or 20 mL H_2O/kg body weight, 120 minutes prior to undertaking 90 minutes of steady-state cycle exercise in dry heat. This exercise task was immediately followed by a 15-minute cycle time trial, during which subjects performed as much work as possible. The pre-exercise urine volume was lower in athletes when glycerol was ingested. Heart rate and body core temperature were lower, while forearm blood flow was higher during the glycerol trial. Despite these changes, skin and muscle temperatures and circulating catecholamine levels were not different between trials. Accordingly, no differences were observed in muscle glycogenolysis, lactate accumulation, adenine nucleotide or PCr degradation when comparing trials. Of note, the work performed during the performance cycle was 5% greater than that during the glycerol trial (Anderson et al. 2001). These results demonstrate that glycerol ingestion results in fluid retention, which is capable of reducing cardiovascular strain and enhancing thermoregulation.

Summary

The magnitude of the effects of heat stress on cardiovascular function during exercise depends on many variables, such as the level of hyperthermia (determined by the environmental temperature and the exercise intensity and duration), hydration status, training status, degree of acclimatisation and body position. However, recent evidence suggests that the cardiovascular alterations during exercise and heat stress are largely mediated by dehydration. .

Exercise in the heat also influences metabolism. Both intramuscular glycogen utilisation and glycolysis are augmented, while lipid utilisation appears to decrease during exercise and heat stress. In addition, high-energy phosphagen metabolism and protein catabolism may, in some circumstances, be increased during exercise in the heat. Apart from changes that take place within the contracting skeletal muscle, liver glucose production is also increased during exercise and heat stress, although this change is not accompanied by any increase in peripheral glucose uptake. As a consequence, the circulating glucose concentration is higher during exercise and thermal stress.

During exercise in the heat a balance between preventing hyperthermia and maintaining an adequate fuel supply to fuel muscle contraction must be maintained. In order to achieve this, athletes need to monitor hydration levels and carbohydrate intake closely leading up to exercise. Daily monitoring of body weight and ensuring that urine is pallid will provide a guide to hydration status. During competition, a 4–8% CHO/fluid/electrolyte solution should be ingested at approximately 400 mL every 15 minutes and such ingestion should be maintained during recovery to ensure fluid and energy replacement. Other dietary modifications, such as increased protein intake, antioxidant supplementation and glycerol hyperhydration, may provide some benefit but further research in these areas is required before definitive recommendations can be made regarding such practices.

References

Anderson MJ, Cotter JD, Garnham, AP, Casley DJ, Febbraio MA. Effect of glycerol-induced hyperhydration on thermoregulation and metabolism during exercise in the heat. *Int J Sports Nutr Ex Metab* 2001;11:320–39.

Angus DJ, Febbraio MA, Lasini D, Hargreaves M. Effect of carbohydrate ingestion on glucose kinetics during exercise in the heat. *J Appl Physiol* 2001;90:601–5.

Armstrong LE, Maresh CM. The induction and decay of heat acclimatisation in trained athletes. *Sports Med* 1991;12:302–12.

Baldwin J, Snow RJ, Carey MF, Febbraio MA. Muscle IMP accumulation during fatiguing submaximal exercise in endurance trained and untrained men. *Am J Physiol* 1999;277:R295–R300.

Below PR, Mora-Rodriguez R, González-Alonso J, Coyle EF. Fluid and carbohydrate ingestion independently improve performance during 1 hr of intense exercise. *Med Sci Sports Exerc* 1995;27:200–10.

Booth J, Marino F, Ward JJ. Improved running performance in hot humid conditions following whole body precooling. *Med Sci Sports Exerc* 1997;29:943–9.

Brück K, Olschewski H. Body temperature related factors diminishing the drive to exercise. *Can J Physiol Pharmacol* 1987;65:1274–80.

Buskirk, ER. Temperature regulation with exercise. Ex Sports Sci Rev 1977;5:45–88.

Candas V, Libert JP, Brandenberger G, Sagot JC, Amaros C, Kahn JM. Hydration during exercise: effects on thermal and cardiovascular adjustments. Eur J Appl Physiol 1986;55:113–22.

Chesley A, Hultman E, Spriet LL. Effects of epinephrine infusion on muscle glycogenolysis during intense aerobic exercise. Am J Physiol 1995;268:E127–E134.

Coggan AR, Coyle EF. Reversal of fatigue following prolonged exercise by carbohydrate infusion or ingestion. J Appl Physiol 1987;63:2388–95.

Constantin-Teodosiu D, Cederblad G, Hultman E. PDC activity and acetyl group accumulation in skeletal muscle during prolonged exercise. *J Appl Physiol* 1992;73:2403–7.

Costill DL, Kramer WF, Fisher A. Fluid ingestion during distance running. *Arch Environ Health* 1970;21:520–5.

Coyle EF, Coggan AR, Hemmert MK, Ivy JI. Muscle glycogen utilisation during prolonged strenuous exercise when fed carbohydrate. J Appl Physiol 1986;61:165–72.

Coyle EF, González-Alonso J. Cardiovascular drift during prolonged exercise: new perspectives. Exerc Sports Sci Rev 2001;29:88–92.

Coyle EF, Montain SJ. Benefits of fluid replacement with carbohydrate during exercise. Med Sci Sports Exerc 1992;24:S324–S330.

Davis JM, Burgess WA, Slentz CA, Bartoli WP, Pate RR. Effects of ingesting 6% and 12% glucose/electrolyte beverages during prolonged intermittent cycling in the heat. Eur J Appl Physiol 1988a;57:563–9.

Davis JM, Lamb DR, Pate RR, Slentz CA, Burgess WA, Bartoli WP. Carbohydrate–electrolyte drinks: effects on endurance cycling in the heat. Am J Clin Nutr 1998b;48:1023–30.

Dolny DG, Lemon PWR. Effect of ambient temperature on protein breakdown during prolonged exercise. *J Appl Physiol* 1988;64:550–5.

Ekelund LG. Circulatory and respiratory adaptations during prolonged exercise of moderate intensity in the sitting position. *Acta Physiol Scand* 1967;69:327–40.

Febbraio MA, Dancey J. Skeletal muscle energy metabolism during prolonged, fatiguing exercise. *J Appl Physiol* 1999;87:2341–7.

Febbraio MA, Murton P, Selig SE, Clark SA, Lambert DL, Angus DJ, Carey MF. Effect of CHO ingestion on exercise metabolism and performance in different ambient temperatures. *Med Sci Sports Exerc* 1996a;28:1380–7.

Febbraio MA, Snow RJ, Hargreaves M, Stathis CG, Martin IK, Carey MF. Muscle metabolism during exercise and heat stress in trained men: effect of acclimation. *J Appl Physiol* 1994a;76:589–97.

Febbraio MA, Snow RJ, Stathis CG, Hargreaves M, Carey MF. Effect of heat stress on muscle energy metabolism during exercise. *J Appl Physiol* 1994b;77:2827–31.

Febbraio MA, Snow RJ, Stathis CG, Hargreaves M, Carey MF. Blunting the rise in body temperature reduces muscle glycogenolysis during exercise in humans. *Exp Physiol* 1996b;81:685–93.

Fink WJ, Costill DL, Van Handel PJ. Leg muscle metabolism during exercise in the heat and cold. *Eur J Appl Physiol* 1975;34:183–90.

Francesconi RP, Hubbard RW. Dietary manipulation and exercise in the heat: thermoregulatory and metabolic effects in rats. *Aviat Space Environ Med* 1986;57:31–5.

Francis KT. Effect of water and electrolyte replacement during exercise in the heat on biochemical indices of stress and performance. *Aviat Space Environ Med* 1979;50:115–19.

Freund BJ, Montain SJ, Young AJ, Sawka MN, DeLuca J, Pandolf KB, Valeri CR. Glycerol hyperhydration: hormonal, renal and vascular fluid responses. *J Appl Physiol* 1995;79:2069–77.

Fritzsche RG, Switzer TW, Hodgkinson BJ, Coyle EF. Stroke volume decline during prolonged exercise is influenced by the increase in heart rate. *J Appl Physiol* 1999;86:799–805.

Galloway SD, Maughan RJ. Effects of ambient temperature on the capacity to perform prolonged cycle exercise in man. *Med Sci Sports Exerc* 1997;29:1240–9.

Gisolfi CV. Influence of acclimatisation and training on heat tolerance and physical endurance. In: Hales JRS, Richards DAB, eds. Heat Stress: Physical Exertion and the Environment. Amsterdam: *Excerpta Medica*, 1987: 355–66.

Gisolfi CV, Wenger CB. Temperature regulation during exercise: old concepts, new ideas. *Exerc Sports Sci Rev* 1984;12:339–72.

González-Alonso J, Calbet JAL, Nielsen B. Metabolic and thermodynamic responses to dehydration-induced reductions in blood flow in exercising humans. *J Physiol* 1999;520:577–89.

González-Alonso J, Mora-Rodriguez R, Below PR, Coyle EF. Dehydration reduces cardiac output and increases systemic and cutaneous vascular resistance during exercise. *J Appl Physiol* 1995;79:1487–96.

González-Alonso J, Mora-Rodriguez R, Below PR, Coyle EF. Dehydration markedly impairs cardiovascular function in hyperthermic endurance athletes during exercise. *J Appl Physiol* 1997;82:1229–36.

Graham TE, Rush JWE, MacLean DA. Skeletal muscle amino acid metabolism and ammonia production during exercise. In: Hargreaves M, ed. *Exercise Metabolism*. Champaign, IL: Human Kinetics, 1995: 131–76.

Greenleaf JE, Brock PJ, Keil LC, Morse JT. Drinking and water balance during exercise and heat acclimation. *J Appl Physiol* 1983;54:414–19.

Hamilton MT, González-Alonso J, Montain SJ, Coyle EF. Fluid replacement and glucose infusion during exercise prevent cardiovascular drift. *J Appl Physiol* 1991;71:871–7.

Hardy JD. Physiology of temperature regulation. *Physiol Rev* 1961;41:521–606.

Hargreaves M, Angus D, Howlett K, Marmy Conus N, Febbraio M. Effect of heat stress on glucose kinetics during exercise. *J Appl Physiol* 1996a;81:1594–7.

Hargreaves M, Costill D, Burke L, McConell G, Febbraio M. Influence of sodium on glucose bioavailability during exercise. *Med Sci Sports Exerc* 1994;26:365–8.

Hargreaves M, Dillo P, Angus D, Febbraio M. Effect of fluid ingestion on muscle metabolism during prolonged exercise. *J Appl Physiol* 1996b;80:363–6.

Hargreaves M, McConell G, Proietto J. Influence of muscle glycogen on glycogenolysis and glucose uptake during exercise in humans. *J Appl Physiol* 1995;78:288–92.

Hespel P, Richter EA. Mechanisms linking glycogen and glycogenolytic rate in perfused contracting rat skeletal muscle. *Biochem J* 1992;284:777–80.

Hessemer V, Langush D, Brük K, Bodeker R, Breidenbach T. Effects of slightly lowered body temperatures on endurance performance in humans. *J Appl Physiol* 1984;57: 1731–7.

Howlett K, Angus DJ, Proietto J, Hargreaves M. Effect of increased blood glucose availability on glucose kinetics during exercise. *J Appl Physiol* 1998a;84:1413–17.

Howlett RA, Parolin ML, Dyck DJ, Hultman E, Jones NL, Heigenhauser GJ, Spriet LL. Regulation of skeletal muscle glycogen phosphorylase and PDH at varying exercise power outputs. *Am J Physiol* 1998b;275:R418–R425.

Jentjens RL, Wagenmakers AJ, Jeukendrup AE. Heat stress increases muscle glycogen use but reduces the oxidation of ingested carbohydrates during exercise. *J Appl Physiol* 2002;92:1562–72.

Jeukendrup AE, Wagenmakers AJM, Stegen JH, Gijsen AP, Brouns F, Saris WHM. Carbohydrate ingestion can completely suppress endogenous glucose production during exercise. *Am J Physiol* 1999;276:E672–E683.

Johnson LN. Glycogen phosphorylase: control by phosphorylation and allosteric effectors. *FASEB J* 1982;6:2274–82.

King DS, Costill DL, Fink WJ, Hargreaves M, Fielding RA. Muscle metabolism during exercise in the heat in unacclimatized and acclimatized humans. *J Appl Physiol* 1985;59:1350–4.

Kirwan JP, Costill DL, Kuipers H, Burrell MJ, Fink WJ, Kovaleski JE, Fielding RA. Substrate utilization in leg muscle of men after heat acclimation. *J Appl Physiol* 1987;63:31–5.

Kjær M. Hepatic fuel metabolism during exercise. In: Hargreaves M, ed. Exercise Metabolism. Champaign, IL: *Human Kinetics*, 1995: 73–97.

Kozlowski S, Brzezinska Z, Kruk B, Kaciuba-Uscilko H, Greenleaf JE, Nazar K. Exercise hyperthermia as a factor limiting physical performance: temperature effect on muscle metabolism. *J Appl Physiol* 1985;59:766–73.

Kruk B, Kaciuba-Uscilco H, Nazar K, Greenleaf JE, Koslowski S. Hypothalamic, rectal, and muscle temperatures in exercising dogs: effect of cooling. *J Appl Physiol* 1985;58:1444–8.

Latzka WA, Sawka MN, Montain SJ, Skrinar GR, Fielding RA, Matott RP, Pandolf KB. Hyperhydration: thermoregulatory effects during compensable exercise–heat stress. *J Appl Physiol* 1997;83:860–6.

Lee DT, Haymes EM. Exercise duration and thermoregulatory responses after whole body precooling. *J Appl Physiol* 1995;79:1971–6.

Levine L, Rose MS, Francesconi RP, Neufer PD, Sawka MN. Fluid replacement during sustained activity in the heat: nutrient solution vs water. *Aviat Space Environ Med* 1991;62:559–64.

Lyons TP, Triedesel ML, Meuli LE, Chick TW. Effects of glycerol-induced hyperhydration prior to exercise in the heat on sweating and core temperature. *Med Sci Sports Exerc* 1990;22:477–83.

MacDougall JD, Reddan WG, Layton CR, Dempsey JA. Effects of metabolic hyperthermia on performance during heavy prolonged exercise. *J Appl Physiol* 1974;36:538–54.

Maughan RJ. Fluid and electrolyte loss and replacement in exercise. In: Harries M, Williams C, Stanish WD, Micheli LJ, eds. *Oxford Textbook of Sports Medicine*. New York: Oxford University Press, 1994: 82–93.

Maughan RJ, Fenn CE, Leiper JB. Effects of fluid, electrolyte and substrate ingestion on endurance capacity. *Eur J Appl Physiol Occup Physiol* 1989;58:481–6.

Maughan RJ, Leiper JB. Sodium intake and post-exercise rehydration in man. *Eur J Appl Physiol* 1995;71:311–19.

Maughan RJ, Leiper JB, Thompson J. Rectal temperature after marathon running. *Br J Sports Med* 1989;19:192–6.

Maxwell NS, Gardner F, Nimmo MA. Intermittent running: muscle metabolism in the heat and effect of hypohydration. *Med Sci Sports Exerc* 1999;31:675–83.

McConell GK, Burge CM, Skinner SL, Hargreaves M. Influence of ingested fluid volume on physiological responses during prolonged exercise. *Acta Physiol Scand* 1997;160:149–56.

McConell G, Fabris S, Proietto J, Hargreaves M. Effects of carbohydrate ingestion on glucose kinetics during exercise. *J Appl Physiol* 1994;77:1537–41.

Millard-Stafford M, Sparling PB, Rosskopf LB, Dicarlo LJ. Carbohydrate–electrolyte replacement improves distance running performance in the heat. *Med Sci Sports Exerc* 1992;24:934–40.

Millard-Stafford M, Sparling PB, Rosskopf LB, Hinson BT, Dicarlo LJ. Carbohydrate–electrolyte replacement during a simulated triathlon in the heat. *Med Sci Sports Exerc* 1990;22:621–8.

Mills PC, Smith NC, Casas I, Harris P, Harris RC, Marlin DJ. Effects of exercise intensity and environmental stress on indices of oxidative stress and iron homeostasis during exercise in the horse. *Eur J Appl Physiol* 1996;74:60–6.

Mittleman K, Ricci M, Bailey SP. Branched-chain amino acids prolong exercise during heat stress in men and women. *Med Sci Sports Exerc* 1995;30:83–91.

Montain SJ, Coyle EF. Influence of graded dehydration on hyperthermia and cardiovascular drift during exercise. *J Appl Physiol* 1992;73:1340–50.

Montain SJ, Sawka MN, Cadarette BS, Quigley MD, McKay JM. Physiological tolerance to uncompensable heat stress: effects of exercise intensity, protective clothing and climate. *J Appl Physiol* 1994;77:216–22.

Montner P, Stark D, Riedelsel ML, Murata G, Robergs RA, Timms M, Chick TW. Pre-exercise glycerol hydration improves cycling endurance time. *Int J Sports Med* 1996;17:27–33.

Murray R, Eddy DE, Murray TW, Paul GL, Seifert JG, Halaby GA. Physiological responses to glycerol ingestion during exercise. *J Appl Physiol* 1991;71:144–9.

Murray R, Eddy DE, Murray TW, Seifert JG, Paul GL, Halaby GA. The effect of fluid and carbohydrate feedings during intermittent cycling exercise. *Med Sci Sports Exerc* 1987;19:597–604.

Nadel ER. Recent advances in temperature regulation during exercise in humans. *Fed Proc* 1985;44:2286–92.

Nielsen B, Savard G, Richter EA, Hargreaves M, Saltin B. Muscle blood flow and muscle metabolism during exercise and heat stress. *J Appl Physiol* 1990;69:1040–6.

Noakes TD, Myburgh KH, Du Plessis J, Lang L, Lambert M, Van Der Riet C, Schall R. Metabolic rate, not percent dehydration, predicts rectal temperature in marathon runners. *Med Sci Sports Exerc* 1991;23:443–9.

Nose H, Mack GW, Shi X, Nadel ER. Role of osmolality and plasma volume during rehydration in humans. *J Appl Physiol* 1988;65:332–6.

Owen MD, Kregel KC, Wall PT, Gisolfi CV. Effects of ingesting carbohydrate beverages during exercise in the heat. *Med Sci Sports Exerc* 1986;18:568–75.

Parkin JM, Carey MF, Zhao S, Febbraio MA. Effect of ambient temperature on human skeletal muscle metabolism during fatiguing submaximal exercise. *J Appl Physiol* 1999;86:902–8.

Robinson S. Temperature regulation during exercise *Pediatrics* 1963;32:691–702.

Rowell LB. Human cardiovascular adjustments to exercise and thermal stress. *Physiol Rev* 1974;54:75–159.

Rowell LB. Human Circulation: *Regulation during Physical Stress*. New York: Oxford University Press, 1986.

Rowell LB, Brengelmann GL, Blackmon JR, Twiss RD, Kusumi F. Splanchnic blood flow and metabolism in heat stressed man. *J Appl Physiol* 1968;24:475–84.

Ryan AJ, Bleiler TL, Carter JE, Gisolfi CV. Gastric emptying during prolonged cycling exercise in the heat. *Med Sci Sports Exerc* 1989;21:51–8.

Sahlin K, Katz A, Broberg S. Tricarboxylic acid cycle intermediates in human muscle during prolonged exercise. *Am J Physiol* 1990;259:C834–C841.

Saltin B, Gagge AP, Bergh U, Stolwijk JAJ. Body temperature and sweating during exhaustive exercise. *J Appl Physiol* 1972;32:635–43.

Saunders PU, Watt MJ, Garnham AP, Spriet LL, Hargreaves M, Febbraio MA. No effect of mild heat stress on the regulation of carbohydrate metabolism at the onset of exercise. *J Appl Physiol* 2001;91:2282–8.

Sawka MN, Young AJ, Latzka WA, Neufer PD, Quigley MD, Pandolf KB. Human tolerance to heat strain during exercise: influence of hydration. *J Appl Physiol* 1992;73:368–75.

Schmidt V, Brück K. Effect of a precooling maneuver on body temperature and exercise performance. *J Appl Physiol* 1981;50:772–8.

Schwellnus MP, Gordon MF, van Zyl GG, Cilliers JF, Grobler HC, Kuyl J, Kohl HW. Effect of a high carbohydrate diet on core temperature during prolonged exercise. *Br J Sports Med* 1990;24:99–102.

Snow RJ, Febbraio MA, Carey MF, Hargreaves M. Heat stress increases ammonia accumulation during exercise. *Exp Physiol* 1993;78:847–50.

Steensberg A, van Hall G, Keller C, Osada T, Schjerling P, Pedersen BK, Saltin B, Febbraio MA. Muscle glycogen content and glucose uptake during exercise in humans: influence of prior exercise and dietary manipulation. *J Physiol* 2002;541: 273–81.

Takamata A, Mack GW, Gillen CM, Jozsi AC, Nadel ER. Osmoregulatory modulation of thermal sweating in humans: reflex effects of drinking. *Am J Physiol* 1995;268: R414–R422.

Tatterson A, Martin DT, Hahn A, Febbraio MA. Effect of heat stress on metabolic and thermoregulatory responses during time trial performance in elite cyclists. *J Sci Med Sport* 2000;3:186–93.

Terrados N, Maughan RJ. Exercise in the heat: strategies to minimize the adverse effects on performance. *J Sports Sci* 1995;13:S55–S62.

Walsh RM, Noakes TD, Hawley JA, Dennis SC. Impaired high-intensity cycling performance time at low levels of dehydration. *Int J Sports Med* 1994;15:392–8.

Yaspelkis III BB, Ivy JL. Effect of carbohydrate supplements and water on exercise metabolism in the heat. *J Appl Physiol* 1991;71:680–7.

Yaspelkis III BB, Scroop GC, Wilmore KM, Ivy JL. Carbohydrate metabolism during exercise in hot and thermoneutral environments. *Int J Sports Med* 1993;14:13–19.

Young AJ, Sawka MN, Levine L, Burgoon PW, Latzka WL, Gonzalez RR, Pandolf KB. Metabolic and thermal adaptations from endurance training in hot and cold water. *J Appl Physiol* 1995;78:793–801.

Young AJ, Sawka MN, Levine L, Cadarette BS, Pandolf KB. Skeletal muscle metabolism during exercise is influenced by heat acclimation. *J Appl Physiol* 1985;59:1929–35.

CHAPTER 11

Exercise at altitude: physiological responses and limitations

Carsten LUNDBY and Bengt SALTIN

Introduction

When Reinhold Messner and Peter Habeler climbed the summit of Mount Everest (8848 m) in 1978 without the use of supplemental oxygen, they proved possible what scientists had proposed impossible. Since then, a little less than 100 climbers have repeated the task. For many, the reduced partial pressure of oxygen at high altitude is the key to attempt higher and higher mountains. Athletes, however, are less enthusiastic about the idea of reduced oxygen availability to their working muscles. In 1968 when the Olympic Games were held in Mexico City at an altitude of 2290 m, there were many complaints and disastrous performances in the longer distances, with Ron Clarke being the most extreme example. When the Games were over, however, two outstanding new records had been set. Bob Beamon jumped a fabulous 8.90 m in the long jump and Lee Evans ran the 400 m dash almost 1 second faster than the previous record. From the above it is obvious that endurance performance is limited at altitude, whereas explosive events where wind resistance plays a role are not.

The most important effect of altitude upon physiological processes is the low oxygen pressure in the ambient air (and thus in the lungs, blood and tissues), known as hypoxia. A more specific term, hypoxaemia, usually refers to a decrease in oxygen *content*. The latter can be induced (e.g. by carbon monoxide hindering oxygen binding). In this chapter, the focus is on hypoxia induced by a reduction in barometric pressure.

The high altitude environment

To understand altitude physiology, one must appreciate the nature of the atmosphere and how humans cope with the reduced partial pressure of oxygen (PO_2). The barometric pressure (P_B) is a measure of the pressure exerted by the weight of air above us. From sea level the atmosphere is approximately 24 km wide, which equals a P_B of 1013 khPa. However, at the summit of Mount Everest (8848 m), the air exerts a pressure that is much less, and accordingly P_B is reduced to approximately 333 khPa or about one-third of P_B at sea level. At 5486 m the pressure of a column of air at the earth's surface equals about one-half of its pressure at sea level (Fig. 11.1). At a given altitude, however, P_B is not exactly the same everywhere. As warm air weighs less than cool air, P_B is air temperature dependent. In summer time, the P_B at the summit of Mount Everest has been measured at 340 khPa in June, compared to 'only' 324 khPa in January. As we shall see later, this makes the climb much more demanding during winter than summer. Moreover, the distribution of warm and cool air in the atmosphere is not uniform, resulting in a slightly increased P_B along the equator compared to the North and South Pole regions for a given altitude.

Although an inverse relationship exists between P_B and altitude, the gas composition of the air is unaffected. The percentages of oxygen, carbon dioxide and nitrogen are always 20.93%, 0.03% and 79.04%, respectively. Only the partial pressure (P) of the gases changes, as it is a function of P_B (gas fraction $\times$ P_B) (Fig. 11.1). The partial pressure of inspired oxygen is moistened by the water vapour in the airways similarly at sea level and altitude. This reduces the oxygen pressure in the alveoli by about 63 khPa, which means relatively more the higher the altitude.

When it comes to the effect of altitude on the human body, the lower Po_2 causes the major difference between sea level and altitude. However, there are also other factors, such as temperature, humidity and radiation, which are affected by altitude. Air temperature is approximately 1°C lower for every 150 m of ascent. A temperature of 15°C at sea level thus corresponds to a temperature of about −40°C at the summit of Mount Everest. The combination of low temperatures and high winds greatly increases the

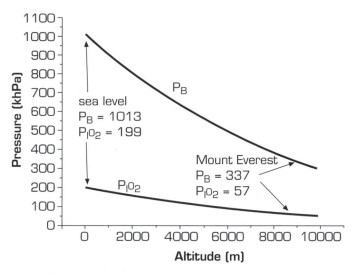

FIG. 11.1 Barometric pressure (P_B) and inspired oxygen pressure (P_IO_2) decreases with increasing altitude

risks of hypothermia and frostbite at altitudes. Because of the cold air, the absolute humidity is extremely low at altitude. This promotes dehydration. Much water is lost via the lungs, to which also the increased ventilation contributes. The atmosphere can absorb less of the ultraviolet light, to which the reduced water content of the air further reduces the absorption of radiation from the sun. These two factors combined expose the individual to a high solar radiation at altitude.

Physiological responses to altitude

Oxygen uptake

Basal oxygen consumption (VO_2) has been reported to be either unchanged or slightly increased with exposure to high altitude. If an increase is observed, it usually only persists for a few days and then returns to sea level values. This transient increase has been explained by the extra oxygen required to increase ventilation, heart rate and other physiological responses that are augmented at the beginning of hypoxic exposure. During submaximal exercise the oxygen uptake is, in essence, as at sea level; however, VO_{2max} decreases with increasing altitude and a given submaximal exercise task will, therefore, elicit a higher percentage of VO_{2max} at altitude. The decrease in VO_{2max} at altitude (Fig. 11.2) is due to the decrease in C_aO_2 and, hence, oxygen delivery.

Despite the many adaptations to increase oxygen delivery, VO_{2max} does not improve with acclimatisation (Lundby & van Hall 2002; Saltin et al. 1968). Endurance capacity, however, gradually increases during acclimatisation. When exercising at 75% of sea level, VO_{2max} endurance increased by 31% from day 2 to day 12 at 4300 m (Maher et al. 1974). The exact mechanism behind this improvement is unknown but a better pH regulation is likely to play a role. The reduction in VO_{2max} is apparent from altitudes of approximately 1000 m and declines further by 8% for every additional 1000 m above sea level (Fulco et al. 1998). There are no gender differences in this response; however, high aerobic fitness levels at sea level have been shown to affect VO_{2max} to a larger extent than in individuals with lower aerobic capacities at altitude (Gore et al. 1996; Lawler et al. 1988; Terrados et al. 1985). The explanation for this is an observed more marked reduction in S_aO_2 in the well-trained individual, thus decreasing oxygen delivery as the peak cardiac output cannot compensate and hence the VO_{2max} is decreased.

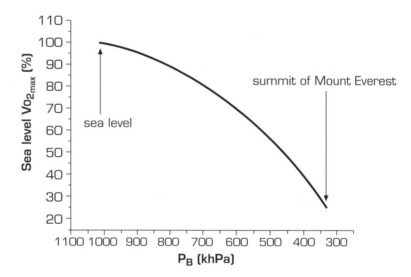

FIG. 11.2 The drop in VO_{2max} with decreasing barometric pressure (P_B) (or increasing altitude)

Lungs

The ventilatory responses to hypoxia were among the first physiological responses investigated; in 1905 Haldane and Priestley reported increased ventilation in response to a decrease either in P_B or in the fraction of inspired oxygen, in order to minimise the drop in alveolar oxygen. The hypoxic ventilatory response (HVR) is present within seconds after hypoxic exposure and is, to a large extent, regulated by the carotid chemoreceptors and, to a lesser extent, by the aortic chemoreceptors (Fitzgerald & Lahiri 1986). The initial increase in ventilation due to chemoreceptor activation is maintained for less than 30 minutes (Weil 1986) and thereafter the regulation of HVR becomes more complex. The increased ventilation causes a profound respiratory alkalosis. The respiratory alkalosis elicits an inhibitory effect on ventilation and the mechanisms that maintain the ventilation high despite the inhibitory effects of an alkaline pH remain to be solved. As pulmonary ventilation is elevated at a given oxygen uptake, alveolar PO_2 (*A–a* gradient) is elevated, which aids in the diffusion of oxygen into the blood in the pulmonary capillaries. Maximal attainable pulmonary ventilation is increased in hypoxic environments and values above 200 L/min are often observed. Since the air density is reduced at altitude, the respiratory work is only marginally affected.

These adaptations in pulmonary ventilation are sufficient to maintain the S_aO_2 close to normal at quite high altitudes. During exercise, however, there is always a drop in S_aO_2 (Fig. 11.3), which is further augmented at peak exercise. Thus, the lungs constitute a major functional limitation to O_2 delivery during exercise at altitude (Wagner 2000).

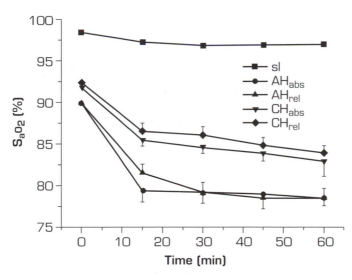

FIG. 11.3 Oxygen saturation (SaO_2) during 60 minute ergometer cycle exercise at sea level (sl), in acute (AH) and chronic (CH) hypoxia (altitude 4100 m), during rest and relative (rel) and absolute (abs) exercise intensities compared to sea level. Unpublished observations, Lundby

Blood

The oxygen–haemoglobin (Hb) dissociation curve has a sigmoidal shape (Fig. 11.4). At sea level where arterial oxygen pressure (P_aO_2) is about 133.5 khPa (100 mmHg), Hb is close to being fully saturated with oxygen (S_aO_2 = 96–98%). Reducing P_aO_2 at rest to 67 khPa (50 mmHg) only reduces S_aO_2 to 87%. However, a further small decrease in P_aO_2 will cause a much larger drop in oxygen binding. The shape of the oxygen–Hb dissociation curve also explains why only minor physiological responses are observed at altitudes below approximately 3000 m. In order to optimise the capacity of the blood to bind oxygen in the lungs, the dissociation curve is shifted to the left, whereby more oxygen will be bound for a given P_aO_2. In the peripheral capillary bed the opposite is the case, that is, more oxygen is unloaded at a given P_aO_2 due to the so-called Bohr effect of changes in pH related to the variation in P_aCO_2. The amount of oxygen available to the cells is the product of oxygen content in the arterial blood (C_aO_2) and blood

TABLE 11.1 Example of how C_aO_2 can increase to levels higher than at sea level after acclimatisation

	SEA LEVEL	ACUTE HYPOXIA	8 WEEKS' HYPOXIA
Arterial Hb (g/L)	140	140	170
Arterial saturation (%)	98	87	87
C_aO_2 (mL/L)	190	160	200

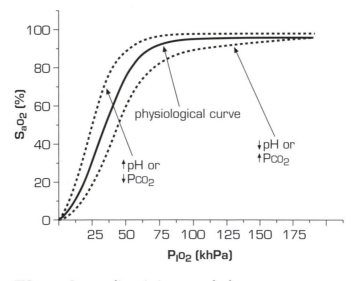

FIG. 11.4 Oxygen dissociation curve for humans

flow to the cells. Assuming a constant blood flow, any increase in C_aO_2 will increase oxygen availability. In humans, several strategies are employed to achieve this at altitude.

Initially, the plasma volume decreases in response to hypoxic exposure in order to elevate Hb, and with acclimatisation over a period of several weeks the plasma volume expands in parallel with the increase in total Hb (Alexander et al. 1967; Hartley et al. 1967). The increase in total Hb occurs gradually as a result of an elevated erythropoiesis (Jelkman 1992; Semenza et al. 1994). Erythropoiesis is controlled by the induction of the glycoprotein erythropoietin (EPO), which is mainly regulated at the mRNA level, probably through the hypoxic-dependent transcription factor hypoxia-induced factor 1 (HIF-1α). With a hypoxic stimulus the basal production of EPO increases by as much as a 100–400-fold (Jelkman 1992; Semenza et al. 1994). The increase in Hb with acclimatisation affects C_aO_2 and, as seen in Table 11.1, C_aO_2 may increase to higher levels than observed at sea level. When returning to sea level the opposite is observed, that is, plasma volume expands quickly and the [Hb] normalises in a few days.

Heart

When acutely exposed to hypoxia, an increase in cardiac output (Q) is observed both at rest and during exercise. This increase is accomplished by an elevated heart rate (HR) and a variable effect of stroke volume (Asmussen & Consolazio 1941; Hannon & Vogel 1977; Saltin et al. 1968). At the simulated altitude of Mount Everest, resting Q was increased from 3 L/min to 9 L/min (Sutton et al. 1988). Depending on the altitude, Q either remains elevated with acclimatisation or decreases to or towards sea level values. There seem to be large individual differences in regard to the altitude at which this occurs. In most humans it seems to be at about 3500 m above sea level. Blood pressure is generally unaffected at low altitudes but from 4000 m an increase in mean arterial pressure of 13.5–27. khPa (10–20 mmHg) is found in most humans (Bender et al. 1988; Wolfel 1993). At maximal exercise in hypoxia a marked decrease in Q is always reported (Pugh et al. 1964; Saltin et al. 1968; Sutton et al. 1988). After 2 weeks at 4300 m Q_{max} had decreased by 22% compared with sea level values. With increasing altitude Q_{max} decreases further during a prolonged stay and was reported to be only 16 L/min at the simulated summit of Mount Everest as compared with 24 L/min at sea level. This decrease in Q_{max} seems to be related to the observed decrease in maximal heart rate (HR_{max}) and to a minor change in stroke volume. Recently, it was shown that HR_{max}

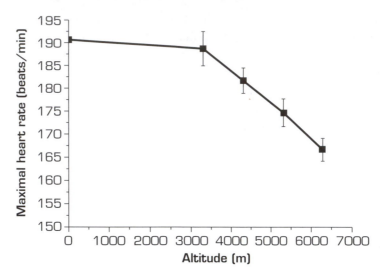

FIG. 11.5 Maximal heart rate at sea level, 3300 m, 4300 m, 5300 m and 6300 m of simulated altitudes. Adapted from Lundby et al. 2001a

decreases at the onset of hypoxia as a function of the degree of hypoxia (Fig. 11.5). Moreover, the response is augmented in individuals with a high physical fitness (Shephard et al. 1988). The mechanism(s) responsible for the reduction has puzzled researchers for many years. The decrease could be caused by:

■ an increase in blood viscosity—however, due to the findings that HR_{max} is decreased within minutes of hypoxic exposure when no changes in haematocrit have yet occurred, this factor seems less likely; also isovolumic normalisation of the haematocrit does not cause changes in Q_{max} at high altitude (Calbet et al. 1999)

■ a myocardial limitation due to the low P_aO_2—against this are the Operation Everest II studies in which myocardial function was found to be unaffected (Reeves et al. 1987)

■ a decrease in sympathetic and/or increase in parasympathetic nervous activity—this could also play a role in the reduction of Q_{max}

Recently, it was shown that sympathetic nervous activity was unrelated to the reduction in HR_{max} (Lundby et al. 2001a, b) and instead the drop in HR could be explained by an elevated parasympathetic activity (Boushel et al. 2001). After several weeks of exposure to 5260 m, HR_{max} could be restored to sea level values by blocking the parasympathetic nervous activity using glycopyrrolate. However, Q_{max} remained unchanged and, accordingly, so did VO_{2max} as stroke volume became reduced (Boushel et al. 2001).

Metabolism

The metabolic response to exercise in hypoxia has long been thought to differ from metabolism at sea level; however, recently the two most well-known beliefs have been challenged. Since the 1930s it has, on numerous occasions, been reported that submaximal and maximal lactate accumulation in the blood decreases from the transition from acute to chronic hypoxia, which is known as the lactate paradox (Fig. 11.6). The finding is regarded as paradoxical since lactate formation is thought to be oxygen-dependent.

Recently, however, results from two studies have challenged the classic view on lactate metabolism in hypoxia. It was shown that lowlanders acclimatised for a long period (9 weeks) were indeed able to attain similar lactate levels at high altitude as compared with sea level (Fig. 11.7, van Hall et al. 2001). The findings were confirmed on climbers in the base camp of Mount Everest. They were examined after 1, 4 and 6 weeks of exposure to 5400 m. Only the 1-week trials elicited a lower lactate concentration, which had returned to sea level values after 6 weeks, indicating that the lactate paradox is a transient phenomenon that vanishes with time spent at altitude (Lundby et al. 2000). The mechanisms underlying the changes that occur with lactate metabolism at high altitude still remain to be resolved.

The reported augmentation of CHO utilisation at a given work load at altitude (Roberts et al. 1996) may not be due to the hypoxia (Lundby & van

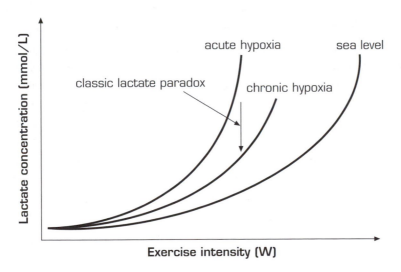

FIG. 11.6 The classic lactate paradox—a reduction in lactate concentration from acute to chronic hypoxic exposure at submaximal as well as at maximal exercise intensities

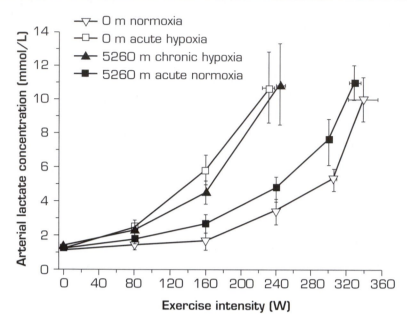

FIG. 11.7 Arterial lactate concentrations at sea level and after 9 weeks of acclimatisation to 5260 m in Danish sea level residents. Adapted from van Hall et al. 2001

Hall 2002). The explanation for the proposed increase in CHO dependency is that it provided the largest ATP yield per mole of oxygen. At altitude, where oxygen supply is limited, it would thus seem favourable to increase CHO utilisation preferentially (Hochachka 1985; Brooks 1992). Of note is the fact that with increasing exercise intensity the contribution of CHO to total energy turnover increases, ultimately providing 100% of the energy at VO_{2max} (Christensen & Hansen 1939). Since VO_{2max} decreases with increasing altitude (Fig. 11.2), a given workload performed at sea level will be relatively higher when performed at altitude. Indeed, it was recently shown that the augmented increase in CHO utilisation at altitude was due to the relative higher exercise intensity and not by hypoxia per se (Fig. 11.8). Substrate utilisation thus seems to be similar to that at sea level; that is, CHO utilisation increases with increasing exercise intensity and is not directly affected by altitude in well-acclimatised subjects.

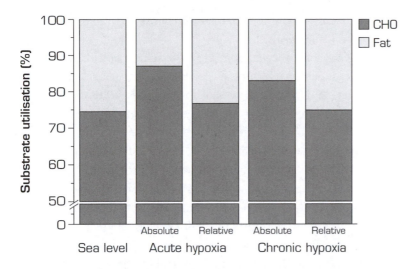

FIG. 11.8 Contribution of CHO and fat to total energy production in Danish sea level residents during 60-minute cycle ergometer exercise at sea level, in acute hypoxia and after 4 weeks' acclimatisation to 4100 m. The exercise in hypoxia was performed at the same relative and same absolute intensities on separate days. Adapted from Lundby & van Hall 2002

Performance

Strength

Angelo Mosso (1898) studied the effect of altitude (4551 m) on lifting weights and found it to be unaffected by hypoxia. These findings have been confirmed on numerous occasions since then, even at the highest altitudes (Caquelard et al. 2000). However, with longer lasting exposure to high altitude, the well-documented decrease in muscle mass will undoubtedly lead to a decrease in muscle strength (see also below).

Anaerobic events

Short-lasting performance in anaerobic events such as sprinting and jumping is also unaffected or improved at altitude. Indeed, due to the reduced air density at altitude, in sport events where performance is related to overcoming air resistance (e.g. in running, skating or cycling) marked improvements in time have been observed. In running, the braking point is in events lasting less than 2 minutes, whereas in cycling a better performance than at sea level can be expected in events lasting up to 1 hour when performed at medium altitude.

Muscle buffering capacity increases at altitude, which could contribute to a larger anaerobic capacity (Gore et al. 2000; Mizuno et al. 1990). The change is observed as early as after 2 weeks and appears to be maintained upon return to sea level for up to 2 weeks. Data are not available for athletes after more extended stays at altitude but findings on mountaineers' arm and leg muscles indicate that it is increased after several months at altitude, but only to a slightly larger extent than at lower altitudes and of shorter duration. In the study by Svedenhag et al. (1997), control groups were included who trained similarly at sea level as those at altitude without any alteration in either lactate dehydrogenase (LDH) isoenzymes or muscle buffering capacity. This finding, as well as the one on the climbers, could indicate that it is the altitude (hypoxia) that induces the changes.

There also appears to be a coupling between the change in anaerobic exercise capacity and running performance. Mizuno and coworkers (1990) tested this hypothesis on cross-country skiers and found a relation between improved running time and change in muscle buffering capacity. An estimation of maximal oxygen deficit also revealed a coupling to performance. In US studies where the concept of living 'high' and training 'low' was tested, no changes were observed of any features of the muscles. They concluded that an improved lactate metabolism or anaerobic exercise capacity were not at play to explain these runners' improved performance (Stray-Gundersen & Levine 1999). Taken together, the anaerobic capacity appears to be increased as a result of exposure to hypoxia, an effect that also is maintained for some time upon return to sea level.

Aerobic events

The praxis of training at altitude was an important integrated part in the preparation for the 1968 Olympic Games held in Mexico City at an altitude of 2100 m above sea level. Several athletes, although struggling in the Games, felt that they had an improved performance when they returned to sea level. One explanation for this could be that, at altitude, total Hb and [Hb] had increased and with the lifetime for red cells of about 100 days or longer, this adaptation would remain for some time also at sea level. There are a multitude of investigations on the topic with a majority of them demonstrating no or trends for an alteration in VO_{2max} after a stay at medium altitude combined with training (see Saltin 1996). At this altitude, the rate of increase in total Hb is in the order of 20 g per week, provided iron is in sufficient supply.

There is another and more important explanation for [Hb] being normal soon after (< 1–3 days) return to sea level after an altitude sojourn, as discussed above. The plasma volume very quickly expands under normobaric conditions. Svedenhag et al. (1997) demonstrated in cross-country skiers, who lived and trained at 2100–2700 m for 4 weeks, that at sea level post-altitude, the plasma volume expanded by 0.4–0.5 L within 48–72 hours, lowering the [Hb] and haematocrit (Hct) levels to pre-altitude levels within a few days. This means a normalised [Hb] and Hct with blood volume being expanded. The enlarged total blood volume will improve filling conditions of the heart and lead to an enlarged stroke volume, cardiac output and peak oxygen delivery during exhaustive exercise and could, thereby, improve performance.

An argument for altitude training being unsuccessful when performing at sea level is that the training intensity and sometimes also the duration of the training are reduced at altitude. The idea has, therefore, been put forward that it is not the training at altitude that is important; instead, it is arterial hypoxia or desaturation per se that causes an elevation in red cell mass. Levine and Stray-Gundersen are the two researchers who have tested this hypothesis the most. The design consists of various combinations of living 'high' (2500–3000 m) and training 'low' (~1200 m) and vice versa. They have summarised their results in a mini-review in 1999. Average runners who, during a month performed standardised training at sea level, were studied first and again at sea level after they had trained for another month at either low (1200 m) or at high (2700 m) altitude, combined with living either low or high. These four alternatives produced no or a small gain in VO_{2max} with those living high and training low obtaining an increase of 1.5 mL/kg/min, reaching a value in the upper 60s. Equally important was the fact that these runners could also perform at a higher steady state VO_2. It should be noted that the term 'training low' is imprecise and not synonymous with no arterial desaturation while training as the 'low' group trained at 1200 m. According to the results by Gore et al. (2000) and others (Fig. 11.3) most well-trained athletes show desaturation when active at this altitude. Thus, the runners in the 'high–low' groups in Levine and Stray-Gundersen's studies experienced some desaturation both when living at altitude and when training 'low'.

In their early studies evaluating the 'high–low' concept no top-level athletes were included. In one later study they were (Chapman et al. 1998). Just after the season when the runners performed well to very well, they were brought to altitude and lived there and trained with low intensity at a high altitude of 2500–2800 m and at high intensity at a lower altitude (1200 m). These athletes improved their VO_{2max} by 1–3% to 74.4 mL/kg/min and an improvement in performance (3000 m time trial) of 1.5% was recorded. This would have made some of these national calibre runners competitive on the international arena. These US-based studies appear to have no flaws. However, the results have not been confirmed by others. Gore and coworkers (Hahn et al. 2001), who in Australia have access to very well-trained endurance athletes, have performed studies with a design similar to the one used by Levine and Stray-Gundersen. They did not observe any elevation in aerobic power after 'living high, training low' as compared with other alternatives of combining living and training at sea level or at altitude.

In the US studies there are non-responders, that is, some do not improve although they live high and train low as reported by the US group. The proposed explanation is that there is an elevation in the red cell mass in the responders, but not in the non-responders, which in turn relates to less of an erythropoietin increase in the non-responders. It is true that there is a difference between these groups in red cell mass. However, [Hb] is the same in responders and non-responders. This would indicate that elevations in blood volume and total amount of haemoglobin, although small, significantly affect aerobic power. Svedenhag et al. (1997) also observed, as mentioned above, a similar expansion of the blood volume of 0.4–0.5 L (and total Hb) post altitude in top endurance athletes with a VO_{2max} above 76 mL/kg/min, but in their study a significant elevation in VO_{2max} was not observed. There was a trend with four out of the seven cross-country skiers having a post-altitude VO_{2max} elevated more than the error of method when measuring VO_{2max}. At the individual level there was also a trend for a coupling between the magnitude of change in total blood volume and VO_{2max}.

This leads to the question whether an enlarged plasma volume enlarges VO_{2max}. In a study by Kanstrup and Ekblom (1982) with infusion of 700 mL of dextran, they observed an elevated stroke volume and cardiac output at peak exercise, but it was not large enough to counteract the lowering of the oxygen-carrying capacity. This resulted in an unchanged systemic oxygen delivery and VO_{2max}. Later studies using only a 300 mL infusion of a plasma expander have demonstrated a 5% elevation in VO_{2max} (Warren et al. 1989). A plasma volume expansion of up to 0.5 L upon return to sea level after training/staying at medium altitude would then be in the range of what may be beneficial for the oxygen delivery and VO_{2max}.

Another observation, which should be commented upon, is that in some studies VO_{2max} remains, or becomes, elevated several weeks after an altitude-training period. Indeed, in Svedenhag's study it was 2.6 mL/kg/min in athletes who already had a mean value of 76 mL/kg/min. At this time point both [Hb] and blood volume are at pre-altitude levels. A physiological explanation for the mechanisms by which this is brought about is therefore difficult to offer other than that more effective training can be performed upon return to sea level, especially in regard to its intensity. However, a 4% elevation in VO_{2max} in already very well-trained athletes is significant in such a short period of time.

Other skeletal muscle adaptations

In addition to the changes observed in some variables related to the anaerobic capacity, other features of the muscle tissue that are important for peak as well as endurance performance could be anticipated to occur (see Saltin 1996). Muscle fibre size and capillarisation have been studied extensively, both in athletes and in climbers. There is a striking similarity in the findings. The number of capillaries per muscle fibre is unaltered by exposure to any altitude. In contrast, muscle fibre size is reduced while at altitude. The hypotrophy is quite pronounced at extreme altitudes but also present during a prolonged stay at a moderate altitude such as 2000 m. With a reduction in muscle fibre size and an unaltered capillary per fibre ratio, an increase occurs in number of capillaries per square millimetre, as well as a reduction in the average diffusion area for a capillary using the Krogh model for estimation. The functional significance of these changes is that, in addition to the reduced diffusion distance, the mean transit time is elongated at a given muscle blood flow, assuming the capillary length is unaltered. These adaptations are critical to optimise oxygen extraction at altitude when oxygen tension in the blood is low but would enhance oxygen delivery to the muscle tissue also at sea level as long as muscle fibre sizes are subnormal. The return to normal muscle fibre size upon return to sea level after a period at altitude has not been studied, but it is likely to be slow as muscle hypertrophy, even with optimal strength training, takes weeks to months.

Muscle mitochondrial capacity is quite stable at altitude (see Saltin 1996). This is the result of studies using morphometric methods to estimate mitochondrial volume, as well as using biochemical assays to determine the V_{max} for mitochondrial enzymes in the respiratory chain, β-oxidation or Krebs cycle. On this topic there is a consensus. In contrast, a small but significant elevation in mitochondrial enzyme activity has been reported in subjects training at simulated altitude or with insufficient blood supply. The study design includes training one leg while using the other leg as a control or the inclusion of a control group training at equivalent exercise intensities at sea level. Not until recently was it possible to explain the contrasting findings. In these latter studies submaximal training loads were used. Based on electromyographic (EMG) amplitude measurements, it was shown that muscle activation was more marked when oxygen availability was reduced. More fast twitch fibres were also recruited, as demonstrated by the muscle glycogen depletion pattern. Thus, the enhancement of the V_{max} for certain mitochondrial enzymes occurred in the fast twitch fibres. These data then confirm that training-induced elevations can be obtained in mitochondrial capacity when training with a subnormoxic amount of oxygen made available to the active muscle. However, the data do not demonstrate that hypoxia is an additional stimulus to the ordinary training stimulus although it appears to modulate motor unit recruitment.

Finally, what about skeletal muscle contractile characteristics or muscle fibre transformation when exposed to hypoxia? The topic is well explored and it does not appear as if the myosin isoforms are sensitive to hypoxia (Saltin 1996). This is based on histochemical staining of myosin ATPase of samples obtained on athletes or climbers in connection with short or even very long stays at various altitudes. Taken together, there are no indications that altitude exposure or training at medium altitude alter the oxidative capacity of the muscles.

Hypoxia houses

The literature on altitude training does not give a basis for a consensus statement. When it comes to the use of hypoxia houses in preparation for sea level performance it is even harder to conclude. The literature is scarce, although hypoxia houses have been used for almost 10 years and in some countries quite extensively. Recently, Hahn, Gore and colleagues (2001) have summarised their own studies and those of other researchers and compared the effects of living in hypoxia houses with that of a combination of a genuine altitude stay, combined with training low. These studies primarily focus on whether living part of a full day (10 hours out of 24) at the equivalent of 1800–2000 m is sufficient to elicit an EPO response followed by an elevation in reticulocytes and red cell mass. EPO is increased by 70–80%, whereas the latter two variables are not increased. Although the lowering of the S_aO_2 is small at this level of hypoxia, it is obviously of a magnitude large enough to enhance EPO production by, and its release from, the kidneys. Why it does not result in a stimulation of red cell mass is not clear. Of note is that the elevation in EPO is transient and not long-lasting as first anticipated would be the case with intermittent hypoxia exposure. The hypoxia is quite mild at 2000 m, with a desaturation of only 1–3%. The present development in the use of hypoxia houses is to expose the athletes to the equivalent of 3000 m or even 4000 m for brief periods of time during the day. As yet, data are only available from acute exposure. This indicates a quite pronounced effect causing haemoconcentration and an EPO response (Rodriguez et al. 1999). Exercise performed during the hypoxia exposure does not augment this effect.

Conclusion

In conclusion it can be stated that in endurance athletes living at medium altitude or in a hypoxia house combined with training at medium or low-to-medium altitude, and especially when the training is rather intense, the VO_{2max} and endurance performance may be enhanced. The mechanisms by which this is brought about are being debated. One possibility is that red cell mass is elevated due to an enlarged blood volume and so is the maximum oxygen uptake, with no change in [Hb]. An alternative possibility is that the anaerobic power is improved primarily related to a larger muscle tissue buffering capacity. The improved prolonged exercise capacity could be related to an improved muscle lactate consuming capacity, as there is an altered LDH isoform pattern when exposed to hypoxia.

References

Alexander JK, Hartley LH, Modelski M, Grover RF. Reduction of stroke volume during exercise in man following ascent to 3100 m altitude. *J Appl Physiol* 1967;23: 849–58.

Asmussen E, Consolazio CF. The circulation in rest and work on Mount Evans (4300 m). *Am J Physiol* 1941;132:555–63.

Bender PR, Groves BM, McCullogh RE, McCullough RG, Huang SY, Hamilton PD, Wagner PD, Cymerman A, Reeves JT. Oxygen transport to exercising leg in chronic hypoxia. *J Appl Physiol* 1988;65:2569–97.

Boushel R, Calbet JAL, Radegran G, Sondergaard H, Wagner PD, Saltin B. Parasympathetic neural activity accounts for the lowering of exercise heart rate at high altitude. *Circulation* 2001;9:15:1785–91.

Brooks GA. Increased glucose dependency in circulatory compensated hypoxia. In: Houston C, Coates J (eds). *Hypoxia and Mountain Medicine.* Burlington, VT: Queen City, 1992.

Calbet JAL, Rådegran G, Boushel R, Søndergård H, Wagner H, Wagner PD, Saltin B. Is acclimatization induced polycythemia an advantage for maximal exercise performance under hypoxic conditions in humans? *FASEB J* 1999;13:LB53.

Caquelard F, Burnet H, Tagliarini F, Cauchy E, Richalet JP, Jammes Y. Effect of prolonged hypobaric hypoxia on human skeletal muscle function and electromyographical events. *Clin Sci (Lond)* 2000;98:329–37.

Chapman RF, Stray-Gundersen J, Levine BJ. Individual variation in response to altitude training. *J Appl Physiol* 1998;85:1448–56.

Christensen EH, Hansen O. Respiratorischen Quotient-Bestimmungen in Ruhe und bei Arbeit. *Skand Arch Physiol* 1939;81:137–51.

Fitzgerald RS, Lahiri S. Reflex responses to chemoreceptor stimulation. In: Cherniack NS, Widdicombe JG (eds). *Handbook of Physiology.* Section 3: *The Respiratory System.* Bethesda, MD: American Physiological Society, 1986.

Fulco CS, Rock PB, Cymerman A. Maximal and submaximal exercise performance at altitude. *Aviat Space Environ Med* 1998;69:793–801.

Gore CJ, Hahn AG, Aughey RJ. Live high: train low changes muscle buffering capacity. International Council of Sport Science and Physical Education 2000 Pre-Olympic Congress, Book of Abstracts, 2000: 64.

Gore CJ, Hahn AG, Scroop GC, Watson DB, Norton KI, Wood RJ, Campbell DP, Emonson DL. Increased arterial desaturation in trained cyclists during maximal exercise at 580 m altitude. *J Appl Physiol* 1996;80:2204–10.

Hahn AG, Gore CJ, Martin DT, Ashenden MJ, Roberts AD, Logan PA. An evaluation of the concept of living at moderate altitude and training at sea level. *Comp Biochem Physiol A Mol Integr Physiol* 2001;128:777–89.

Haldane JS, Priestley JG. The regulation of lung-ventilation. *J Physiol (Lond)* 1905;32: 225–66.

Hannon JP, Vogel A. Oxygen transport during early altitude acclimatization: a perspective study. *Eur J Appl Physiol* 1977;36:285–97.

Hartley LH, Alexander JK, Modelski M, Grover RF. Subnormal cardiac output at rest and during exercise in residents at 3100 m altitude. *J Appl Physiol* 1967;23: 839–48.

Hochachka PW. Exercise limitations at high altitude: the metabolic problem and search for its solution. In: Gilles R (ed). *Circulation, Respiration, and Metabolism.* Berlin: Springer-Verlag, 1985.

Jelkman W. Erythropoietin: structure, control of production, and function. *Physiol Rev* 1992;72:449–89.

Kanstrup IL, Ekblom B. Acute hypervolemia, cardiac performance and aerobic power during exercise. *J Appl Physiol* 1982;52:1186–91.

Lawler J, Powers SK, Thompson D. Linear relationship between VO_{2max} and VO_{2max} decrement during exposure to acute hypoxia. *J Appl Physiol* 1988;64:1486–92.

Lundby C, Saltin B, van Hall G. The 'lactate paradox', a transient phenomenon with acclimatization to severe hypoxia in lowlanders. *Acta Scand Physiol* 2000;170: 265–9.

Lundby C, Araoz M, van Hall G. Peak heart rate decreases with increasing levels of acute hypoxia. *High Alt Med Biol* 2001a;2:369–76.

Lundby C, Møller P, Kanstrup IL, Olsen NV. Heart rate response to hypoxic exercise: role of dopamine D2-receptors and effect of oxygen supplementation. *Clin Sci (Lond)* 2001b;101:377–83.

Lundby C, van Hall G. Substrate utilization in sea level residents during exercise in acute hypoxia and after 4 weeks of acclimatization to 4100 m. *Acta Physiol Scand* 2002;176:1–7.

Maher JT, Jones LG, Hartley LH. Effects of high altitude exposure on submaximal endurance capacity of men. *J Appl Physiol* 1974;37:895–8.

Mizuno M, Juel C, Bro-Rasmussen T, Schibye B, Rasmussen B, Saltin B. Limb skeletal muscle adaptation in athletes after training at altitude. *J Appl Physiol* 1990;68: 496–502.

Mosso A. *Der Mensch auf den Hochalpen.* Leipzig: Verlag von Veit & Comp, 1898.

Pugh LG. Cardiac output in muscular exercise at 5800 m (19 000 ft). *J Appl Physiol* 1964;19:441–7.

Reeves JT, Groves BM, Sutton JR, Wagner PD, Cymerman A, Malconian MK, Rock PB, Young PM, Houston CS. Operation Everest II: preservation of cardiac function at extreme altitude. *J Appl Physiol* 1987;63:531–9.

Roberts AC, Reeves JT, Butterfield GE, Mazzeo RS, Sutton JR, Wolfel EE, Brooks GA. Altitude and β-blockade augments glucose utilization during submaximal exercise. *J Appl Physiol* 1996;80:605–15.

Rodriguez FA, Casas H, Casas M, Pages T, Rama R, Ricart A, Ventura JL, Ibanez J, Viscor G. Intermittent hypobaric hypoxia stimulates erythropoiesis and improves aerobic capacity. *Med Sci Sports Exerc* 1999;31:264–8.

Saltin B. Exercise and the environment: focus on altitude. *Res Quarterly Exerc Sport* 1996;67:1–10.

Saltin B, Grover RF, Blomqvist CG, Hartley LH, Johnson RL. Maximal oxygen uptake and cardiac output after 2 weeks at 4300m. *J Appl Physiol* 1968;25:400–9.

Semenza GL, Roth PH, Fang HM, Wang GL. Transcriptional regulation of genes encoding glycolytic enzymes by hypoxia-inducible-factor 1. *J Biol Chem* 1994; 269(23):575–763.

Shephard RJ, Bouhlel E, Vandewalle H, Monod H. Peak oxygen intake and hypoxia: influence of physical fitness. *Int J Sports Med* 1988;9:279–83.

Stray-Gundersen J, Levine B. 'Living high and training low' can improve sea level performance in endurance athletes. *Br J Sports Med* 1999;33:150–1.

Sutton JR, Reeves JT, Wagner PD, Groves BM, Cymerman A, Malconian MK, Rock PB, Young PM, Walter SD, Houston CS. Operation Everest II: oxygen transport during exercise at extreme simulated altitude. *J Appl Physiol* 1988;64:1309–21.

Svedenhag J, Piehl-Aulin K, Skog C, Saltin B. Increased left ventricular muscle mass after long-term altitude training in athletes. *Acta Physiol Scand* 1997;161:63–70.

Terrados N, Mizuno M, Andersen H. Reduction in maximal oxygen uptake at low altitudes; role of training status and lung function. *Clin Physiol* 1985;5:75–9.

Van Hall G, Calbet JAL, Sondergaard H, Saltin B. The re-establishment of the normal blood lactate response to exercise in humans after prolonged acclimatization to altitude. *J Physiol* 2001;536:963–75.

Wagner PD. Reduced maximal cardiac output at altitude—mechanisms and significance. *Resp Physiol* 2000;120:1–11.

Warren GL, Cureton KJ. Modelling the effect of alterations in hemoglobin concentration on VO$_{2max}$. *Med Sci Sport Exerc* 1989;21:526–31.

Weil JV. Ventilatory control at high altitude. In: Cherniack NS, Widdicombe JG (eds). *Handbook of Physiology*. Section 3: *The Respiratory System*. Bethesda, MD: American Physiological Society, 1986.

Wolfel EE. Sympatho-adrenal and cardio-vascular adaptations to hypoxia. In: Sutton JR, Houston CS, Coates G (eds). *Hypoxia and Molecular Medicine*. Burlington, VT: Queen City Press, 1993.

CHAPTER 12

Gender differences in sport

Anne L. FRIEDLANDER

Introduction

As long as sports records have been kept for both men and women, there have been differences between the genders in performance. Over the past 50 years, gender differences in world record times in most events have narrowed as sports participation by women has become more socially acceptable and prevalent. However, since the late 1980s the closing of the gender gap has begun to slow and, although all sports continue to see improvements in the records for both men and women, the percentage differences between genders in most events have not decreased. For example, the average percentage difference in 1960 for the various sports listed in Table 12.1 was 21.1%. By 1980, that percentage gender difference had fallen to 10.6%, but over the last 20 years it has crept back up to 11.2%. Those numbers may not be representative of all levels of competition, but more comparable training and coaching opportunities at higher levels of competition suggest that elite male and females athletes are closer in maximal performance than their recreational counterparts. Therefore, world record times usually represent the smallest differences between genders (Brooks et al. 2000). Fewer females than males still participate in most sports but the stability of the gender differences between 6% and 15% over the past two decades suggests that the divergences reflect actual physiological distinctions rather than social and environmental influences.

The purpose of this chapter is to summarise the gender-based physiological and metabolic differences that contribute to the gender

TABLE 12.1 Progression of percentage differences[a] between genders in world record times of selected events over the last 40 years

EVENT	1960	1970	1980	1990	2001	2001 WORLD RECORD (MEN)	2001 WORLD RECORD (WOMEN)
Running							
100 m run	13	11.4	9.3	5.7	7.2	9.79	10.49
1500 m run	NA	17.4	10	11	11.7	3:26.00	3:50.46
Marathon	63	42.2	13.3	11	10.4	2:05.42	2:18.47
4 × 100 m relay	12.4	12.0	9.4	9.5	10.6	37.40	41.37
4 × 400 m relay	NA	19.3	13.1	10.8	12.1	2:54.20	3:15.17
Swimming							
100 m freestyle	9.9	13.4	10.8	13	12.4	47.84	53.77
400 m freestyle	11.8	9.1	6.5	7.5	10.9	3:40.17	4:03.85
Other							
High jump	16.2	16.2	14.8	14.3	14.7	2.45[b]	2.09[b]
Average difference	21.1	17.6	10.6	10.4	11.2		

(a) Differences were calculated as: ([larger − smaller]/men) × 100.
(b) Units are metres (all others are time).

separation in sports performance. In addition, the proposal that women will eventually outperform men in endurance events will be evaluated.

In the sections that follow, it is important to remember that considerable variation in the characteristics discussed exist within each gender. In fact, the differences between the mean values for men and women in variables such as percentage body fat often seem small in comparison to the range of values within each gender. Also, mean values for men and women representing the entire population often show greater divergence than comparisons made between elite male and female athletes participating in the same sport. Therefore, the comparisons that follow are for the general population unless otherwise specified.

Gender differences prior to puberty

Normative data from the 1985 US School Population Fitness Survey indicates that up to age 10 years, girls in the highest percentage of fitness do better than the fittest boys on some tests such as the 50-yard (45.7-m) dash or the 2-mile (3.2-km) walk. Some girls may outperform boys because their earlier growth spurt affords them greater strength and better coordination than prepubescent boys. However, data compiled for the President's Council on Physical Fitness and Sports suggests that the majority of boys can outperform girls on most of the fitness tests. The better performance in the boys is at least partly a result of boys being more active than girls, a difference that continues into adulthood (Schoenborn & Barnes 2002). During puberty, gender differences in performance begin to widen. For example, whereas boys increase the number of pull-ups they can do from age 10–17 years, the number of pull-ups that girls can do decreases over that same age range.

Morphological differences

Body size and dimensions

During puberty, evolving differences in body size and body proportions that will later distinguish men and women become apparent. Elevated concentrations of gonadotrophic hormones increase levels of androgens in males, which promote greater increases in muscle mass and body size. On average, women are approximately 10% shorter and 17% smaller than men

(Brooks et al. 2000). Women also have shorter legs even for their height, which can limit their peak force development and speed due to shorter lever arms and stride length (Shephard 2000). Shorter femurs combined with wider hips can lead to a slightly lower centre of gravity. A lower centre of gravity is often associated with better balance, so the shorter legs in combination with the overall shorter stature of women may be beneficial in events such as gymnastics that require good balance (Atwater 1988; Sanborn & Jankowski 1994). However, the lower body proportions of females also can lead to an increased Q angle (femur angle off vertical), which is thought to increase the risk of knee injuries. Contraction of the quadriceps at an angle tends to pull the patella more laterally, causing a disruption in normal joint tracking (Wells 1991). The narrower shoulders in women reduce strength production of the upper body, but have the advantage of producing less drag in swimming events. For events such as running and cycling where the body is moved against gravity, the smaller overall body size of women does have the advantage of requiring less force to displace the lighter body mass (Shephard 2000). A summary of gender differences and their potential effect on performance are listed in Table 12.2.

TABLE 12.2 Gender differences and the possible impact on performance of those differences

WOMEN COMPARED TO MEN	IMPACT ON PERFORMANCE
Anthropometric	
Body size: smaller, shorter	Decreased speed and power
Less muscle mass	Decreased strength and power
Higher percentage body fat	Decreased jumping ability and speed
	Increased buoyancy
Shorter legs, wider hips	Better balance
	Greater risk for knee problems
	Reduced speed
Cardiovascular	
Smaller heart, smaller ventricular volume	Decreased stroke volume and cardiac output + Decreased oxygen transport = lower VO_{2max}
Decreased haematocrit, haemoglobin, red blood cells	
Substrate use	
Increased lipid use, decreased CHO use	Better whole body endurance
Decreased protein use	Preservation of muscle mass
Muscle	
Higher percentage type I (slow oxidative) fibres (?)	Better muscular endurance
Delayed fatigue, higher ATP/ADP ratio	
Greater muscle blood flow (?)	

Body composition

Upon maturity, significant differences in body composition between men and women emerge. The total muscle mass and muscle fibre cross-sectional area in women is approximately 60–85% that of men and is accompanied by similar decrements in maximal strength (Bassey et al. 1996; Cureton et al. 1988; Heyward et al. 1986). Due to a disproportionally greater amount of muscle mass in the upper body of men relative to women, gender differences in strength are usually larger for the upper than the lower body (Brooks et al. 2000). Even in elite athletes, differences in strength are substantially greater than those seen in endurance events. For example, the current world record for weight-lifting is 357.5 kg versus 275.5 kg (snatch and jerk combined) for men and women in the 69-kg weight class, respectively, a difference of 28%.

Women also have a higher percentage of body fat than do men (about 10% higher) and percentage body fat tends to increase in parallel with age for both men and women at least until the start of menopause in women (Wells 1991). The larger amount of body fat in women is a result of both greater essential fat and non-essential (storage) fat. Essential fat is required for normal physiological and reproductive function and is predominantly contained in the heart, lungs, nervous system and gender-specific tissues such as breasts. Women require 10–12% of their body weight as essential fat compared to only 3% for men. The remainder of the difference is accounted for by greater amounts of storage fat in women. Gender differences in body fat are smaller in highly trained athletes. For example, the percentage difference in body fat in male and female elite distance runners has been estimated to be in the range of 2–6% versus 10–12% for sedentary individuals (Wells 1991). Fat also tends to accumulate more in the hips and thigh regions (gynoidal pattern obesity) in premenopausal women, whereas it tends to develop in the abdominal region (androidal obesity) in men (Ley et al. 1992). Individuals with androidal obesity patterns are more sensitive to exercise-stimulated weight loss but are also at higher risk for cardiovascular disease and type II diabetes (at least within gender) (Depres et al. 1988).

Higher body fat percentages in women have a negative impact on sports requiring speed or jumping but may assist in long-distance swimming events by providing increased buoyancy and heat insulation. In addition, because adipose tissue is not metabolically active, it contributes to the lower maximal oxygen consumption (VO_{2max}) in comparably trained male and female athletes. A study by Cureton and Sparling (1980) demonstrated that 65% of the difference in VO_{2max} between training-matched male and female athletes could be eliminated by adding the body fat weight equivalent of the women to the male athletes. The relative importance of body size and fat mass can be seen when aerobic capacity is corrected for those parameters. For example, when oxygen consumption is expressed in absolute terms (litres O_2 consumed per min), gender differences are of the order of 40%. However, the difference falls to approximately 20% and to less than 10% when adjusted for body weight (mL/kg/min) and lean mass (mL/kg lean mass/min), respectively (Brooks et al. 2000; Carter et al. 2001b). Much of the remaining difference (~10%) can be accounted for by the cardiovascular characteristics described below.

Cardiovascular differences

Along with greater increases in body size and muscle mass, elevated concentrations of androgens during puberty in men cause greater hypertrophy of the heart compared to women even when corrected for body size. Testosterone has been shown to bind directly to cardiac tissue (McGill & Sheridan 1981) and testosterone supplementation has been shown to increase heart weights in gonadectomised male rats (McGill & Sheridan 1981; Schaible et al. 1984). Smaller heart size contributes to the smaller stroke volume, lower maximal cardiac output (Q_{max}) and higher submaximal heart rates observed in women relative to men (Ogawa et al. 1992). Although endurance training increases left-ventricular end-diastolic volume in women as it does in men, the differences in left ventricular size between genders remain even in highly trained athletes (George et al. 1995). In addition, women generally have lower haematocrit (42% vs 47%) and haemoglobin levels (13.8 vs 15.8 g/dL), which has been attributed to iron loss during menses, lower dietary intake of iron-rich foods and/or lower levels of androgens (Brooks et al. 2000; Sanborn & Jankowski 1994). Although the oxygen-binding capacity of haemoglobin (1.34 mL O_2/g) does not differ between genders, the lower amount of haemoglobin reduces the oxygen content (C_aO_2) of blood in women.

The issue of what ultimately limits the VO_{2max} is still being debated but most believe that oxygen delivery $Q(C_aO_2)$], rather than oxygen extraction by the tissues, is critical. Therefore, as described above, the lower cardiac output and lower oxygen content of the blood combine to decrease oxygen transport and, thus, VO_{2max} in women. The relative importance of haemoglobin content as a determinant of maximal capacity was investigated in a study by Cureton et al. (1986). When haemoglobin content was equated experimentally in matched male and female subjects, percentage differences in VO_{2max} expressed in mL/kg/min fell from 11.5% to 3.8% (Cureton et al. 1986). It is likely that the remaining separation between genders in the experiment could be accounted for by the differences in cardiac output. In contrast, Ogawa et al. (1992) estimated that, in physically fit individuals, 86–95% of the gender differences in weight-normalised VO_{2max} could be accounted for by a greater maximal cardiac output in the men resulting from a higher stroke volume.

Cardiovascular changes with training

When similar endurance training regimens are followed, most show that men and women have similar relative increases in VO_{2max} and submaximal work performance (Drinkwater 1984; Eddy et al. 1977; Mitchell et al. 1992). For example, Rubal et al. (1987) demonstrated that 10 weeks of running in previously sedentary men and women was sufficient to cause parallel increases of 20% in VO_{2max} and similar (but non-significant) increases in the left ventricular mass and end-diastolic volume. However, some training studies have elicited greater gains in VO_{2max} in women compared to men, perhaps reflecting a lower initial fitness level of the women used in those studies (Carter et al. 2001b; Friedlander et al. 1997, 1998). Regardless of the magnitude, the pattern of adaptation and types of changes are similar in men and women. As in men, trained women have larger left ventricles, stroke volumes and cardiac outputs, and lower resting heart rates compared to sedentary controls (George et al. 1995; Ogawa et al. 1992; Rubal et al. 1987). Female athletes and women undergoing long-term endurance training programs have also been shown to have elevated arteriovenous oxygen differences (Cunningham & Hill 1975; Ogawa et al. 1992), which may be partially reflective of increased vascularisation of the endurance-trained muscle (Ingjer & Brodal 1978; Saltin et al. 1977). Since women seem to exhibit the same capacity for cardiovascular adaptation to training, existing gender differences in cardiovascular performance must be a result of differences in initial baseline values and/or the quality and quantity of training.

Muscle morphology and histology

The disproportionate increase in muscle mass during puberty in males compared to females is reflected in widening differences in maximal strength into adulthood (Glenmark et al. 1994). Most investigators have shown that the strength to cross-sectional area ratio is similar between genders, suggesting that the observed gender differences in strength are simply a function of muscle quantity. In contrast, others have suggested that lesser strength can also be attributed to a greater fat content within the muscle tissue of women, resulting in a lower strength to cross-sectional area ratio in women (Forsberg et al. 1991). However, fat infiltration (non-contractile area) may be more related to physical activity levels than gender per se (Kent-Braun et al. 2000). The lower absolute accumulation of skeletal muscle mass in women does not seem to be a function of architectural characteristics (i.e. muscle fibre arrangement) but more likely a result of hormonal differences or inherent limits to the muscle fibre growth capacity (Abe et al. 1998).

The gender differences in skeletal muscle may not be simply quantitative but qualitative as well. Women have smaller cross-sectional areas of both type I and type II fibres compared to men (Coggan et al. 1992; Costill et al. 1976) but some studies suggest that the ratio of type I:type II fibre area may also be greater in women (Brooke & Engel 1969; Carter et al. 2001c). In addition, some (Brooke & Engel 1969; Kuipers et al. 1989; Simoneau & Bouchard 1989), but not all (Carter et al. 2001c; Costill et al. 1976, 1979), investigations have found a higher proportion of type I fibres in women relative to men in biopsies of the gastrocnemius, vastus lateralis and biceps brachii muscles. Female muscle tissue may also have a higher ratio of oxidative to glycolytic enzymes than that of men (Lundberg et al. 1985; Nygaard 1981; Simoneau & Bouchard 1989). Finally, Green et al. (1984) suggest that men may have higher glycolytic and oxidative enzyme activity but lower activity of enzymes critical for fat oxidation (3-hydroxyacyl-CoA dehydrogenase), thus suggesting that women may have a greater capacity for fat use relative to other substrates.

The histochemical data is by no means consistent, but there does seem to be evidence to suggest that the muscle tissue of women may be better suited for endurance-type activities than for high-intensity power activities. Such an idea is appealing as it could serve as a partial explanation for gender differences in the metabolic and muscle fatigue characteristics.

Muscle changes with training

Some short-term resistance training studies indicate that men and women are capable of attaining similar absolute and relative gains in strength, fibre area, muscle cross-sectional area and muscle volume (Cureton et al. 1988; O'Hagan et al. 1995). In contrast, Ivey et al. (2000) demonstrated that high-volume, high-intensity resistance training results in greater relative and absolute gains in muscle volume in men compared to women. The latter finding is supported by cross-sectional studies in power lifters that show men may have a greater capacity for muscle hypertrophy than women. In addition, hypertrophy of type II muscle groups in men may occur to a greater extent, whereas in women hypertrophy may occur less in total and in a way that is distributed more evenly between the type I and type II fibres (Alway et al. 1989; Bell & Jacobs 1990).

The discrepancy between the short-term intervention studies and cross-sectional studies suggests that the extent to which muscle hypertrophies within each gender may be dependent on the duration of the stimulus. It is likely that the ultimate capacity for muscle hypertrophy in women is limited by the reduced anabolic stimulus resulting from lower circulating androgens. Certainly in women, as with men, anecdotal evidence suggests that the use of exogenous anabolic steroids can greatly increase normal capacity for muscle hypertrophy.

In contrast to resistance exercise, endurance training seems to elicit similar muscular adaptations between genders. Increased oxidative capacity of muscle in response to endurance training in men has been well documented (Henriksson 1977; Holloszy & Coyle 1984; Hultman 1995). In a recent study by Carter et al. (2001c), both men and women demonstrated no change in fibre area or distribution, but did show similar increases in muscle oxidative potential following 7 weeks of endurance training. As in men, endurance training in women increases the number of capillaries per muscle fibre (Saltin et al. 1977) and this ratio does not seem to differ between men and women of similar training status (Bell & Jacobs 1990).

Metabolism and substrate use

Data on gender differences in substrate utilisation suggests that, at rest and for given relative submaximal exercise intensities, women oxidise a higher proportion of fat relative to carbohydrate (CHO) than do men as determined by lower respiratory exchange ratio (RER) values (Carter et al. 2001b; Friedlander et al. 1998; Tarnopolsky et al. 1990). Furthermore, reduced net glycogen utilisation and lower blood lactate concentrations have been observed in women compared to men while exercising at similar relative intensities (Friedlander et al. 1998; Tarnopolsky et al. 1990). However, not all investigations have demonstrated differences in substrate utilisation (Costill et al. 1979). Moreover, any such differences are likely to be negated during high-intensity exercise when glycogenolysis is the predominant energy pathway (Froberg & Pedersen 1984) or when the individuals are highly trained (Costill et al. 1979; Friedmann & Kindermann 1989).

The common wisdom used to explain gender differences in substrate use is that women use more fat because they have a more abundant supply. However, there is little data to support such a contention, with substantial data contrary to this hypothesis. Comparisons of normal weight and obese men and women suggest that individuals with higher body fat actually oxidise *less* lipid at rest and during submaximal exercise (Harms et al. 1995; Keim et al. 1996). Thus, lipid oxidative capacity seems to determine fat accumulation rather than the opposite. Because fat oxidation appears to be inversely related to body fat content in both men and women, it seems unlikely that gender differences in substrate selection could be a result of the higher body fat in women.

The ovarian hormones (oestrogen and progesterone) have been proposed as potential regulators of substrate utilisation (Bunt 1990; Hatta et al. 1988; Kendrick et al. 1987). Oestrogen may alter glucose metabolism by decreasing gluconeogenesis and insulin-binding capacity (Bunt 1990). Progesterone also has been shown to influence glucose flux by decreasing glucose uptake and oxidation in adipose tissue, decreasing hepatic gluconeogenesis, increasing hepatic glycogen storage, and decreasing peripheral insulin sensitivity (Kalkhoff 1982). In contrast, the ovarian hormones seem to have opposing effects on lipid metabolism with oestrogen working to mobilise and oxidise free fatty acids (FFAs) and progesterone promoting FFA storage (Bunt 1990; Kalkhoff 1982). Hackney et al. (1994) observed higher levels of lipid oxidation in women who were in the mid-luteal phase of their menstrual cycle compared to the mid-follicular phase. The differences were observed at rest, and at 35% and 65% of VO_{2peak}, but at 75% of VO_{2peak} the differences disappeared. Similarly, Graham et al. (1986) reported differences in plasma FFA and lactate concentrations between amenorrhoeic and eumenorrhoeic women during rest and mild exercise (at 30% of VO_{2max}), but not during moderate (60% VO_{2max}) or intense (90% of VO_{2max}) exercise. As previously noted, at the higher exercise intensities, it is likely that glycolytic flux governs substrate selection and the impact of mitigating factors such as menses, training and nutritional status are reduced or abolished completely.

The influence of oestrogen on CHO metabolism in humans has been investigated using short-term hormone treatment protocols. Ruby et al. (1997) used labelled glucose to demonstrate that the rate of glucose appearance was reduced in response to short-term oestrogen treatment in amenorrhoeic females. In addition, short-term treatment with oestradiol in men has been shown to decrease glucose turnover and increase glucose concentration but not to affect whole body substrate use during exercise (Carter et al. 2001a). Because oestrogen may have a suppressive effect on hepatic gluconeogenesis, women may be more similar to men in terms of glucose metabolism during the follicular phase of the menstrual cycle when hormonal levels are lowest.

Ovarian hormones may act in combination with other circulating hormones to modulate the substrate selection during rest and exercise in women. For example, men have higher circulating levels of catecholamines than do women at the same relative exercise intensities (Carter et al. 2001b; Friedlander et al. 1998; Tarnopolsky et al. 1990). Higher circulating epinephrine concentrations in men could increase the rate of muscle glycogenolysis as would the observed higher pre-exercise muscle glycogen concentrations in men (Hargreaves et al. 1985). In addition, women have higher circulating levels of growth hormone at rest and exercise, which could augment lipid mobilisation and oxidation (Wideman et al. 1999). Gender differences in receptor availability and affinity may also be important in determining substrate utilisation in response to circulating hormone levels. For example, insulin receptor binding has been shown to be greater and more similar to observations of binding in men when women were in their follicular rather than luteal phase of the menstrual cycle (Bertoli et al. 1980; De Pirro et al. 1978).

Muscle fatigue and endurance

It is not surprising based on the characteristics described above that there is strong evidence to support gender differences in muscle fatigue and endurance capacity. Fatigue can be defined as a decrement in the ability to sustain a predetermined force or tension, and several studies have shown that females resist fatigue and have greater muscular endurance than do men (Fulco et al. 1999; Maughan et al. 1986; West et al. 1995). The female advantage in fatigue resistance seems to be greatest at lower intensities and gradually disappears as the contraction protocols used in various studies approach maximum (Hicks et al. 2001). Although the mechanisms remain to be elucidated, several theories have been proposed (for a more extensive review see Hicks et al. 2001).

Firstly, an increased proportion of type I fibres in women could play a role. If a higher percentage of the contraction is being sustained by type I fibres in women, one would expect an increased fatigue resistance.

Secondly, women's increased dependence on lipid as a fuel source, because of a greater proportion of type I fibres, an increased relative oxidative capacity or hormonal differences, could result in glycogen sparing and thus increased muscular endurance. Indeed, the administration of oestradiol has been shown to postpone muscle and liver glycogen depletion in male rats and prolong running times in oophorectomised female rats (Kendrick et al. 1987; Rooney et al. 1993). However, it is likely that such a mechanism is more important in long-term glycogen depleting exercise (Froberg & Pedersen 1984) than the short-term, single muscle contraction protocols often used to study fatigue characteristics of muscle (Fulco et al. 1999; Maughan et al. 1986; West et al. 1995).

A third mechanism commonly used to explain the female advantage in fatigue resistance is related to the gender differences in strength and muscle mass. Because women have less muscle, comparisons made between men and women at the same relative percentage of maximum voluntary contraction result in women working at a lower absolute workload. This makes interpretation of some studies difficult because the higher ATP and oxygen demands for the men could have contributed to shorter endurance times (Maughan et al. 1986; Miller et al. 1993; West et al. 1995). Similarly, the greater force generated in males could result in more vascular occlusion in the working muscle and a resultant reduction in oxygen availability and metabolic by-product removal during contraction (Hicks et al. 2001).

A recent study by Fulco et al. (1999) questions the importance of absolute strength as an explanation of gender differences in fatigue. In the Fulco study, men and women were matched on maximal strength of the adductor pollicis muscle so that they were working at the same absolute and relative workloads. Under such conditions, gender differences persisted with maximal voluntary contraction force falling approximately twofold slower and recovering faster in the women (Fig. 12.1; Fulco et al. 1999). These differences were not only evident in the mean values but the women in each matched pair showed improved fatigue resistance as well (Fig. 12.2). The authors suggest that a greater proportion of type I fibres and/or a higher oxidative to glycolytic capacity could have resulted in a greater regeneration of ATP and decreased production of inhibitory waste products such as hydrogen ions, ADP and inorganic phosphate.

Despite similar absolute work rates in the study of Fulco et al. (1999), blood flow to the working muscle may still have been elevated in the women. The flow-mediated diameter of the brachial artery in women has been shown to be responsive to circulating oestradiol levels and to

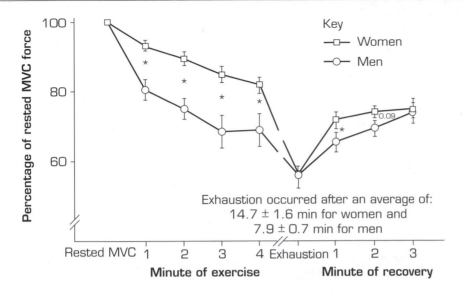

FIG. 12.1 Percentage of maximal voluntary contraction (MVC) force of rested muscle for men and women during the first 4 minutes of intermittent static adductor pollicis contractions, at exhaustion, and during 3 minutes of recovery. For each minute of exercise, the percentage of rested MVC force was markedly higher ($P < 0.01$) for women compared with men. After declining to a similar level of MVC force at exhaustion, MVC rose faster for women than men during the first minute of recovery ($P < 0.05$) (from Fulco et al. 1999)

be greater during the luteal phase than the flow-mediated diameter in men (Hashimoto et al. 1995). In addition, male-to-female transsexuals undergoing long-term oestrogen treatment show improved nitroglycerine-stimulated vasodilation in the brachial artery. However, it is still unclear whether differences in blood flow could be a significant contributor to gender differences in fatigue characteristics.

Oestrogens may work to delay fatigue by reducing free radical damage within the muscle tissue. The potential connection between fatigue, free radicals and oestrogen has been reviewed previously (Tiidus 1999). Briefly, an association between the development of fatigue and a build-up of oxygen radicals has been established in vivo and in vitro (Tiidus 1999). Vitamin E supplementation and infusion of a hydroxyl radical scavenger were shown to prolong swimming times in rats and delay the onset of fatigue in contracting dog muscle, respectively (Barclay & Hansel 1991; Novelli et al. 1990). Tiidus (1999) and others suggest that the presence of free radicals may shorten time to exercise-induced fatigue within a single bout of exercise by disrupting

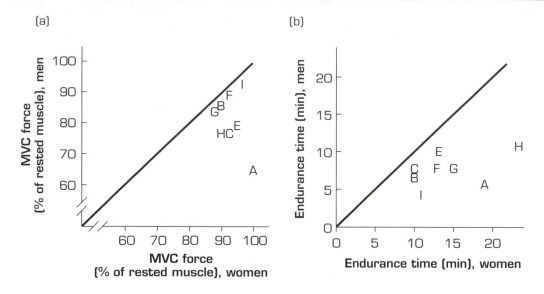

FIG. 12.2 (a) Adductor pollicis muscle maximal voluntary contraction (MVC) force after the first minute of submaximal adductor pollicis muscle contractions in each pair (A–I) of men and women matched for initial muscle strength. Each woman maintained a higher percentage of MVC force than each man. (b) Adductor pollicis muscle endurance time to exhaustion for the nine pairs of men and women matched for MVC force of rested muscle. For each matched pair, each woman had a longer endurance time than each man (from Fulco et al. 1999)

function of the sarcoplasmic reticulum, thus inhibiting uptake and/or release of calcium. Further, the more prolonged decrement in muscle force observed hours to days following an excessive bout of exercise may be a result of tissue inflammation caused by free radical muscle damage (Tiidus 1999).

Oestrogen may successfully reduce fatigue because it has been shown to have antioxidant properties. Oestrogen is capable of preventing the oxidative modifications of low-density lipoproteins and other lipoprotein fractions in vitro, perhaps by inhibiting superoxide production (Arteaga et al. 1998; Bekesi et al. 2000). In vivo, vitamin-E deficient female rats showed less muscle damage following treadmill running than did vitamin-E deficient male rats (Amelink et al. 1991). It has been hypothesised that oestradiol may be able to act as a substitute for vitamin E because both molecules have hydroxyl groups in similar positions on their A rings, which can be oxidised and reduced in the presence of free radicals. Other steroid hormones that do not have such a structure have shown no antioxidant capabilities (Tiidus 1999).

Exercising when oestrogens are high: an advantage?

Based on the hypothesised effects of oestrogen on fat utilisation and the prevention of fatigue described previously, one might expect endurance performance to be enhanced in women during the luteal phase of the menstrual cycle when oestrogen levels are higher. Evidence presented in isolated muscle groups in vivo is promising but by no means conclusive. Young women have been shown to have higher peak force during isometric contractions of the adductor pollicis and improved strength and fatigue resistance in the quadriceps when oestrogen was at peak levels compared to other times during the menstrual cycle (Phillips et al. 1996; Sarwar et al. 1996). Women taking oral contraceptives did not show cyclical changes in the performance parameters. However, studies in older women have not supported the relationship between oestrogen and muscle performance (Bassey et al. 1996; Seeley et al. 1995). Data collected from whole-body performance studies investigating the impact of the menstrual cycle phase is even less impressive. With all the records that have been kept and all of the studies that have been undertaken, there is still debate on whether there are menstrual variations in athletic performance (Dibrezzo et al. 1991; Lebrun et al. 1995; Nicklas et al. 1989). Therefore, despite measurable differences in individual muscle performance or in animal studies, the impact of menstrual phase on actual performance in humans is minimal at best. It could be that increased water retention, dysmenorrhoea (menstrual discomfort), slight elevation in body temperature or changes in motivation may overwhelm any small benefit at the individual muscle level that could be obtained from normal cycle variations in oestrogen levels.

Could women outperform men?

The possibility that women could outperform men in distance events is an appealing notion and one that has been previously proposed (Bam et al. 1997; Speechly et al. 1996; Whipp & Ward 1992). Some of the most intriguing data on this subject comes from two South African laboratories where the ultra-distance Comrades marathon is a popular event. Both groups found that when men and women competitors were matched on their training level and performance at distances of 42–56 km, the women outperformed the men at a distance of 90 km (Bam et al. 1997; Speechly et al. 1996). The women, who were smaller and had lower maximal aerobic capacity, prevailed because they were able to sustain a higher fractional percentage of their VO_{2max} throughout the 90-km race (Speechly et al. 1996). These studies, along with others showing better endurance in women performing submaximal exercise (Froberg & Pedersen 1984) and greater fatigue resistance of muscle in females compared to matched men (Fulco et al. 1999), are intriguing and the mechanisms responsible for the differences certainly warrant further study.

Matching genders is difficult and may account for some of the discrepancies present in the literature: it is difficult to know whether to match by selecting male and female subjects with identical characteristics or select them to be typical for the pool being investigated. Matching the genders is critical when the study is trying to identify the mechanisms that account for differences in performance. However, when it comes to actual performance, the bottom line is how are the top men and the top women currently performing. For example, although the results of the studies from South Africa (Bam et al. 1997; Speechly et al. 1996) look promising, the results are somewhat deceiving: the marathon distance world record times for men are still faster than women at that distance (Table 12.1) so the men who were selected for the studies were less accomplished within their gender than the women. Because the record for the fastest woman in the Comrades marathon is still approximately 15% lower than that of the fastest man, we must assume that the better performance in the second half of the race by the female runners is not sufficient to overcome the slower pace of the first half. Apparently, extending the race further does not help either. For example, in even longer events, such as the Western States 100-mile (161-km) race held in northern California, the fastest man outpaced the fastest women by 11% in 2001 (16:38:30 h vs 18:33:34 h).

Because ultra-distance events are still relatively new (women first started racing in the Comrades marathon in 1975), it could be that the races have yet to attract a large enough pool of female competitors to challenge the men. However, it may also be that the gender differences in body composition, muscle mass and cardiovascular capacity are too substantial to overcome with the greater fatigue resistance and enhanced fat oxidation experienced by women even in ultra-endurance events. It is also possible that in endurance events that are long enough to require supplemental CHO consumption during the race, the benefits of increased fat oxidation may be negated both because of the exogenous fuel source and because glycogen use slows as stores are depleted (which may eventually equate men and women). At this point, only time and further research will tell.

Conclusion

Over the past 50 years, sports performance has been improving gradually for both men and women. Initially during that time period, the rate of improvement for women exceeded that of men and there was a narrowing of world record times in many sports. However, over the past two decades the closing of the gap between genders has slowed, stopped or even reversed. Although some predicted, that based on the progression of records, women would outperform men in endurance events by 1998 (Whipp & Ward 1992), there is no indication that we are nearing such an achievement. Differences in gender performance have remained in the range of 6–15% for most events over the past 20 years and it is likely that the differences are reflective of physiological and metabolic distinctions between genders. Smaller body size, more body fat, less muscle mass and decreased maximal oxygen transport put women at a disadvantage in activities requiring speed, power or high-intensity work. However, women have shown higher fat utilisation, glycogen sparing, muscle fatigue resistance and an ability to sustain a higher percentage of maximal capacity, all of which should confer an advantage in prolonged endurance events. Whether the advantages will eventually overcome the disadvantages in a way that will allow women to outperform men in select events remains to be seen.

References

Abe T, Brechue WF, Fujita S, Brown JB. Gender differences in FFM accumulation and architectural characteristics of muscle. *Med Sci Sports Exerc* 1998;30:1066–70.

Alway SE, Grumbt WH, Gonyea WJ, Stray-Gundersen J. Contrasts in muscle and myofibers of elite male and female bodybuilders. *J Appl Physiol* 1989;67:24–31.

Amelink GJ, van der Waals W, Wokke JH, van Asbeck BS, Bar PR. Exercise-induced muscle damage in the rat: the effect of vitamin E deficiency. *Pflugers Arch* 1991;419:304–9.

Arteaga E, Rojas A, Villaseca P, Bianchi M, Arteaga A, Duran D. In vitro effects of estradiol, progesterone, testosterone, and of combined estradiol/progestin on low density lipoprotein (LDL) oxidation in postmenopausal women. *Menopause* 1998;5:16–23.

Atwater AE. Biomechanics and the female athlete. In: Puhl J, Brown CH, Voy RO, eds. *Sports Science Perspectives for Women*. Champaign, IL: Human Kinetics Books, 1988.

Bam J, Noakes TD, Juritz J, Dennis SC. Could women outrun men in ultramarathon races? *Med Sci Sports Exerc* 1997;29:244–7.

Barclay JK, Hansel M. Free radicals may contribute to oxidative skeletal muscle fatigue. *Can J Physiol Pharmacol* 1991;69:279–84.

Bassey EJ, Mockett SP, Fentem PH. Lack of variation in muscle strength with menstrual status in healthy women aged 45–54 years; data from a national survey. *Eur J Appl Physiol Occup Physiol* 1996;73:382–6.

Bekesi G, Kakucs R, Varbiro S, Racz K, Sprintz D, Feher J, Szekacs B. In vitro effects of different steroid hormones on the superoxide anion production of human neutrophil granulocytes. *Steroids* 2000;65:889–94.

Bell DG, Jacobs I. Muscle fibre area, fibre type and capillarization in male and female bodybuilders. *Can J Sport Sci* 1990;15:115–19.

Bertoli A, De Pirro R, Fusco A, Greco AV, Magnatta R. Differences in insulin receptors between men and menstruating women and influence of sex hormones in insulin binding during menstrual cycle. *J Clin Endocrinol* 1980;50:246–50.

Brooke MH, Engel WK. The histographic analysis of human muscle biopsies with regard to fiber types 1. Adult male and female. *Neurology* 1969;19:221–33.

Brooks GA, Fahey TD, White TP, Baldwin K. *Exercise Physiology: Human Bioenergetics and its Applications.* 3rd edn. Mountain View, CA: Mayfield, 2000.

Bunt J. Metabolic actions of estradiol: significance for acute and chronic exercise responses. *Med Sci Sports Exerc* 1990;22:286–90.

Carter S, McKenzie S, Mourtzakis M, Mahoney DJ, Tarnopolsky MA. Short-term 17 beta-estradiol decreases glucose Ra but not whole body metabolism during endurance exercise. *J Appl Physiol* 2001a;90:139–46.

Carter SL, Rennie C, Tanopolosky MA. Substrate utilization during exercise in men and women after endurance training. *Am J Physiol Endocrinol Metab* 2001b;280: E898–E907.

Carter SL, Rennie CD, Hamilton SJ, Tarnopolsky MA. Changes in skeletal muscle in males and females following endurance training. *Can J Physiol Pharmacol* 2001c;79:386–92

Coggan AR, Spina RJ, King DS, Rogers MA, Brown M, Nemeth PM, Holloszy JO. Histochemical and enzymatic comparison of the gastrocnemius muscle of young and elderly men and women. *J Gerontol* 1992;47:B71–B76.

Costill DL, Daniels J, Evans W, Fink W, Krahenbuhl G, Saltin B. Skeletal muscle enzymes and fiber composition in male and female track athletes. *J Appl Physiol* 1976;40:149–54.

Costill DL, Fink WJ, Getchell LH, Ivy JL. Lipid metabolism in skeletal muscle of endurance-trained males and females. *J Appl Physiol* 1979;47:787–91.

Cunningham DA, Hill JS. Effect of training on cardiovascular response to exercise in women. *J Appl Physiol* 1975;39:891–5.

Cureton K, Bishop P, Hutchinson P, Newland H, Vickery S, Zwiren L. Sex differences in maximal oxygen uptake. Effect of equating haemoglobin concentration. *Eur J Appl Physiol Occup Physiol* 1986;54:656–60.

Cureton KJ, Collins MA, Hill DW, McElhannon FM. Muscle hypertrophy in men and women. *Med Sci Sports Exerc* 1988;20:338–44.

Cureton KJ, Sparling PB. Distance running performance and metabolic responses to running in men and women with excess weight experimentally equated. *Med Sci Sports Exerc* 1980;12:288–94.

De Pirro R, Fusco A, Bertoli A, Greco AV, Lauro R. Insulin receptors during menstrual cycle in normal women. *J Clin Endocrinol Metab* 1978;47:1387–9.

Depres JP, Tremblay AN, Nadeau A, Bouchard C. Physical training and changes in regional adipose tissue distribution. *Acta Medica Scand* 1988;723:203–12.

Dibrezzo R, Fort I, Brown B. Relationships among strength, endurance, weight and body fat during three phases of the menstrual cycle. *J Sports Med Phys Fitness* 1991;31:89–94.

Drinkwater BL. Women and exercise: physiological aspects. *Exerc Sports Sci Rev* 1984;12:21–51.

Eddy DO, Sparks KL, Adelizi DA. The effects of continuous and interval training in women and men. *Eur J Appl Physiol* 1977;37:83–92.

Forsberg AM, Nilsson E, Werneman J, Bergstrom J, Hultman E. Muscle composition in relation to age and sex. *Clin Sci* 1991;81:249–56.

Friedlander AL, Casazza GA, Horning MA, Huie MJ, Brooks GA. Training-induced alterations of glucose flux in men. *J Appl Physiol* 1997;82:1360–9.

Friedlander AL, Casazza GA, Horning MA, Huie M, Piancentini MF, Trimmer J, Brooks GA. Training-induced alterations in carbohydrate metabolism: women respond differently than men. *J Appl Physiol* 1998;85:1175–86.

Friedmann B, Kindermann W. Energy metabolism and regulatory hormones in women and men during endurance exercise. *Eur J Appl Physiol* 1989;59:1–9.

Froberg K, Pedersen PK. Sex differences in endurance capacity and metabolic response to prolonged, heavy exercise. *Eur J Appl Physiol* 1984;52:446–50.

Fulco CS, Rock PB, Muza SR, Lammi E, Cymerman A, Butterfield G, Moore LG, Braun B, Lewis SF. Slower fatigue and faster recovery of the adductor pollicis muscle in women matched for strength with men. *Acta Physiol Scand* 1999;167:233–9.

George KP, Wolfe LA, Burggraf GW, Norman R. Electrocardiographic and echocardiographic characteristics of female athletes. *Med Sci Sports Exerc* 1995;27:1362–70.

Glenmark B, Hedberg G, Kaijser L, Jansson E. Muscle strength from adolescence to adulthood—relationship to muscle fibre types. *Eur J Appl Physiol Occup Physiol* 1994;68:9–19.

Graham TE, Van Dijk JP, Viswanathan M, Giles KA, Bonen A, George JC. Exercise metabolic responses in men and eumenorrheic and amenorrheic women. In: Saltin B, ed. *Biochemistry of Exercise VI*. Champaign, IL: Human Kinetics, 1986: 2227–8.

Green HJ, Fraser IG, Ranney DA. Male and female differences in enzyme activities of energy metabolism in vastus lateralis muscle. *J Neurol Sci* 1984;65:323–31.

Hackney AC, McCracken-Compton MA, Ainsworth B. Substrate responses to submaximal exercise in the midfollicular and midluteal phase of the menstrual cycle. *Int J Sport Nutr* 1994;4:299–308.

Hargreaves M, McConell G, Proietto J. Influence of muscle glycogen on glycogenolysis and glucose uptake during exercise in humans. *J Appl Physiol* 1985;78:288–92.

Harms CA, Cordain L, Stager JM, Sockler JM, Harris M. Body fat mass affects postexercise metabolism in males of similar lean body mass. *Med Exerc Nutr Health* 1995;4:33–9.

Hashimoto M, Akishita M, Eto M, Ishikawa M, Kozaki K, Toba K, Sagara Y, Taketani Y, Orimo H, Ouchi Y. Modulation of endothelium-dependent flow-mediated dilatation of the brachial artery by sex and menstrual cycle. *Circulation* 1995;92:3431–5.

Hatta H, Atomi Y, Shinohara S, Yamamoto Y, Yamada S. The effects of ovarian hormones on glucose and fatty acid oxidation during exercise in female ovariectomized rats. *Horm Metab Res* 1988;20:609–11.

Henriksson J. Training induced adaptation of skeletal muscle and metabolism during submaximal exercise. *J Physiol* 1977;270:661–75.

Heyward VH, Johannes-Ellis SM, Romer JF. Gender differences in strength. *Res Quart* 1986;57:154–9.

Hicks AL, Kent-Braun J, Ditor DS. Sex differences in human skeletal muscle fatigue. *Exerc Sports Sci Rev* 2001;29:109–12.

Holloszy JO, Coyle EF. Adaptations of skeletal muscle to endurance exercise and their metabolic consequences. *J Appl Physiol* 1984;56:831–8.

Hultman E. Fuel selection, muscle fibre. *Proceed Nutr Soc* 1995;54:107–21.

Ingjer F, Brodal P. Capillary supply of skeletal muscle fibers in untrained and endurance trained women. *Eur J Appl Physiol* 1978;38:291–9.

Ivey FM, Roth SM, Ferrell RE, Tracy BL, Lemmer JT, Hurlbut DE, Martel GF, Siegel EL, Fozard JL, Metter EJ, Fleg JL, Hurley BF. Effects of age, gender, and myostatin genotype on the hypertropic response to heavy resistance strength training. *J Gerontol* 2000;55A:M641–M648.

Kalkhoff RK. Metabolic effects of progesterone. *Am J Obstet Gynecol* 1982;142:735–8.

Keim NL, Belko AZ, Barbieri TF. Body fat percentage and gender: associations with energy expenditure, substrate utilization, and mechanical work efficiency. *Int J Sport Nutr* 1996;6:356–69.

Kendrick ZV, Steffen CA, Rumsey WL, Goldberg DI. Effect of estradiol on tissue glycogen metabolism in exercised oopherectomized rats. *J Appl Physiol* 1987;63:492–6.

Kent-Braun JA, Ng AV, Young K. Skeletal muscle contractile and noncontractile components in young and older women and men. *J Appl Physiol* 2000;88:662–8.

Kuipers H, Janssen GME, Bosman F, Frederick PM, Geurten P. Structural and ultrastructural changes in skeletal muscle associated with long-distance training and running. *Int J Sports Med* 1989;10:S156–S159.

Lebrun CM, McKenzie DC, Prior JC, Taunton JE. Effects of menstrual cycle phase on athletic performance. *Med Sci Sports Exerc* 1995;27:437–44.

Ley C, Lees B, Stevenson J. Sex and menopause-associated changes in body-fat distribution. *Am J Clin Nutr* 1992;55:950–4.

Lundberg B, Esbjornsson M, Hedberg G, Jansson E. Skeletal muscle fiber types and physical performance. A 10 year follow up study. *Clinical Phys* 1985;5:167.

Maughan RJ, Harmon M, Leiper JB, Sale DG, Delman A. Endurance capacity of untrained males and females in isometric and dynamic muscular contractions. *Eur J Appl Physiol Occup Ther* 1986;55:395–400.

McGill HC, Sheridan PJ. Nuclear uptake of sex-steroid hormones in the cardiovascular system of the baboon. *Circ Res* 1981;48:238–44.

Miller AEJ, MacDougall JD, Tarnopolsky MA, Sale DG. Gender differences in strength and muscle fibre characteristics. *Eur J Appl Physiol* 1993;66:254–62.

Mitchell JH, Tate C, Raven PB. Acute response and chronic adaptation to exercise in women. *Med Sci Sports Exerc* 1992;24(suppl.):S258–S269.

Nicklas BJ, Hackney AC, Sharp RL. The menstrual cycle and exercise: performance, muscle glycogen, and substrate responses. *Int J Sports Med* 1989;10:264–9.

Novelli GP, Braciotti G, Falsini S. Spin-trappers and vitamin E prolong endurance to muscle fatigue in mice. *Free Radic Biol Med* 1990;8:9–13.

Nygaard E. Skeletal muscle fibre characteristics in young women. *Acta Physiol Scand* 1981;112:299–304.

Ogawa T, Spina RJ, Martin WH, Kohrt WM, Schechtman KB, Holloszy JO, Ehsani AA. Effects of aging, sex, and physical training on cardiovascular responses to exercise. *Circulation* 1992;86:494–503.

O'Hagan FT, Sale DG, MacDougall JD, Garner SH. Response to resistance training in young women and men. *Int J Sports Med* 1995;16:314–21.

Phillips SK, Sanderson AG, Birch K, Bruce SA, Woledge RC. Changes in maximal voluntary force of human adductor pollicis muscle during the menstrual cycle. *J Physiol* 1996;496:551–7.

President's Council on Physical Fitness and Sports. 1985 *National School Population Fitness Survey*, Washington, DC: US Department of Health & Human Services, Public Health Service, Office of the Assistant Secretary for Health, 1986.

Rooney TP, Kendrick ZV, Carlson J, Ellis GS, Matakevich B, Lorusso SM, McCall JA. Effect of estradiol on the temporal pattern of exercise-induced tissue glycogen depletion in male rats. *J Appl Physiol* 1993;75:1502–6.

Rubal BJ, Al-Muhailani AR, Rosentsweig J. Effects of physical conditioning on the heart size and wall thickness of college women. *Med Sci Sports Exerc* 1987;19: 423–9.

Ruby BC, Robergs RA, Waters DL, Burge M, Mermier C, Stolarczyk L. Effects of estradiol on substrate turnover during exercise in amenorrheic females. *Med Sci Sports Exerc* 1997;29:1160–9.

Saltin B, Henriksson J, Nygaard E, Anderson P. Fiber types and metabolic potentials of skeletal muscles in sedentary man and endurance runners. *Ann NY Acad Sci* 1977;301:3–29.

Sanborn CF, Jankowski CM. Physiologic considerations for women in sport. *Clin Sports Med* 1994;13:315–27.

Sarwar R, Niclos B, Rutherford OM. Changes in strength, relaxation rate and fatiguability during the human menstrual cycle. *J Physiol* 1996;493:267–72.

Schaible TF, Malhotra A, Ciambrone G, Scheuer J. The effects of gonadectomy on left ventricular function and cardiac contractile proteins in male and female rats. *Circ Res* 1984;54:38–49.

Schoenborn CA, Barnes PM. Leisure-time physical activity among adults: United States, 1997–98. *Advance Data* 2002;325:1–16.

Seeley DG, Cauley JA, Grady D, Browner WS, Nevitt MC, Cummings SR. Is postmenopausal estrogen therapy associated with neuromuscular function or falling in the elderly? Study of Osteoporotic Fractures Research Group. *Arch Intern Med* 1995;155:293–9.

Shephard RJ. Exercise and training in women. Part 1: influence of gender on exercise and training responses. *Can J Appl Physiol* 2000;25:19–34.

Simoneau JA, Bouchard C. Human variation in skeletal muscle fiber-type proportion and enzyme activities. *Am J Physiol* 1989;257:E567–E572.

Speechly DP, Taylor SR, Rogers GG. Differences in ultra-endurance exercise in performance-matched male and female runners. *Med Sci Sports Exerc* 1996;28: 359–65.

Tarnopolsky LJ, MacDougall JD, Atkinson SA, Tarnopolsky MA, Sutton JR. Gender differences in substrate for endurance exercise. *J Appl Physiol* 1990;68:302–8.

Tiidus PM. Nutritional implications of gender differences in metabolism: estrogen and oxygen radicals: oxidative damage, inflammation, and muscle function. In: Tarnopolsky M, ed. *Gender Differences in Metabolism.* New York: CRC Press, 1999: 265–81.

Wells CL. *Women, Sport, and Performance: a Physiologic Perspective.* 2nd edn. Champaign, IL: Human Kinetics, 1991.

West W, Hicks A, Clements L, Dowling J. The relationship between voluntary electromyogram, endurance time and intensity of effort in isometric handgrip exercise. *Eur J Appl Physiol Occup Ther* 1995;71:301–5.

Whipp BJ, Ward SA. Will women soon outrun men? *Nature* 1992;355:25.

Wideman L, Weltman JY, Shah N, Story S, Veldhuis JD, Welman A. Effects of gender on exercise-induced growth hormone release. *J Appl Physiol* 1999;87:1154–62.

Index

Page numbers in **bold** print refer to main entries. Page numbers in *italics* refer to figures and tables.